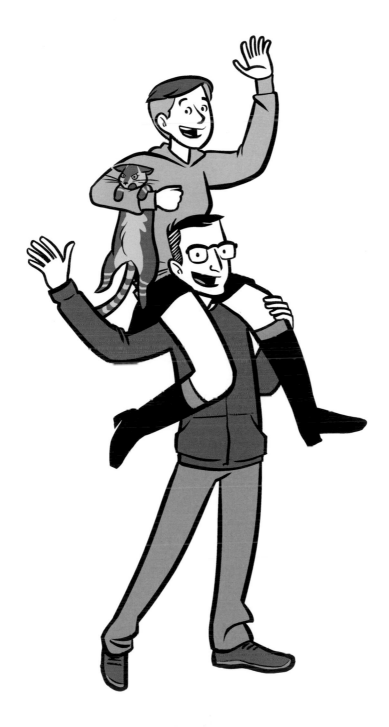

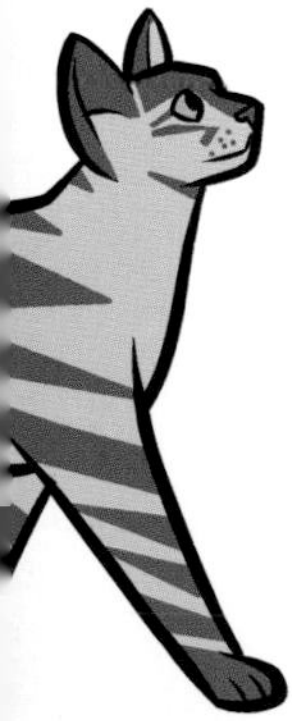

– Drawn to Sex –

Our Bodies and Health

created by

Erika Moen &
Matthew Nolan

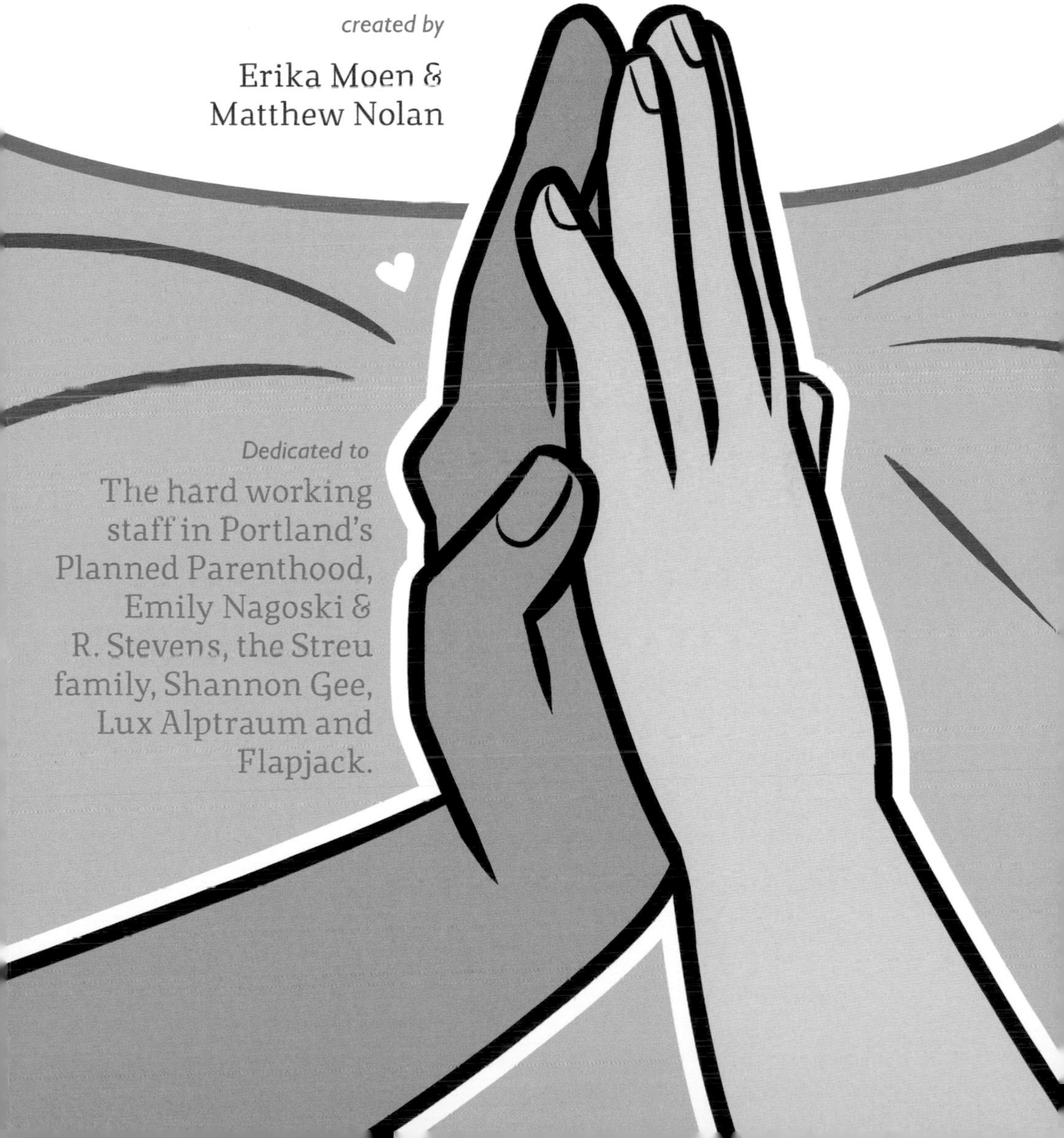

Dedicated to

The hard working staff in Portland's Planned Parenthood, Emily Nagoski & R. Stevens, the Streu family, Shannon Gee, Lux Alptraum and Flapjack.

Published by Erika Moen Comics & Illustration, LLC
Helioscope Studio
333 SW 5th Ave, Suite 500
Portland, OR 97204
Matthew Nolan, creator • Erika Moen, creator

OhJoySexToy.com
Patreon.com/Erikamoen
Twitter.com/ErikaMoen
Instagram.com/Fuckyeaherikamoen/
Facebook.com/ErikaMoenComics
Erikamoen.com

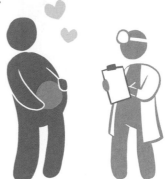

Published by Limerence Press
Limerence Press is an imprint of Oni-Lion Forge Publishing Group, LLC
1319 SE Martin Luther King Jr. Blvd., Suite 240,
Portland, OR 97214
James Lucas Jones, president & publisher • Sarah Gaydos, editor in chief • Charlie Chu, e.v.p. of creative & business development • Brad Rooks, director of operations • Amber O'Neill, special projects manager • Harris Fish, events manager • Margot Wood, director of marketing & sales • Devin Funches, sales & marketing manager • Katie Sainz, marketing manager • Tara Lehmann, publicist • Troy Look, director of design & production • Kate Z. Stone, senior graphic designer • Sonja Synak, graphic designer • Hilary Thompson, graphic designer • Sarah Rockwell, junior graphic designer • Angie Knowles, digital prepress lead • Vincent Kukua, digital prepress technician • Jasmine Amiri, senior editor • Shawna Gore, senior editor • Amanda Meadows, senior editor • Robert Meyers, senior editor, licensing • Grace Bornhoft, editor • Zack Soto, editor • Chris Cerasi, editorial coordinator • Steve Ellis, vice president of games • Ben Eisner, game developer • Michelle Nguyen, executive assistant • Jung Lee, logistics coordinator

Joe Nozemack, publisher emeritus

LimerencePress.com
Twitter.com/LimerencePress
Onipress.com | Lionforge.com
Facebook.com/onipress | Facebook.com/lionforge
Twitter.com/onipress | Twitter.com/lionforge
Instagram.com/onipress | Instagram.com/lionforge

First edition: November 2020
ISBN 13: 978-1-62010-791-1
ISBN 10: 1-62010-791-0

PRINTED IN CHINA.

Library of Congress Control Number: 2020937765
1 2 3 4 5 6 7 8 9 10

Index

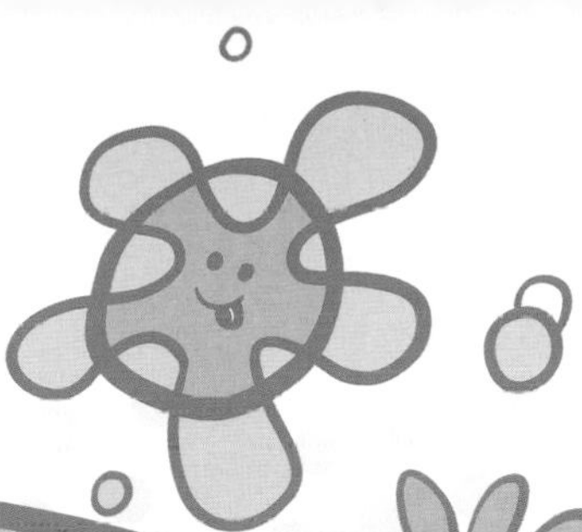

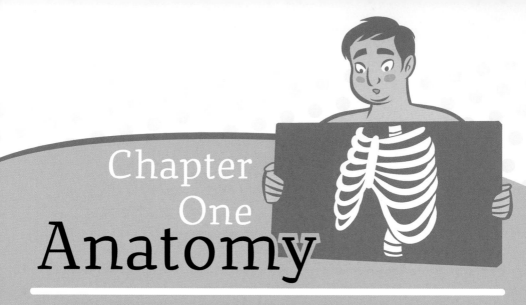

Chapter One
Anatomy

Hello and welcome to our second book! A book all about your bod!

Drawn to Sex is a collection of comics from our long-running webcomic, *Oh Joy Sex Toy*. Over the years we've made a ton of silly, informative, and helpful strips all about the world of sex. We've made so many, in fact, that we've finally been able to create a series of books just for the educational comics. In our first book, *The Basics*, we set out to make a good sex education foundation, but there were a ton of things we didn't have room to include. Things like: how your body actually works, how it sometimes doesn't work, how pregnancy happens, and what an STI even is.

So, say hello to *Drawn to Sex: Our Bodies and Health!* This second book contains comics about biology by us (Matt and Erika, hi!) and by a bunch of knowledgeable friends we recruited to take part in this project. This book is a short, silly, fast starting point on subjects that can be complicated and intimidating in the real world. Use this collection as a first-glance tool, to introduce you to bigger concepts and names that you can do deeper research on.

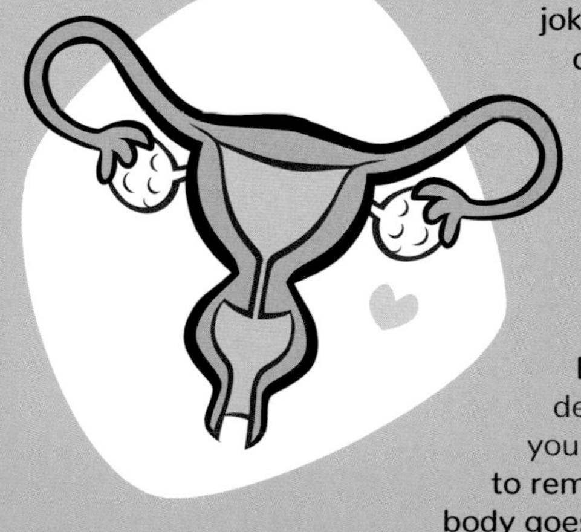

We're sex-nerd-comic-artists who love our dad jokes and dick puns, *buuuuut* we're not your doctor. While we do our best to give up-to-date, medically accurate information in our comics, our advice will become dated and medicine and treatments will change. So, when health things *do* come up in your life, do way more research and talk with actual experts on those subjects!

Emergencies aside, we hope our book will help demystify some of your questions surrounding your body and sex; and at the very least, it's here to remind you that you're normal – even when your body goes wack-a-boo.

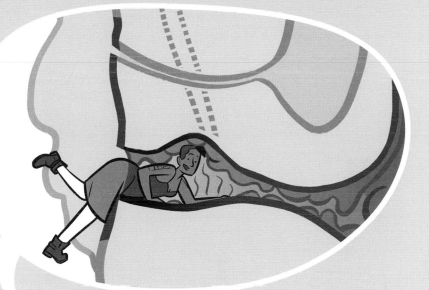

Vulva & Vagina

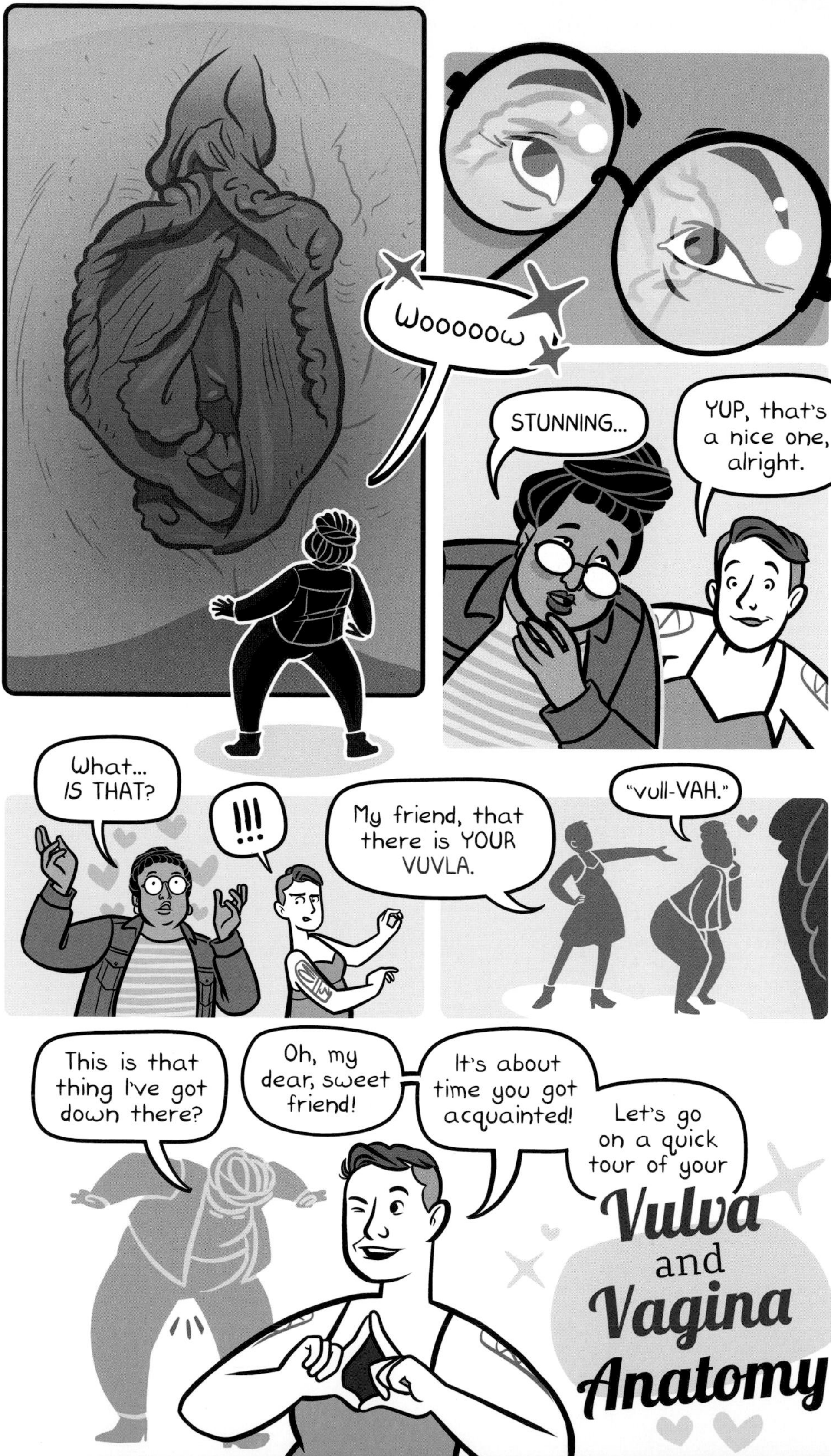
Woooooow
STUNNING...
YUP, that's a nice one, alright.
What... IS THAT?
!!!
My friend, that there is YOUR VUVLA.
"vull-VAH."
This is that thing I've got down there?
Oh, my dear, sweet friend!
It's about time you got acquainted!
Let's go on a quick tour of your
Vulva and Vagina Anatomy

There's a LOT more information than we have the space to include here, so please do more research on your own at **plannedparenthood.org** and **scarleteen.com**.

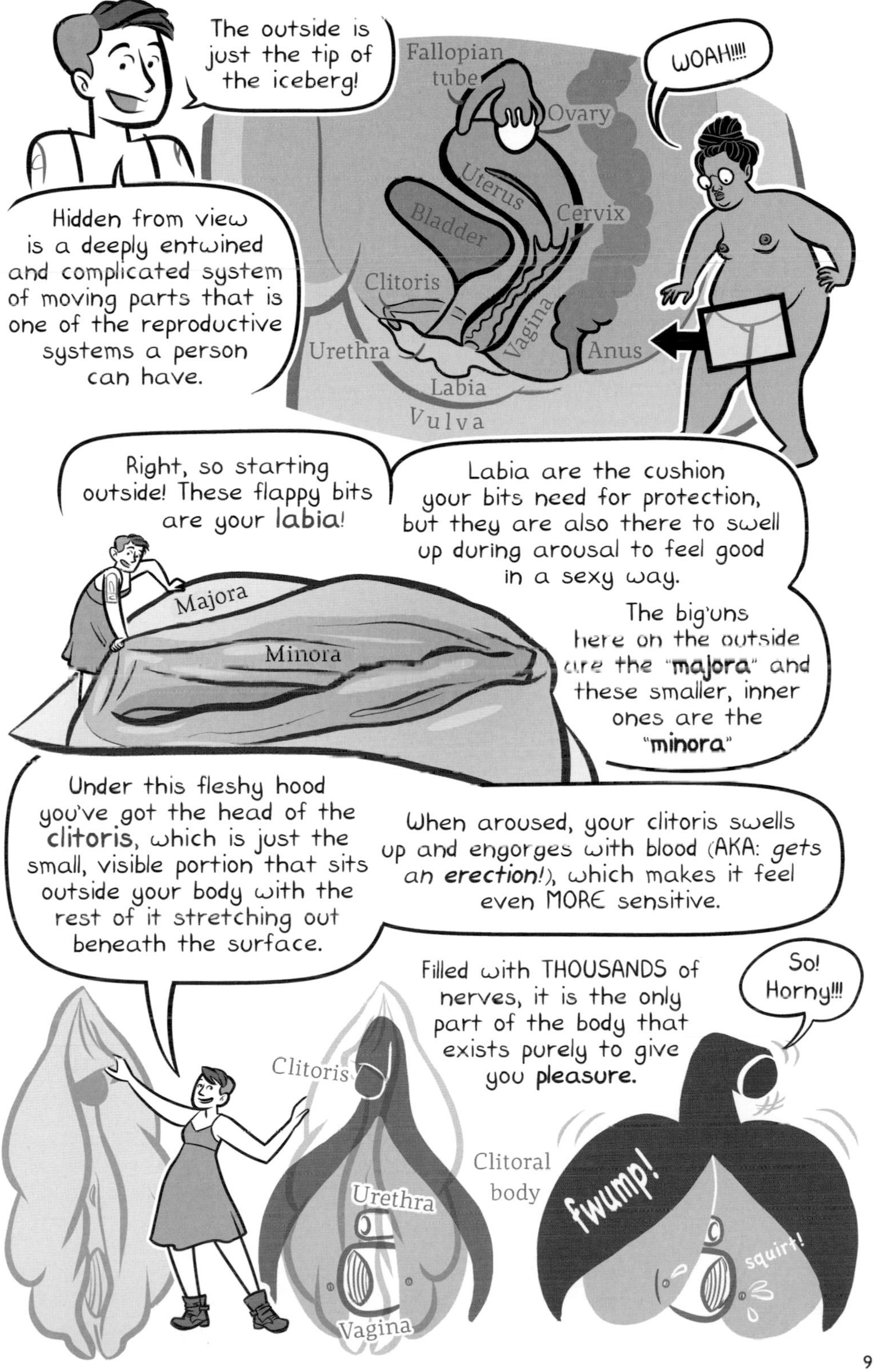

The outside is just the tip of the iceberg!
Fallopian tube
Ovary
Uterus
Bladder
Cervix
Clitoris
Vagina
Urethra
Anus
Labia
Vulva
WOAH!!!!
Hidden from view is a deeply entwined and complicated system of moving parts that is one of the reproductive systems a person can have.
Right, so starting outside! These flappy bits are your **labia**!
Labia are the cushion your bits need for protection, but they are also there to swell up during arousal to feel good in a sexy way.
Majora
Minora
The big'uns here on the outside are the "**majora**" and these smaller, inner ones are the "**minora**"
Under this fleshy hood you've got the head of the **clitoris**, which is just the small, visible portion that sits outside your body with the rest of it stretching out beneath the surface.
When aroused, your clitoris swells up and engorges with blood (AKA: *gets an **erection!***), which makes it feel even MORE sensitive.
Filled with THOUSANDS of nerves, it is the only part of the body that exists purely to give you **pleasure**.
So! Horny!!!
Clitoris
Clitoral body
Urethra
Vagina
fwump!
squirt!

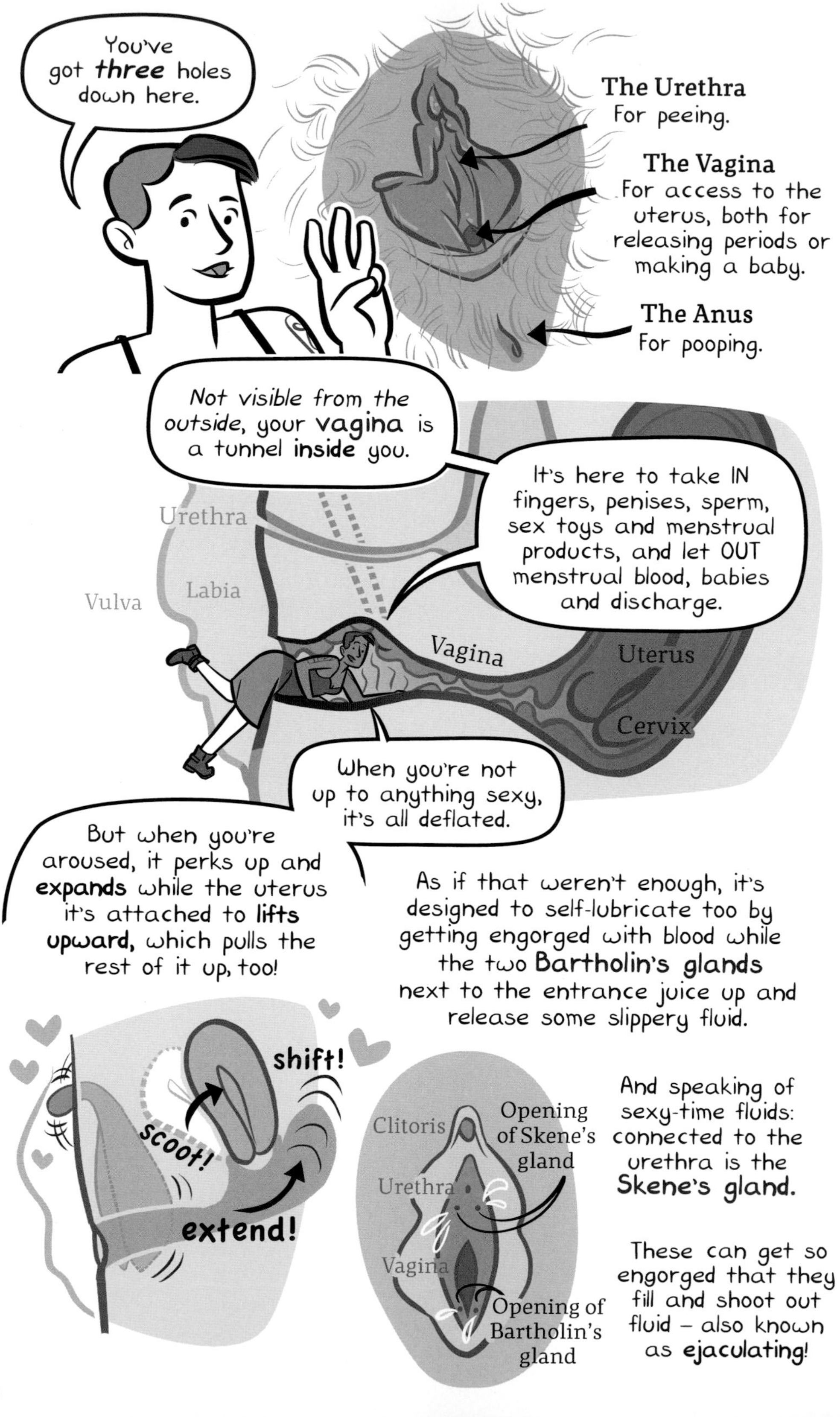

You've got **three** holes down here.
The Urethra
For peeing.
The Vagina
For access to the uterus, both for releasing periods or making a baby.
The Anus
For pooping.
Not visible from the outside, your **vagina** is a tunnel **inside** you.
It's here to take IN fingers, penises, sperm, sex toys and menstrual products, and let OUT menstrual blood, babies and discharge.
Urethra
Vulva
Labia
Vagina
Uterus
Cervix
When you're not up to anything sexy, it's all deflated.
But when you're aroused, it perks up and **expands** while the uterus it's attached to **lifts upward,** which pulls the rest of it up, too!
As if that weren't enough, it's designed to self-lubricate too by getting engorged with blood while the two **Bartholin's glands** next to the entrance juice up and release some slippery fluid.
shift!
scoot!
extend!
Clitoris
Opening of Skene's gland
Urethra
Vagina
Opening of Bartholin's gland
And speaking of sexy-time fluids: connected to the urethra is the **Skene's gland.**
These can get so engorged that they fill and shoot out fluid – also known as **ejaculating**!

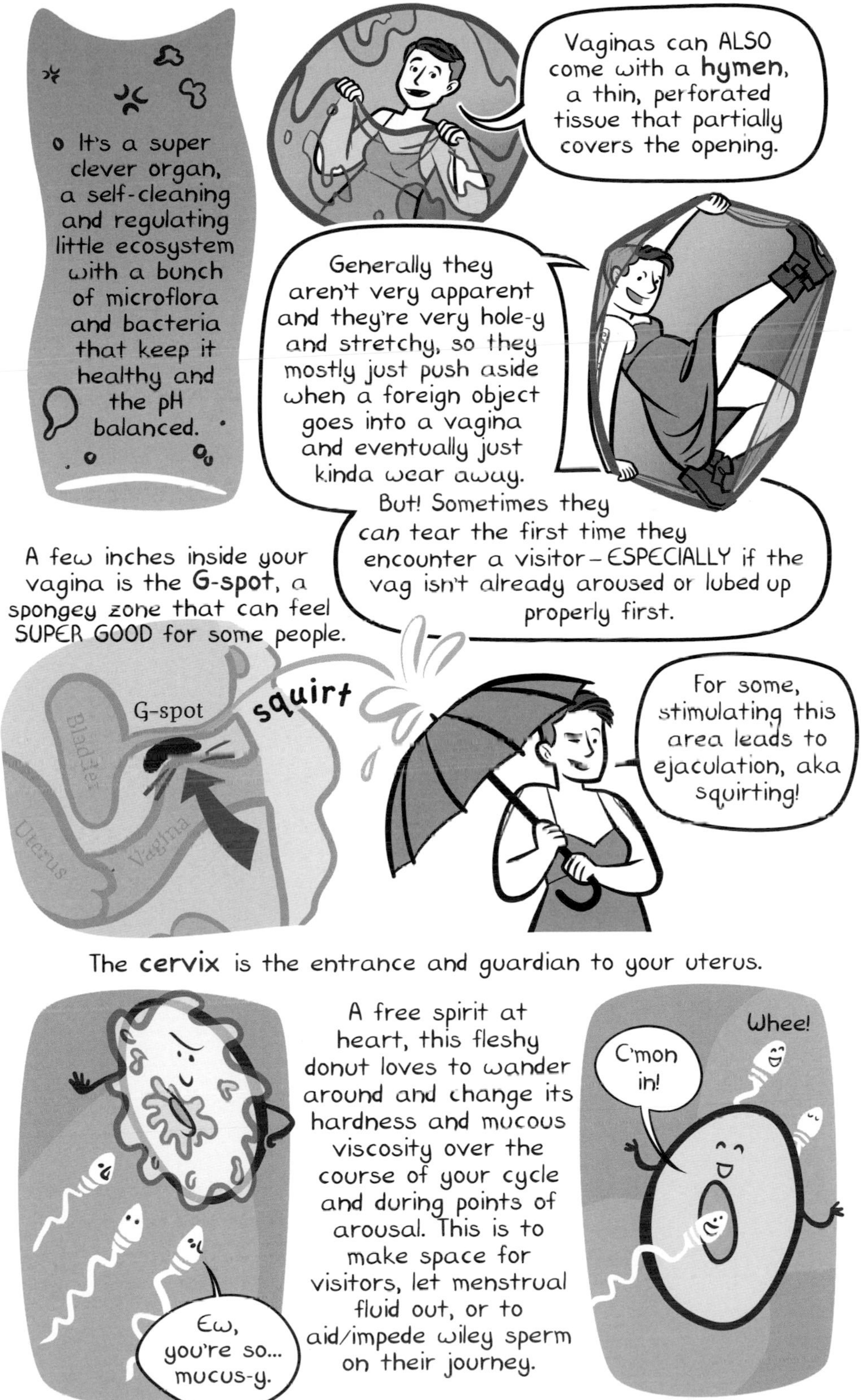
It's a super clever organ, a self-cleaning and regulating little ecosystem with a bunch of microflora and bacteria that keep it healthy and the pH balanced.
Vaginas can ALSO come with a hymen, a thin, perforated tissue that partially covers the opening.
Generally they aren't very apparent and they're very hole-y and stretchy, so they mostly just push aside when a foreign object goes into a vagina and eventually just kinda wear away.
But! Sometimes they can tear the first time they encounter a visitor—ESPECIALLY if the vag isn't already aroused or lubed up properly first.
A few inches inside your vagina is the G-spot, a spongey zone that can feel SUPER GOOD for some people.
G-spot
Bladder
Uterus
Vagina
squirt
For some, stimulating this area leads to ejaculation, aka squirting!
The cervix is the entrance and guardian to your uterus.
Ew, you're so... mucus-y.
A free spirit at heart, this fleshy donut loves to wander around and change its hardness and mucous viscosity over the course of your cycle and during points of arousal. This is to make space for visitors, let menstrual fluid out, or to aid/impede wiley sperm on their journey.
C'mon in!
Whee!

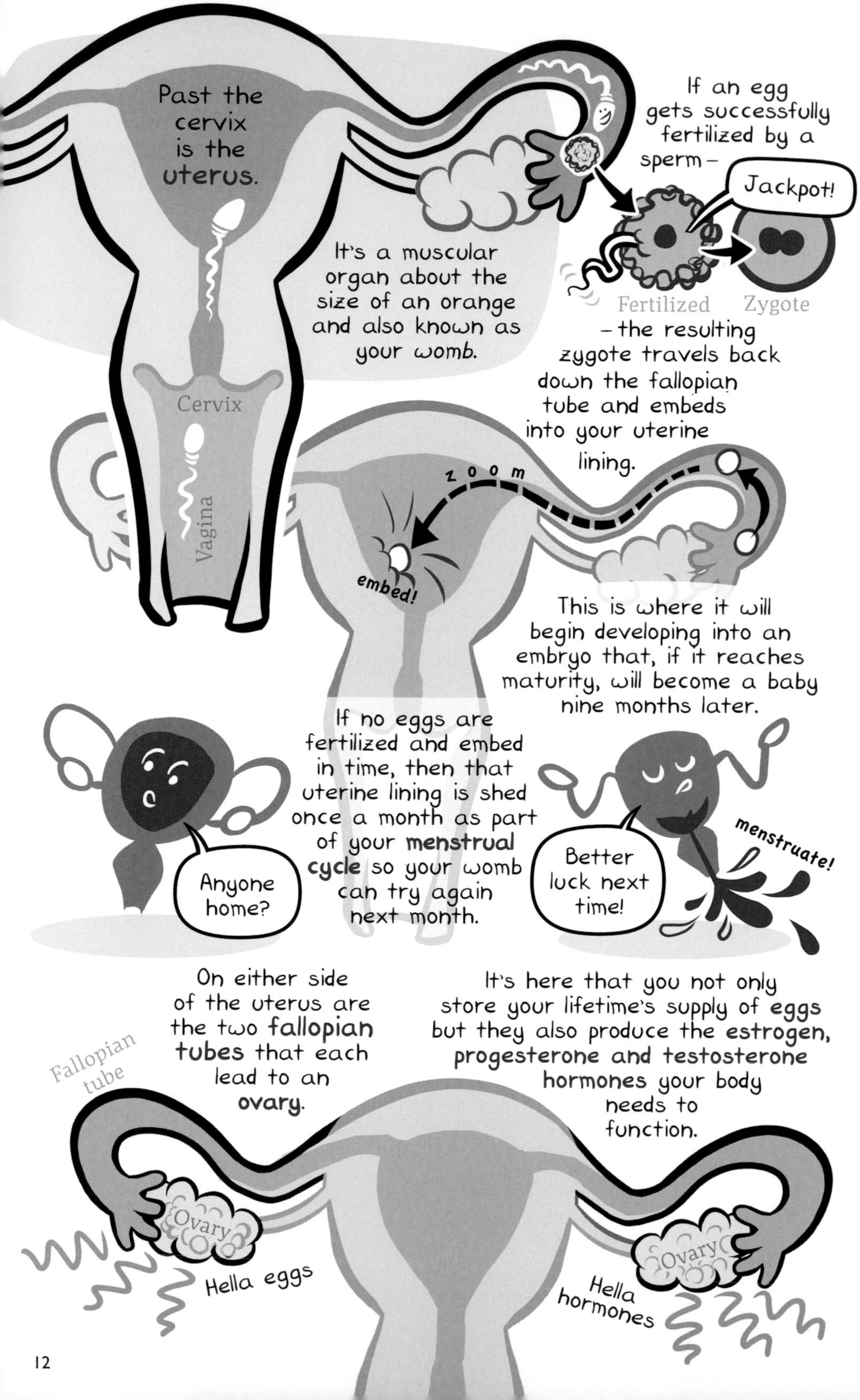
Past the cervix is the uterus.
It's a muscular organ about the size of an orange and also known as your womb.
Cervix
Vagina
If an egg gets successfully fertilized by a sperm –
Jackpot!
Fertilized
Zygote
– the resulting zygote travels back down the fallopian tube and embeds into your uterine lining.
zoom
embed!
This is where it will begin developing into an embryo that, if it reaches maturity, will become a baby nine months later.
If no eggs are fertilized and embed in time, then that uterine lining is shed once a month as part of your menstrual cycle so your womb can try again next month.
Anyone home?
Better luck next time!
menstruate!
On either side of the uterus are the two fallopian tubes that each lead to an ovary.
It's here that you not only store your lifetime's supply of eggs but they also produce the estrogen, progesterone and testosterone hormones your body needs to function.
Fallopian tube
Ovary
Ovary
Hella eggs
Hella hormones

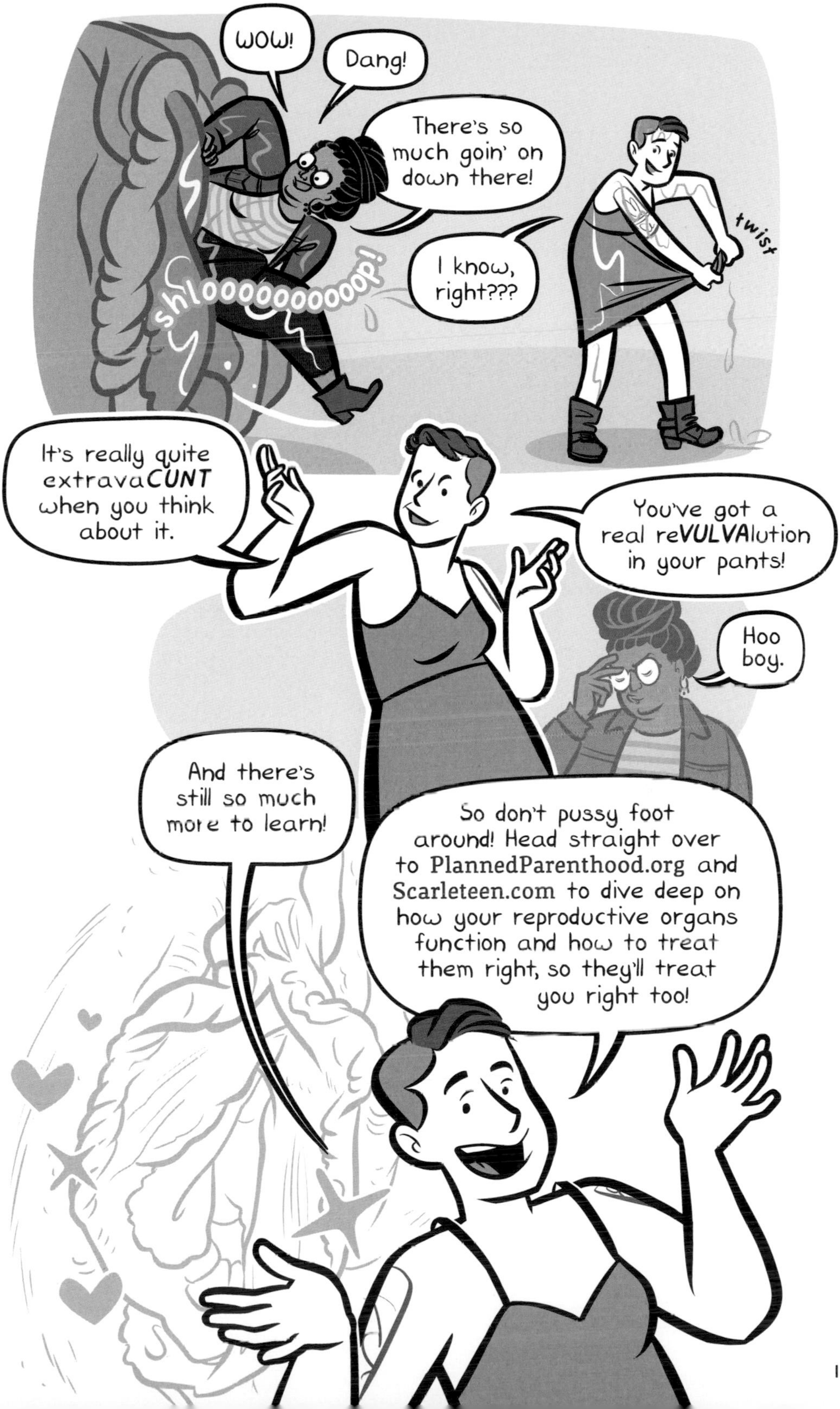
WOW!
Dang!
There's so much goin' on down there!
shlooooooooooop!
I know, right???
twist
It's really quite extravaCUNT when you think about it.
You've got a real reVULVAlution in your pants!
Hoo boy.
And there's still so much more to learn!
So don't pussy foot around! Head straight over to PlannedParenthood.org and Scarleteen.com to dive deep on how your reproductive organs function and how to treat them right, so they'll treat you right too!

DROOP
ZWOOP

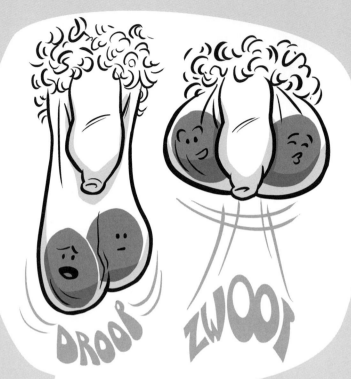

Penis & Scrotum

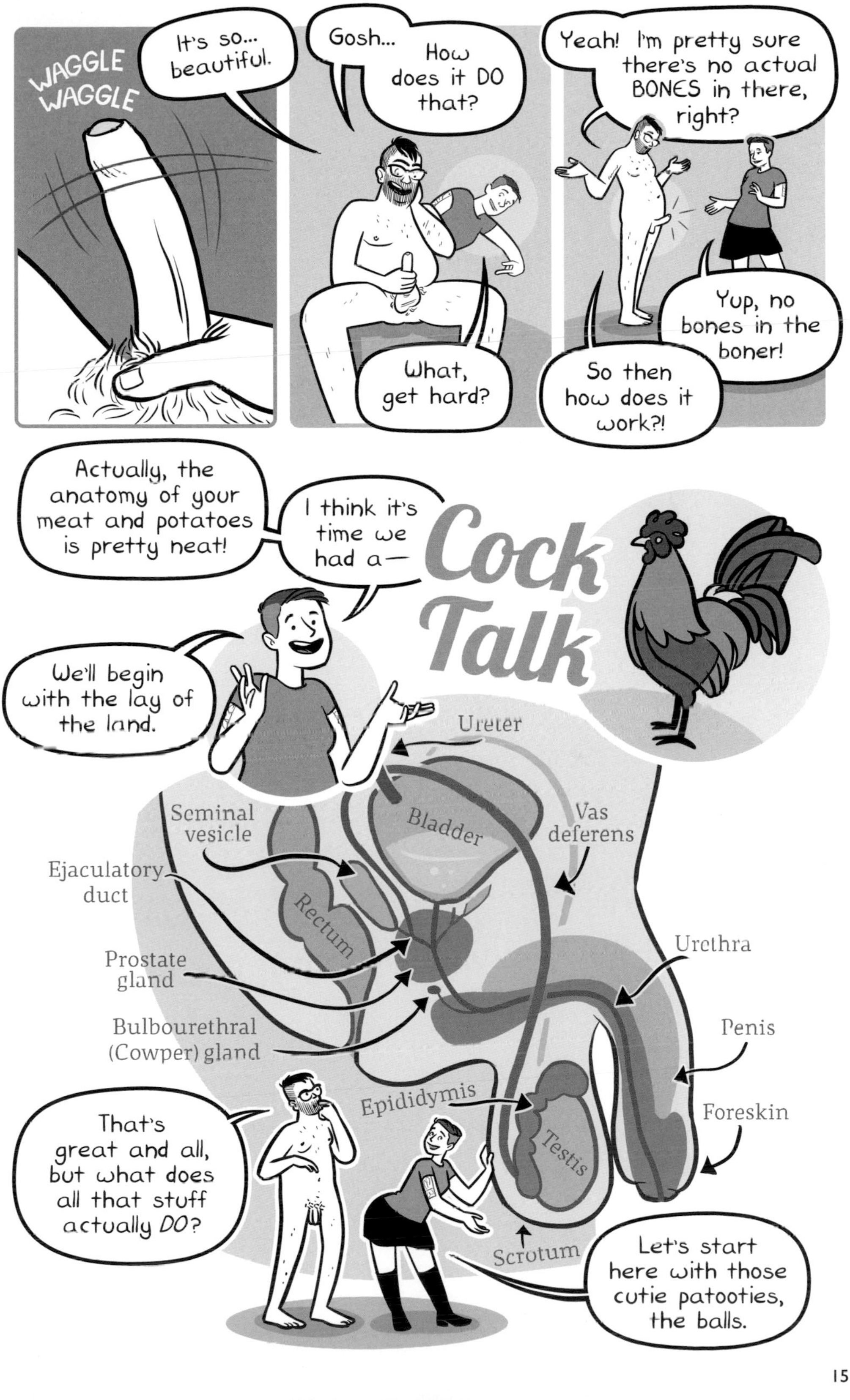
WAGGLE WAGGLE
It's so... beautiful.
Gosh...
How does it DO that?
What, get hard?
Yeah! I'm pretty sure there's no actual BONES in there, right?
Yup, no bones in the boner!
So then how does it work?!
Actually, the anatomy of your meat and potatoes is pretty neat!
I think it's time we had a—
Cock Talk
We'll begin with the lay of the land.
Ureter
Seminal vesicle
Bladder
Vas deferens
Ejaculatory duct
Rectum
Prostate gland
Urethra
Bulbourethral (Cowper) gland
Penis
Epididymis
Testis
Foreskin
Scrotum
That's great and all, but what does all that stuff actually DO?
Let's start here with those cutie patooties, the balls.

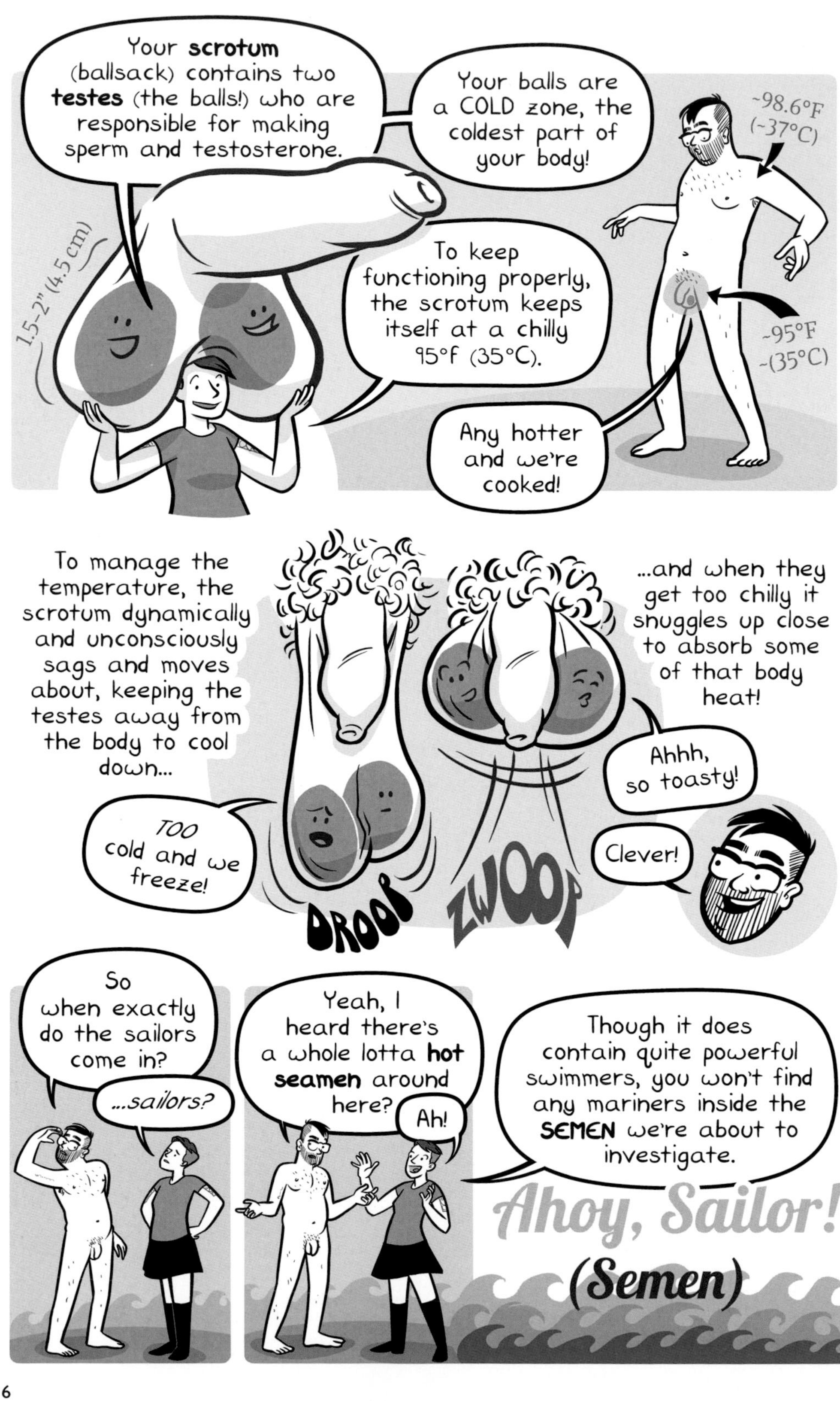
Your **scrotum** (ballsack) contains two **testes** (the balls!) who are responsible for making sperm and testosterone.
Your balls are a COLD zone, the coldest part of your body!
~98.6°F (~37°C)
1.5–2" (4.5 cm)
To keep functioning properly, the scrotum keeps itself at a chilly 95°F (35°C).
~95°F ~(35°C)
Any hotter and we're cooked!
To manage the temperature, the scrotum dynamically and unconsciously sags and moves about, keeping the testes away from the body to cool down...
...and when they get too chilly it snuggles up close to absorb some of that body heat!
Ahhh, so toasty!
TOO cold and we freeze!
Clever!
DROOP
ZWOOP
So when exactly do the sailors come in?
...sailors?
Yeah, I heard there's a whole lotta **hot seamen** around here?
Ah!
Though it does contain quite powerful swimmers, you won't find any mariners inside the **SEMEN** we're about to investigate.
Ahoy, Sailor!
(Semen)

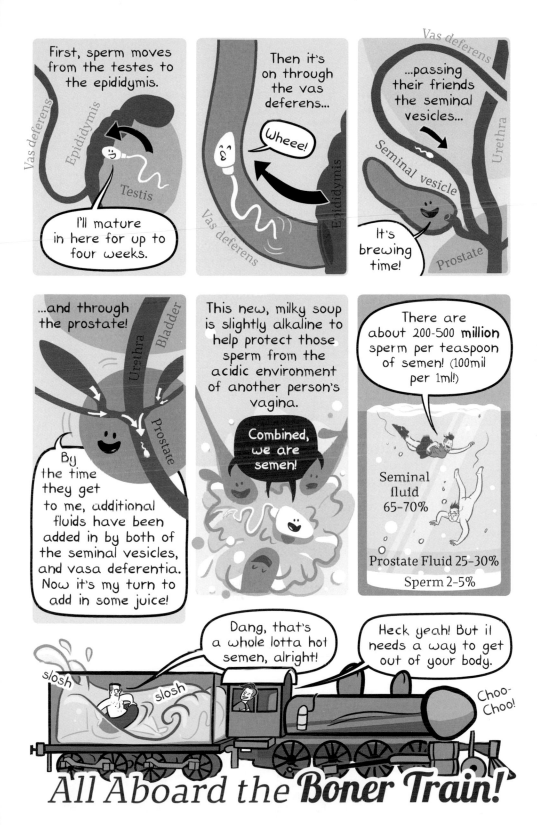

First, sperm moves from the testes to the epididymis.

Vas deferens

Epididymis

Testis

I'll mature in here for up to four weeks.

Then it's on through the vas deferens...

Wheee!

Vas deferens

Epididymis

Vas deferens

...passing their friends the seminal vesicles...

Seminal vesicle

Urethra

It's brewing time!

Prostate

...and through the prostate!

Urethra

Bladder

Prostate

By the time they get to me, additional fluids have been added in by both of the seminal vesicles, and vasa deferentia. Now it's my turn to add in some juice!

This new, milky soup is slightly alkaline to help protect those sperm from the acidic environment of another person's vagina.

Combined, we are semen!

There are about 200-500 **million** sperm per teaspoon of semen! (100mil per 1ml!)

Seminal fluid 65-70%

Prostate Fluid 25-30%

Sperm 2-5%

Dang, that's a whole lotta hot semen, alright!

Heck yeah! But it needs a way to get out of your body.

slosh

slosh

Choo-Choo!

All Aboard the Boner Train!

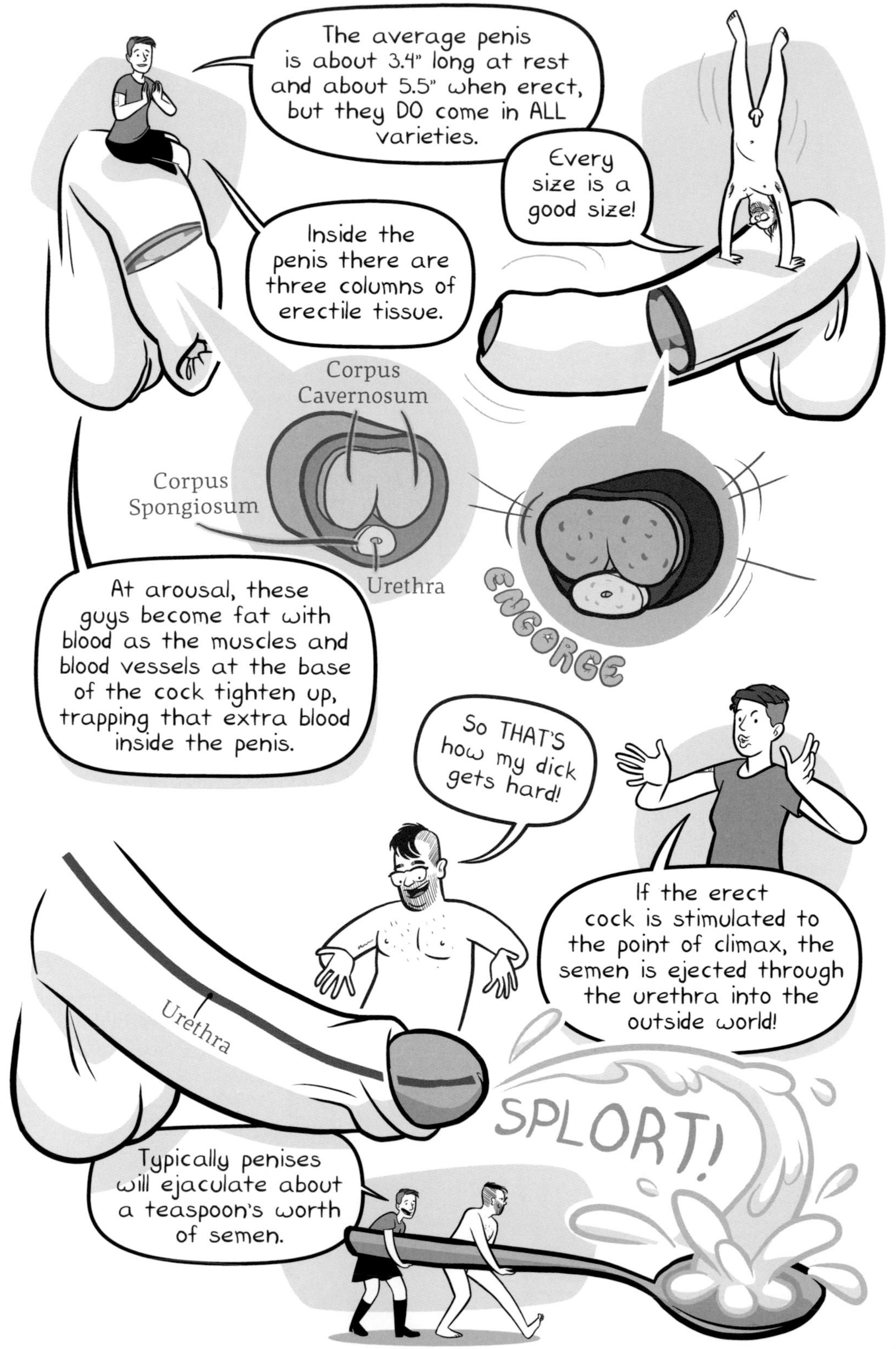
The average penis is about 3.4" long at rest and about 5.5" when erect, but they DO come in ALL varieties.
Every size is a good size!
Inside the penis there are three columns of erectile tissue.
Corpus Cavernosum
Corpus Spongiosum
Urethra
ENGORGE
At arousal, these guys become fat with blood as the muscles and blood vessels at the base of the cock tighten up, trapping that extra blood inside the penis.
So THAT'S how my dick gets hard!
If the erect cock is stimulated to the point of climax, the semen is ejected through the urethra into the outside world!
Urethra
SPLORT!
Typically penises will ejaculate about a teaspoon's worth of semen.

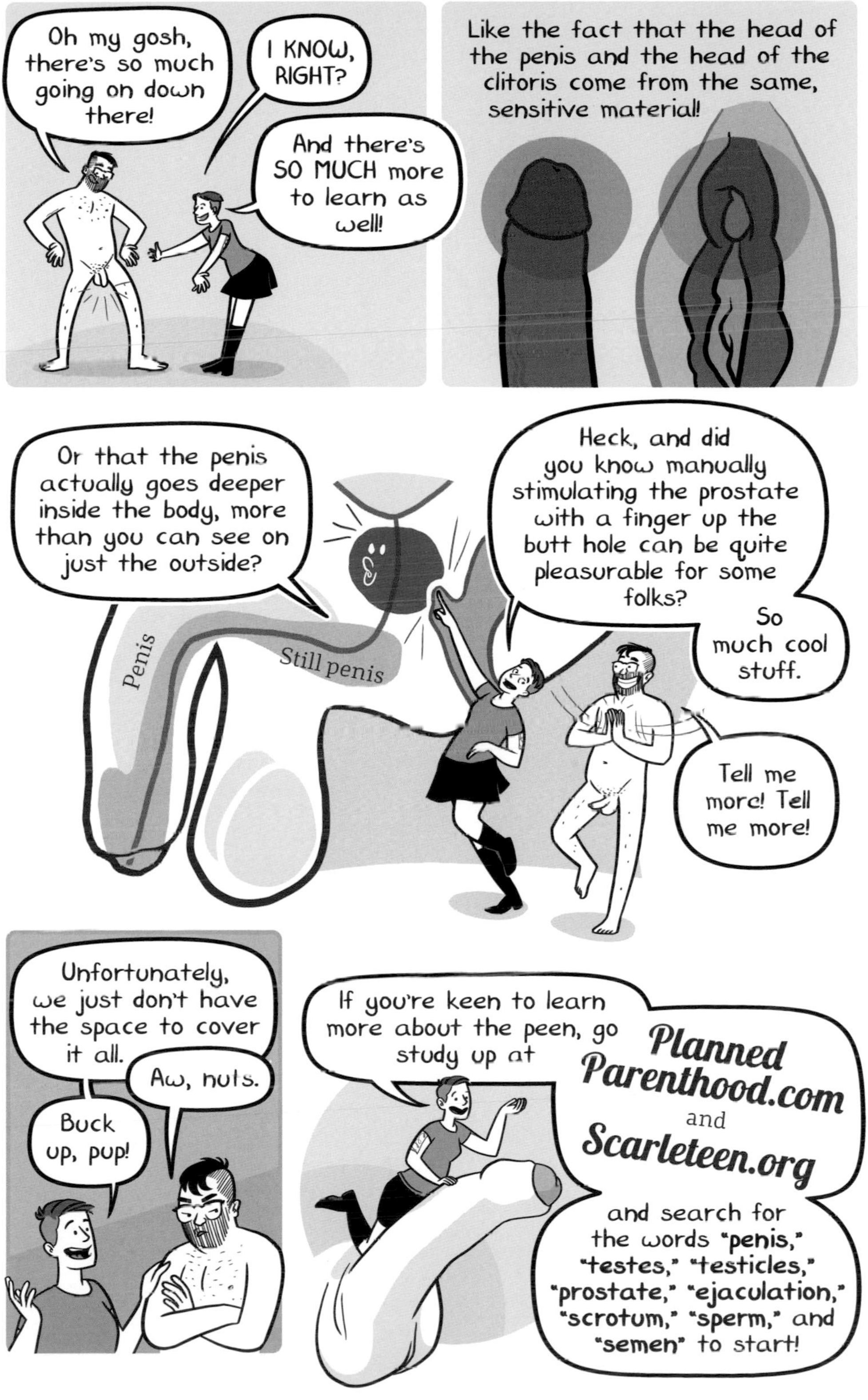

Oh my gosh, there's so much going on down there!
I KNOW, RIGHT?
And there's SO MUCH more to learn as well!
Like the fact that the head of the penis and the head of the clitoris come from the same, sensitive material!
Or that the penis actually goes deeper inside the body, more than you can see on just the outside?
Penis
Still penis
Heck, and did you know manually stimulating the prostate with a finger up the butt hole can be quite pleasurable for some folks?
So much cool stuff.
Tell me more! Tell me more!
Unfortunately, we just don't have the space to cover it all.
Aw, nuts.
Buck up, pup!
If you're keen to learn more about the peen, go study up at
Planned Parenthood.com
and
Scarleteen.org
and search for the words "penis," "testes," "testicles," "prostate," "ejaculation," "scrotum," "sperm," and "semen" to start!

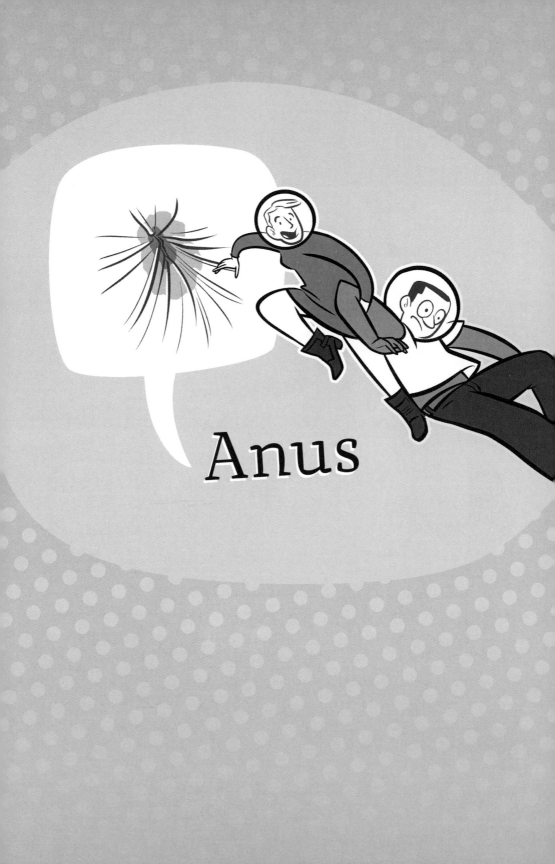

Anus

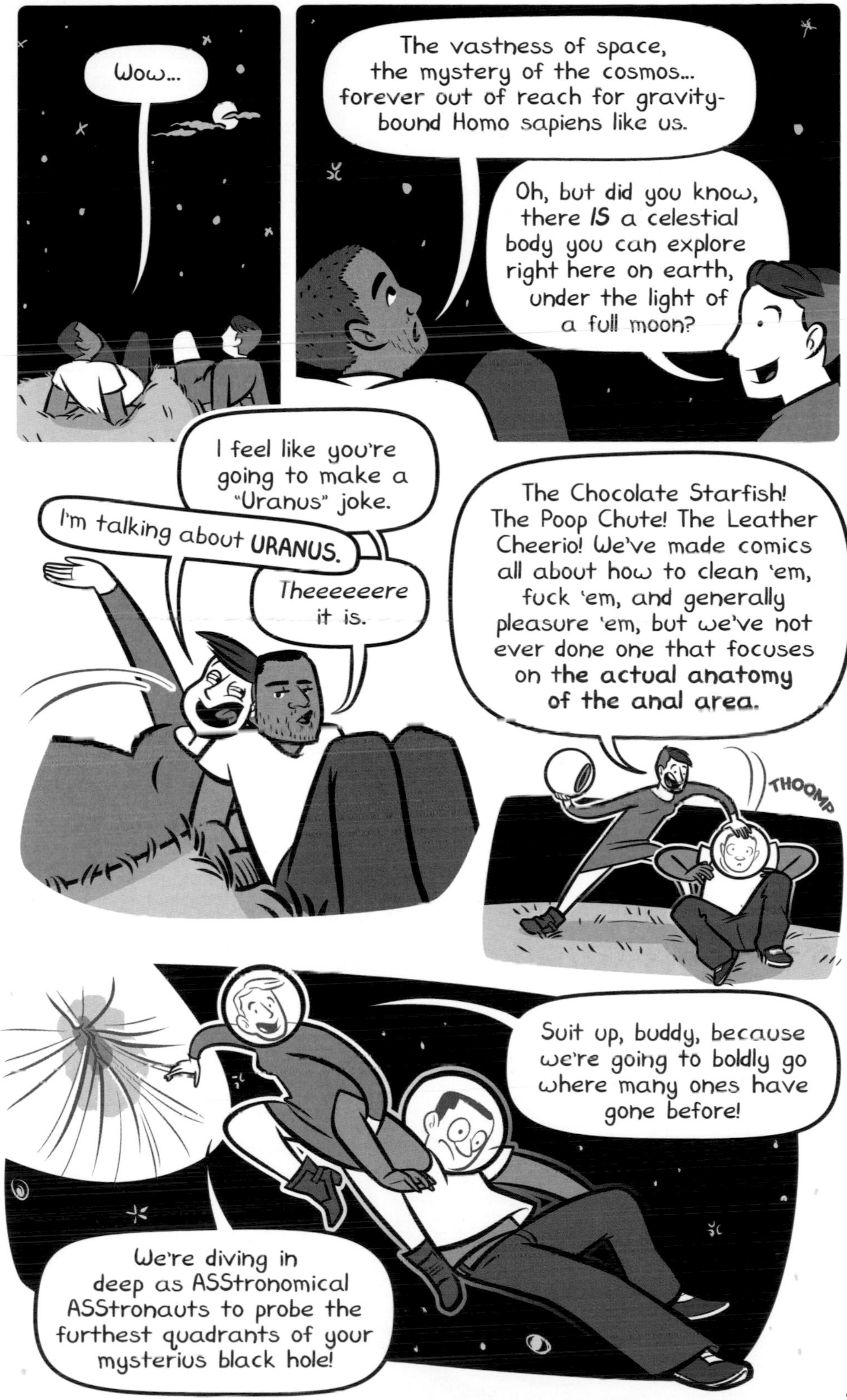
Wow...
The vastness of space, the mystery of the cosmos... forever out of reach for gravity-bound Homo sapiens like us.
Oh, but did you know, there IS a celestial body you can explore right here on earth, under the light of a full moon?
I feel like you're going to make a "Uranus" joke.
I'm talking about URANUS.
Theeeeeere it is.
The Chocolate Starfish! The Poop Chute! The Leather Cheerio! We've made comics all about how to clean 'em, fuck 'em, and generally pleasure 'em, but we've not ever done one that focuses on the actual anatomy of the anal area.
THOOMP
Suit up, buddy, because we're going to boldly go where many ones have gone before!
We're diving in deep as ASStronomical ASStronauts to probe the furthest quadrants of your mysterius black hole!

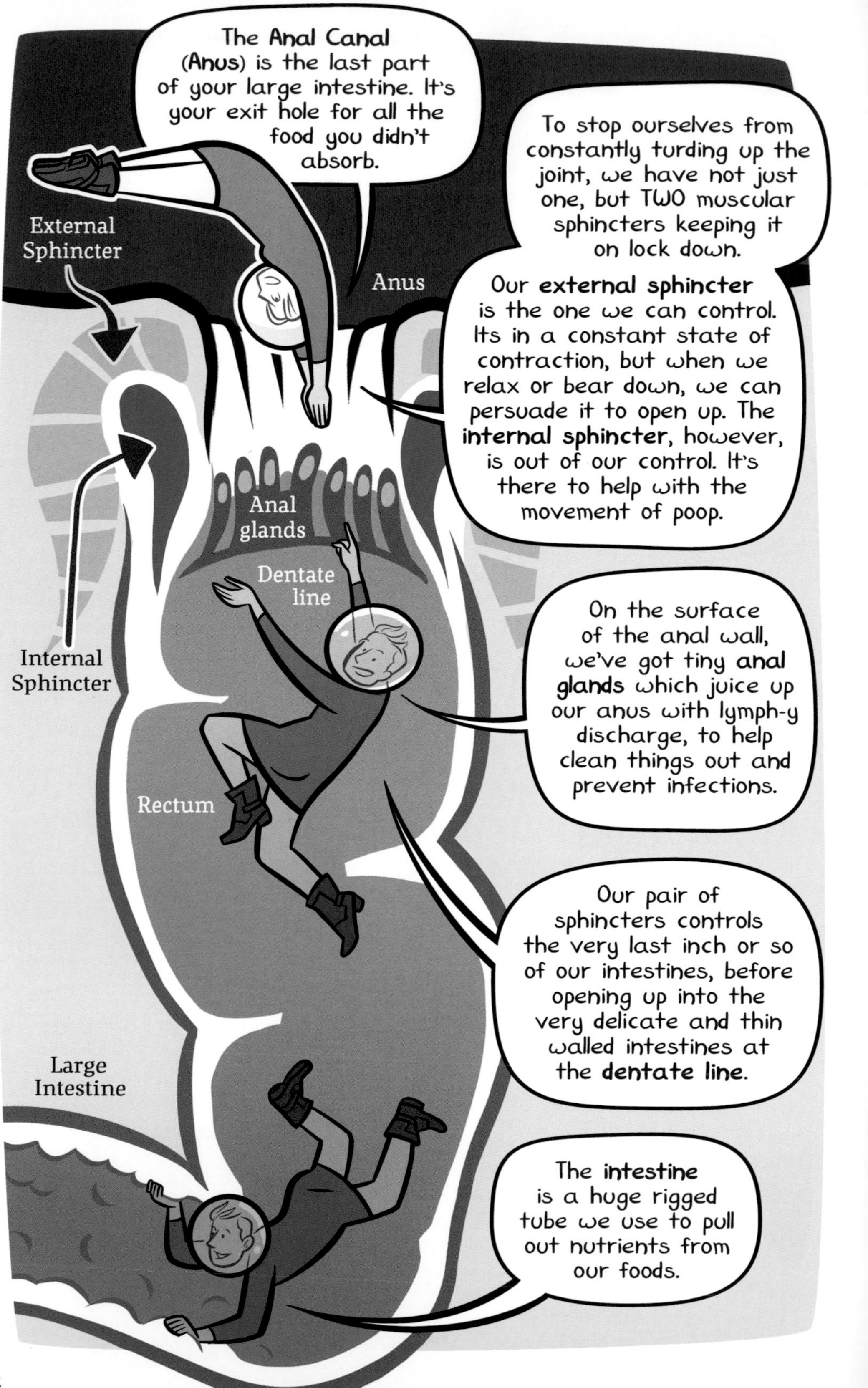
The **Anal Canal** (**Anus**) is the last part of your large intestine. It's your exit hole for all the food you didn't absorb.
To stop ourselves from constantly turding up the joint, we have not just one, but TWO muscular sphincters keeping it on lock down.
Our **external sphincter** is the one we can control. Its in a constant state of contraction, but when we relax or bear down, we can persuade it to open up. The **internal sphincter**, however, is out of our control. It's there to help with the movement of poop.
On the surface of the anal wall, we've got tiny **anal glands** which juice up our anus with lymph-y discharge, to help clean things out and prevent infections.
Our pair of sphincters controls the very last inch or so of our intestines, before opening up into the very delicate and thin walled intestines at the **dentate line**.
The **intestine** is a huge rigged tube we use to pull out nutrients from our foods.
External Sphincter
Anus
Anal glands
Dentate line
Internal Sphincter
Rectum
Large Intestine

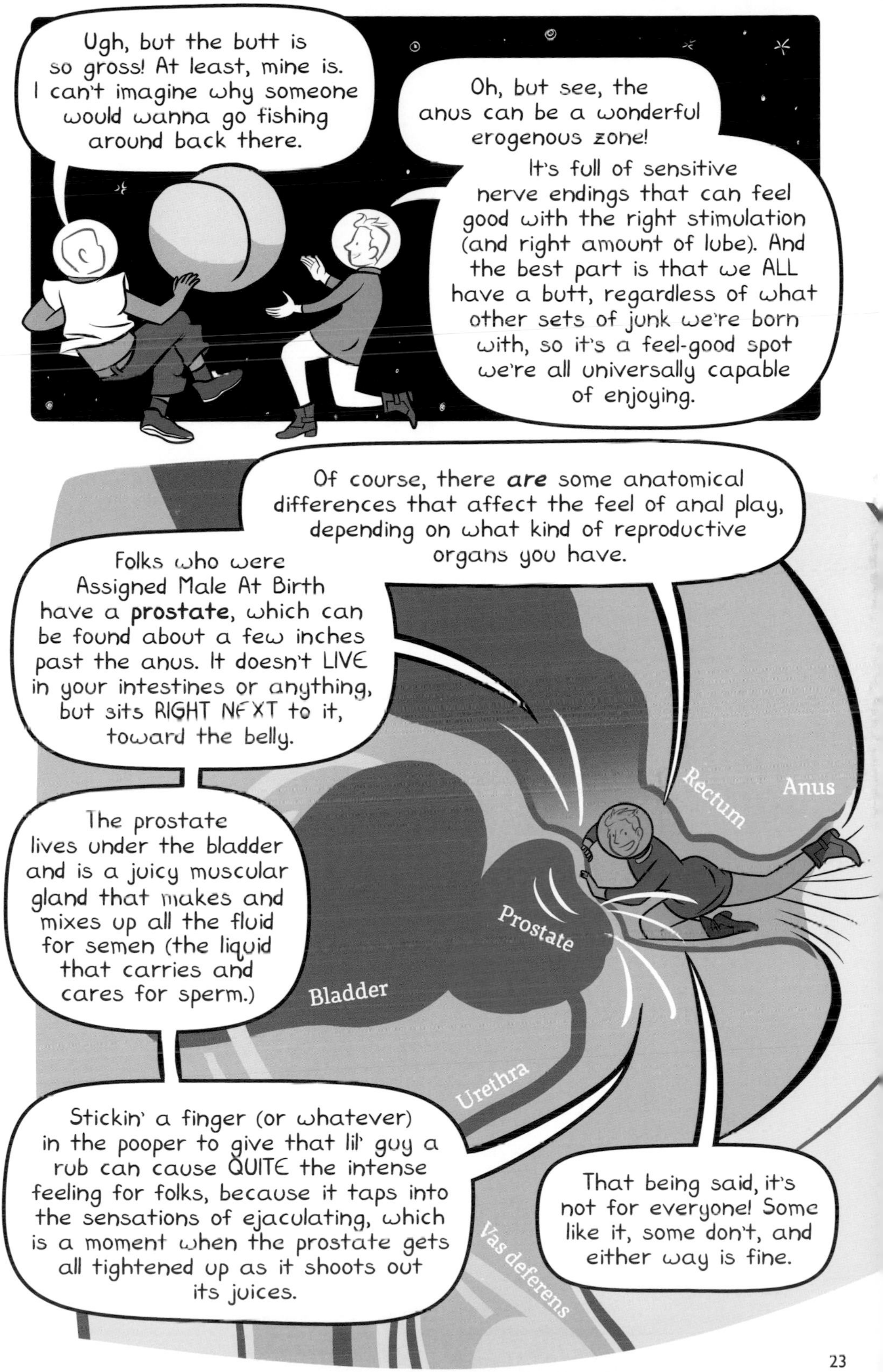
Ugh, but the butt is so gross! At least, mine is. I can't imagine why someone would wanna go fishing around back there.
Oh, but see, the anus can be a wonderful erogenous zone!
It's full of sensitive nerve endings that can feel good with the right stimulation (and right amount of lube). And the best part is that we ALL have a butt, regardless of what other sets of junk we're born with, so it's a feel-good spot we're all universally capable of enjoying.
Of course, there **are** some anatomical differences that affect the feel of anal play, depending on what kind of reproductive organs you have.
Folks who were Assigned Male At Birth have a **prostate**, which can be found about a few inches past the anus. It doesn't LIVE in your intestines or anything, but sits RIGHT NEXT to it, toward the belly.
The prostate lives under the bladder and is a juicy muscular gland that makes and mixes up all the fluid for semen (the liquid that carries and cares for sperm.)
Rectum
Anus
Prostate
Bladder
Urethra
Vas deferens
Stickin' a finger (or whatever) in the pooper to give that lil' guy a rub can cause QUITE the intense feeling for folks, because it taps into the sensations of ejaculating, which is a moment when the prostate gets all tightened up as it shoots out its juices.
That being said, it's not for everyone! Some like it, some don't, and either way is fine.

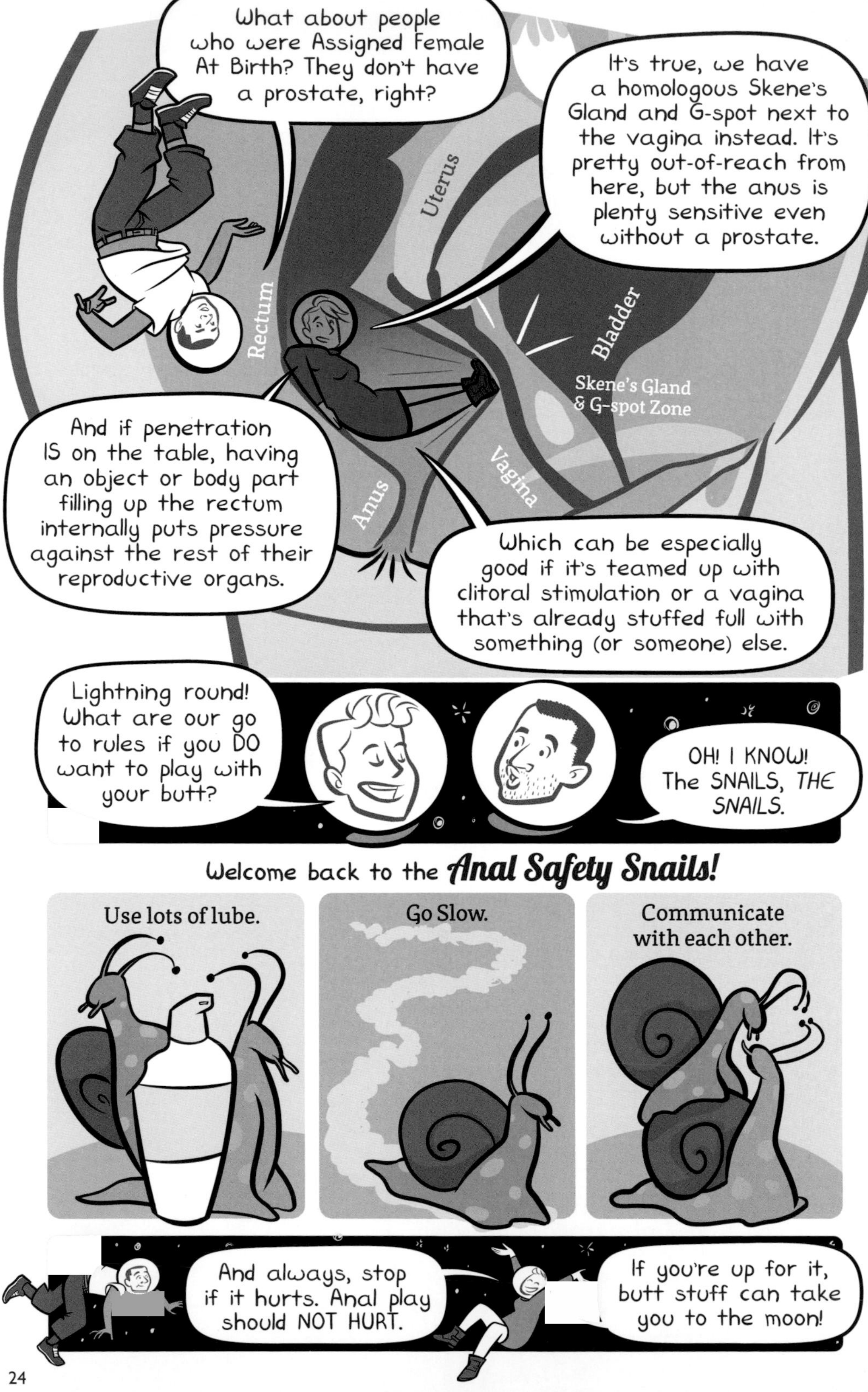

What about people who were Assigned Female At Birth? They don't have a prostate, right?
It's true, we have a homologous Skene's Gland and G-spot next to the vagina instead. It's pretty out-of-reach from here, but the anus is plenty sensitive even without a prostate.
Uterus
Rectum
Bladder
Skene's Gland & G-spot Zone
Vagina
Anus
And if penetration IS on the table, having an object or body part filling up the rectum internally puts pressure against the rest of their reproductive organs.
Which can be especially good if it's teamed up with clitoral stimulation or a vagina that's already stuffed full with something (or someone) else.
Lightning round! What are our go to rules if you DO want to play with your butt?
OH! I KNOW! The SNAILS, *THE SNAILS.*
Welcome back to the ***Anal Safety Snails!***
Use lots of lube.
Go Slow.
Communicate with each other.
And always, stop if it hurts. Anal play should NOT HURT.
If you're up for it, butt stuff can take you to the moon!

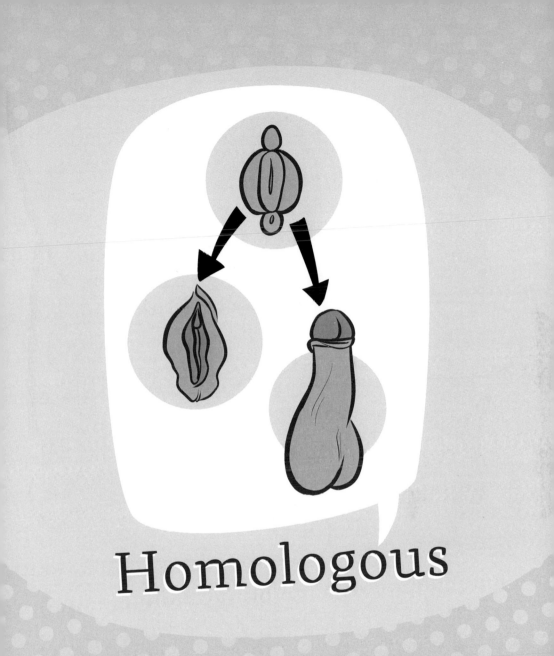

Homologous

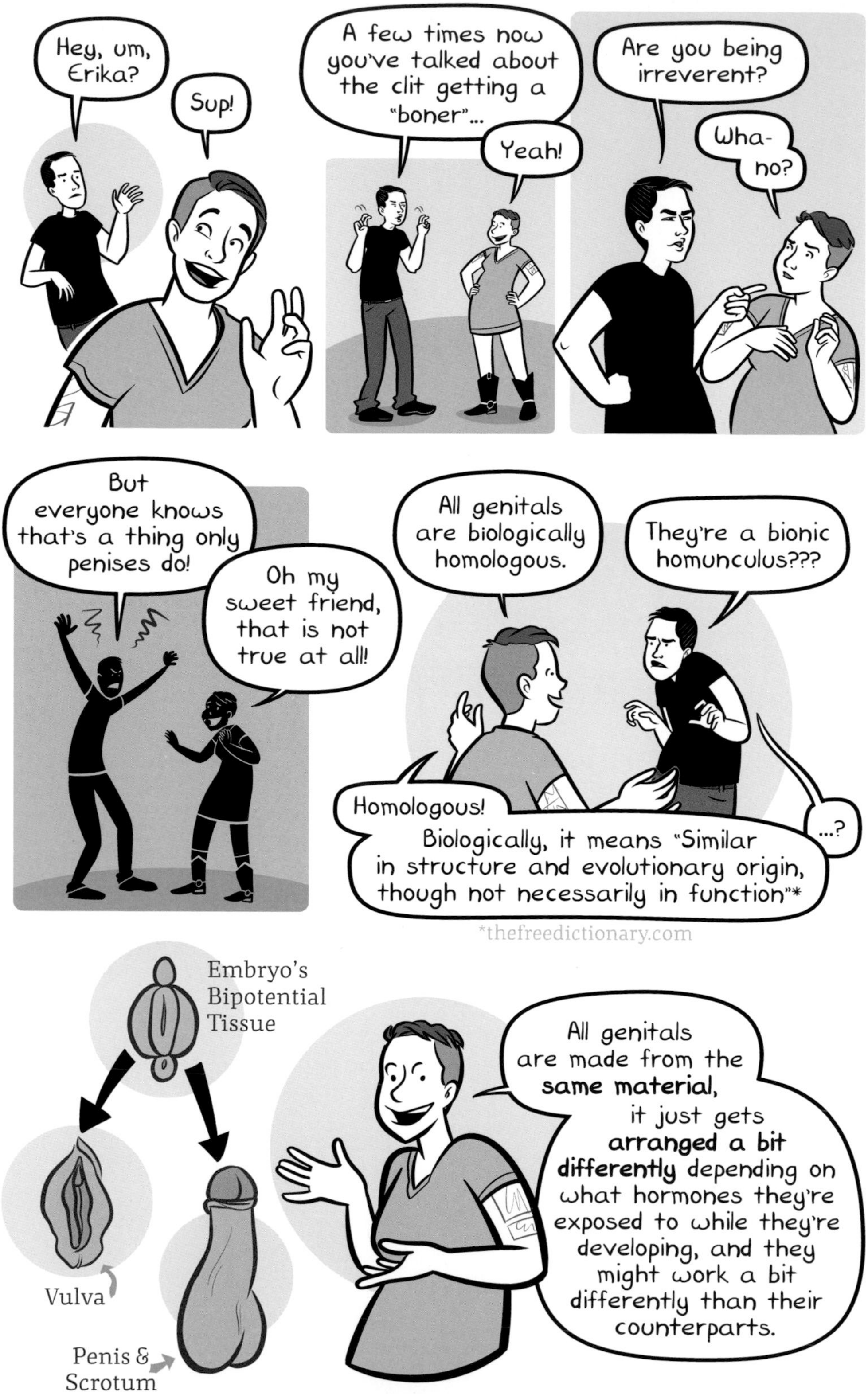
Hey, um, Erika?
Sup!
A few times now you've talked about the clit getting a "boner"...
Yeah!
Are you being irreverent?
Wha- no?
But everyone knows that's a thing only penises do!
Oh my sweet friend, that is not true at all!
All genitals are biologically homologous.
They're a bionic homunculus???
Homologous!
Biologically, it means "Similar in structure and evolutionary origin, though not necessarily in function"*
...?
*thefreedictionary.com
Embryo's Bipotential Tissue
Vulva
Penis & Scrotum
All genitals are made from the **same material,** it just gets **arranged a bit differently** depending on what hormones they're exposed to while they're developing, and they might work a bit differently than their counterparts.

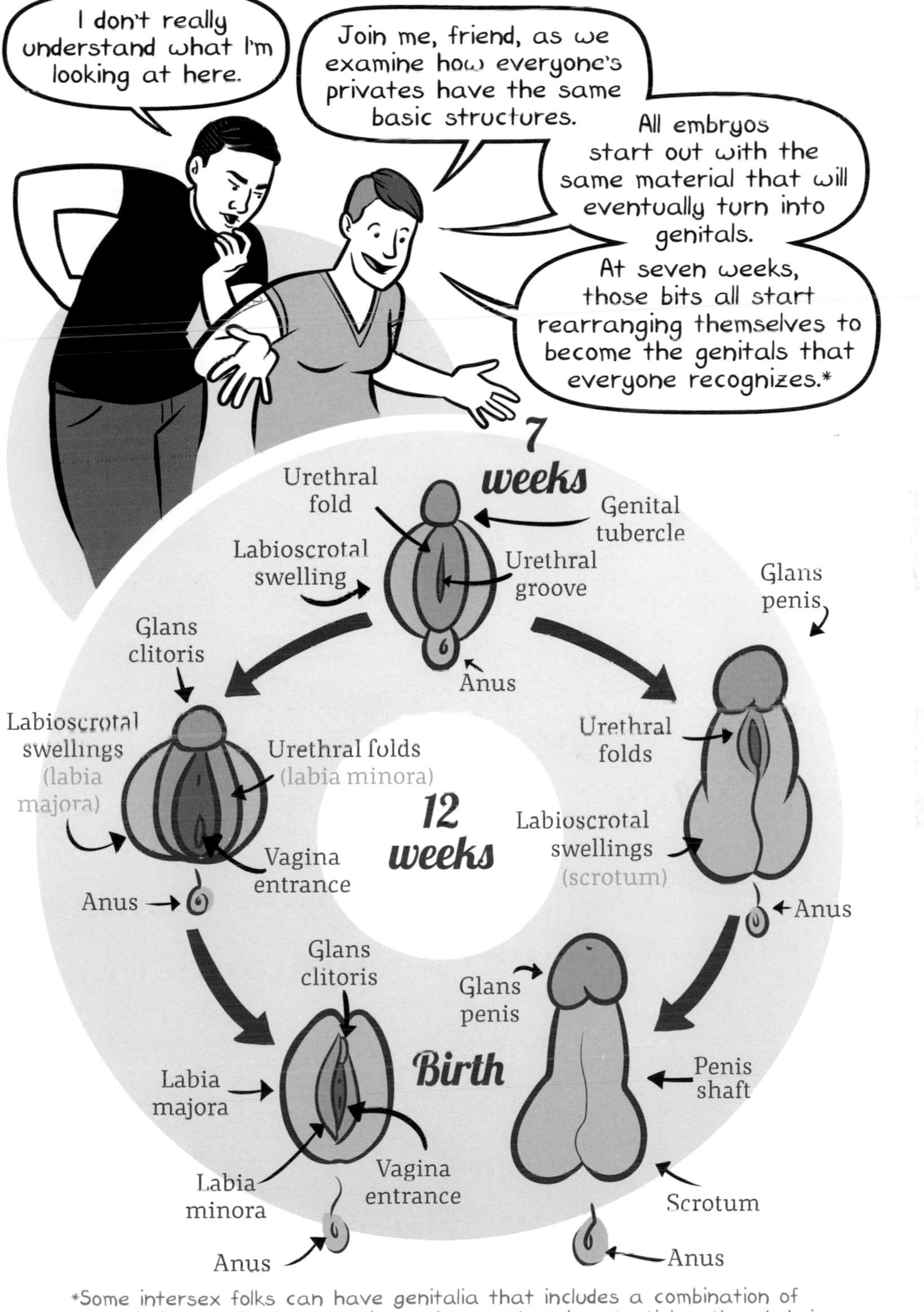
I don't really understand what I'm looking at here.
Join me, friend, as we examine how everyone's privates have the same basic structures.
All embryos start out with the same material that will eventually turn into genitals.
At seven weeks, those bits all start rearranging themselves to become the genitals that everyone recognizes.*
7 weeks
Urethral fold
Genital tubercle
Labioscrotal swelling
Urethral groove
Anus
Glans penis
Glans clitoris
Labioscrotal swellings (labia majora)
Urethral folds (labia minora)
Vagina entrance
Anus
12 weeks
Urethral folds
Labioscrotal swellings (scrotum)
Anus
Glans clitoris
Birth
Labia majora
Labia minora
Vagina entrance
Anus
Glans penis
Penis shaft
Scrotum
Anus

*Some intersex folks can have genitalia that includes a combination of characteristics attributed to typical vulvas and penises/testicles, though being intersex definitely does not always show up in an externally visible way.

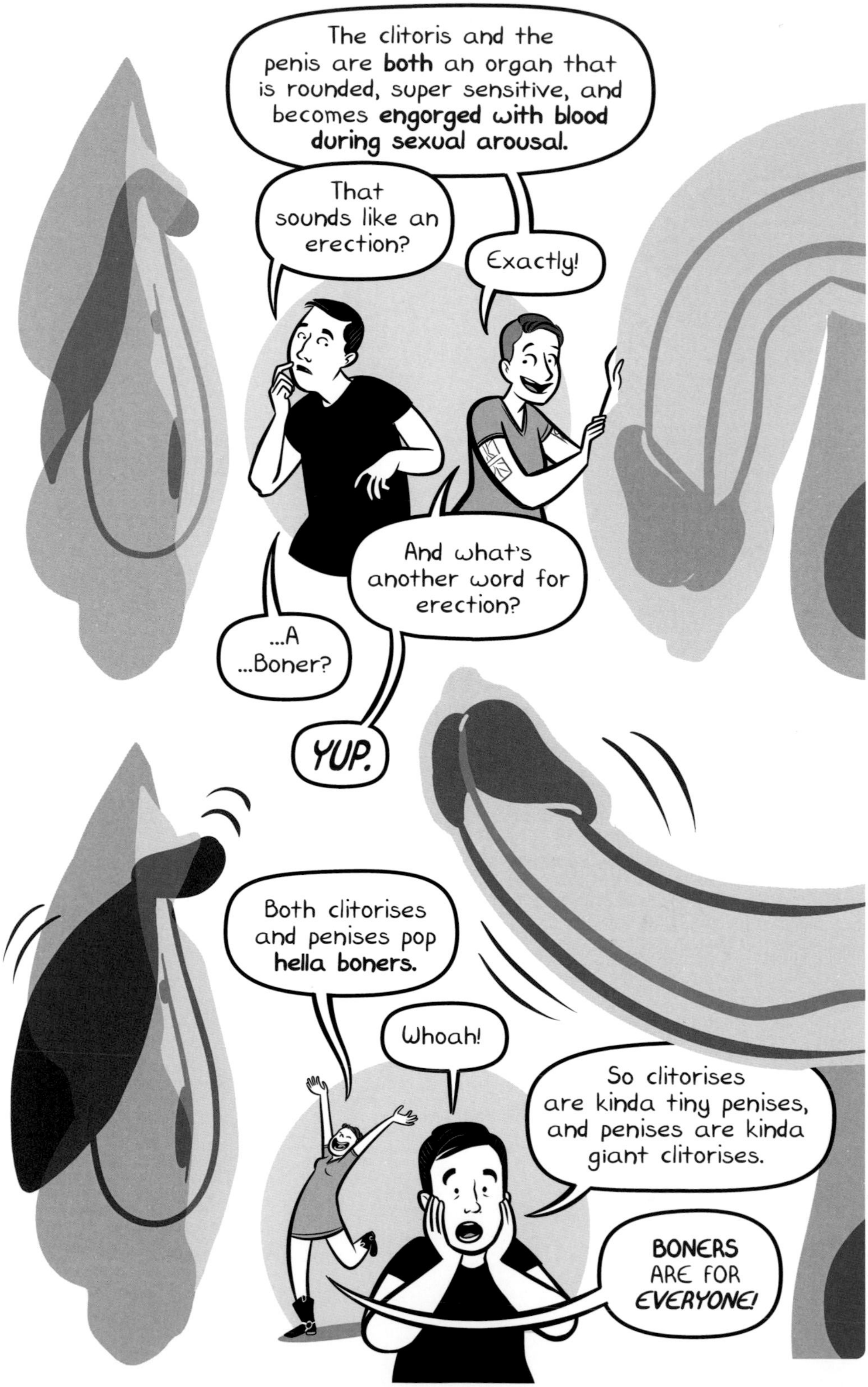
The clitoris and the penis are **both** an organ that is rounded, super sensitive, and becomes **engorged with blood during sexual arousal.**
That sounds like an erection?
Exactly!
And what's another word for erection?
...A ...Boner?
YUP.
Both clitorises and penises pop **hella boners.**
Whoah!
So clitorises are kinda tiny penises, and penises are kinda giant clitorises.
BONERS ARE FOR *EVERYONE!*

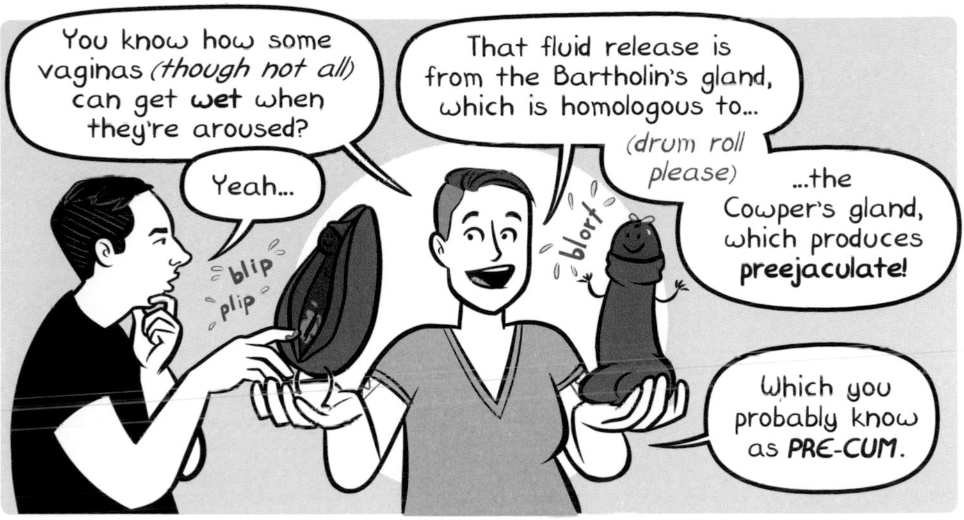
You know how some vaginas *(though not all)* can get **wet** when they're aroused?
Yeah...
blip
plip
That fluid release is from the Bartholin's gland, which is homologous to...
(drum roll please)
blort
...the Cowper's gland, which produces **preejaculate!**
Which you probably know as **PRE-CUM**.

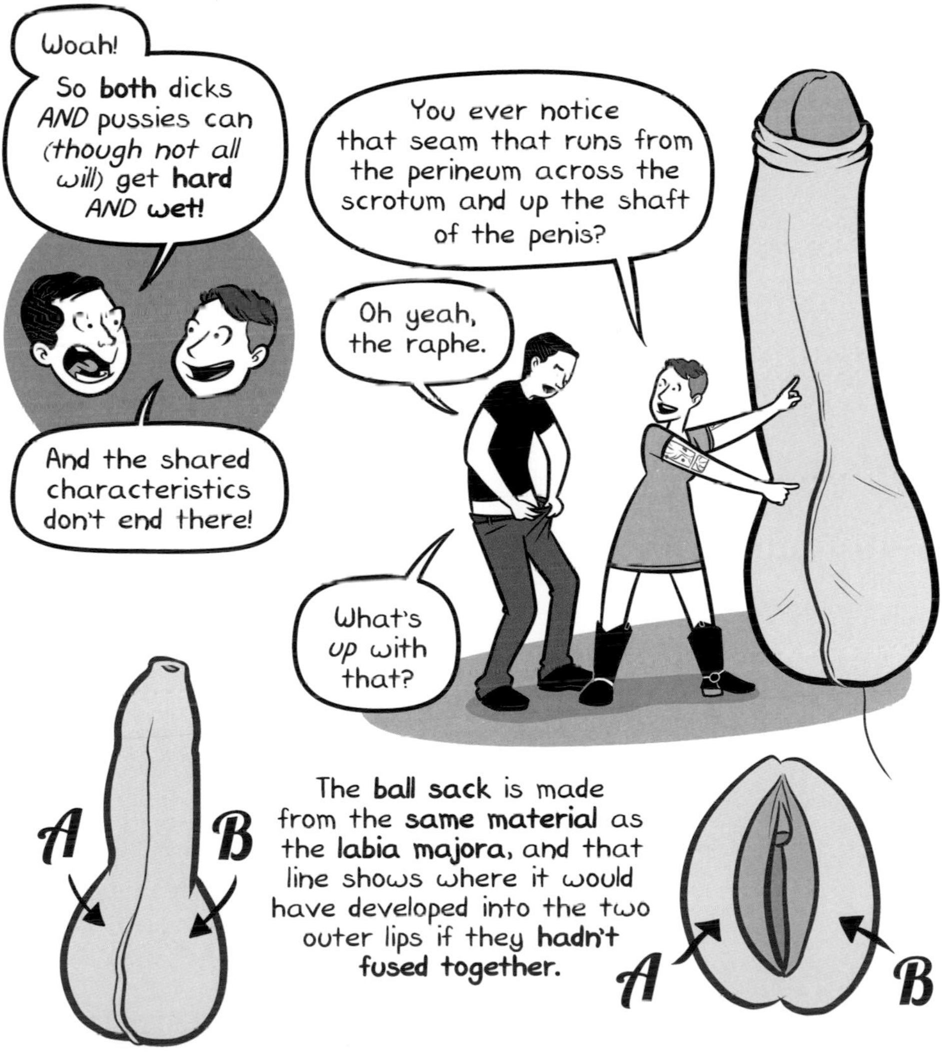
Woah!
So **both** dicks *AND* pussies can (*though not all will*) get **hard** *AND* **wet!**
And the shared characteristics don't end there!
You ever notice that seam that runs from the perineum across the scrotum and up the shaft of the penis?
Oh yeah, the raphe.
What's *up* with that?
A
B
The **ball sack** is made from the **same material** as the **labia majora**, and that line shows where it would have developed into the two outer lips if they **hadn't fused together.**
A
B

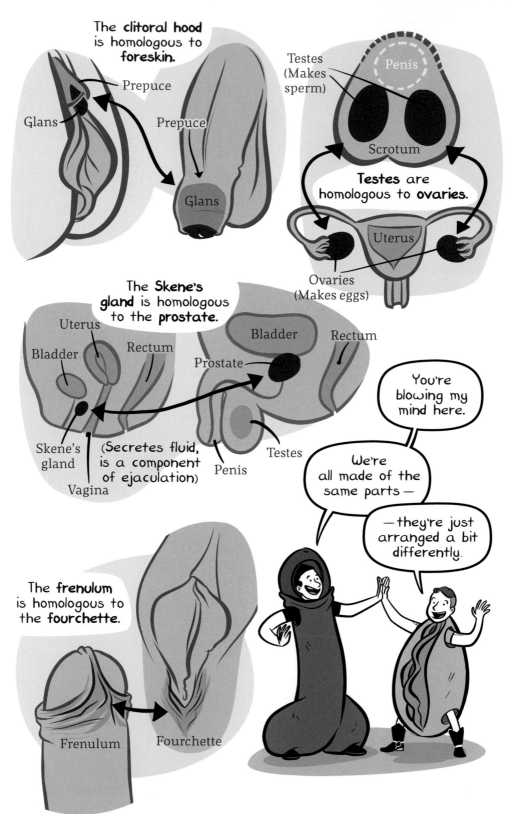

The **clitoral hood** is homologous to **foreskin**.

Prepuce
Glans
Prepuce
Glans

Testes (Makes sperm)
Penis
Scrotum
Testes are homologous to **ovaries**.
Uterus
Ovaries (Makes eggs)

The **Skene's gland** is homologous to the **prostate**.

Uterus
Bladder
Rectum
Bladder
Prostate
Rectum
Skene's gland
(Secretes fluid, is a component of ejaculation)
Penis
Testes
Vagina

You're blowing my mind here.

We're all made of the same parts—

—they're just arranged a bit differently.

The **frenulum** is homologous to the **fourchette**.

Frenulum
Fourchette

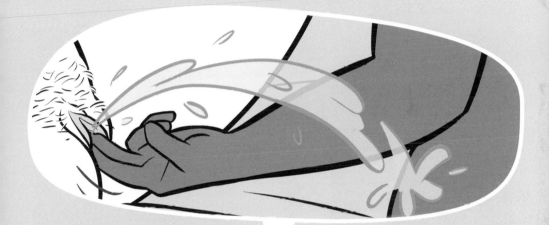

Squirting

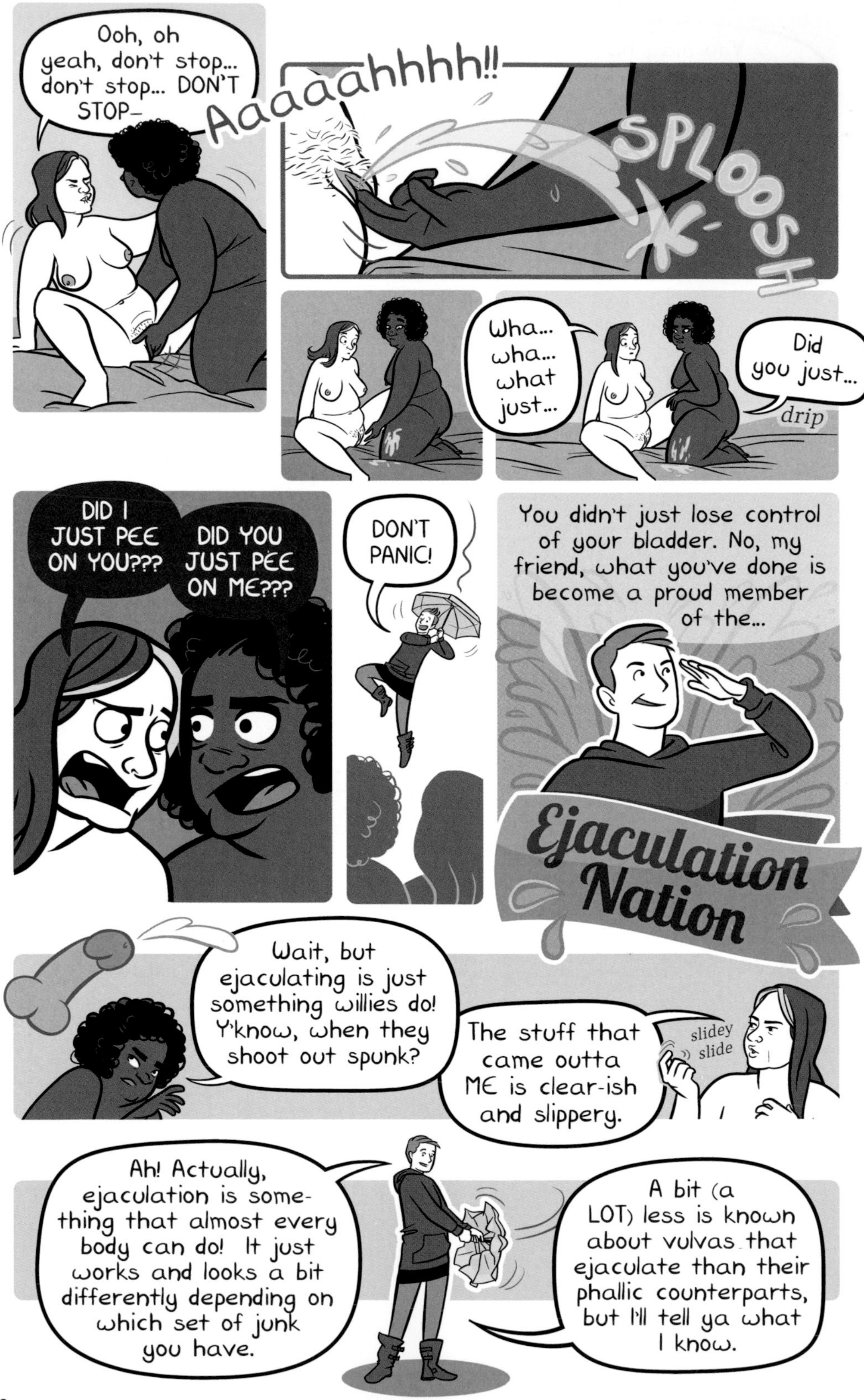

Ooh, oh yeah, don't stop... don't stop... DON'T STOP–
Aaaaahhhh!!
SPLOOSH
Wha... wha... what just...
Did you just...
drip
DID I JUST PEE ON YOU???
DID YOU JUST PEE ON ME???
DON'T PANIC!
You didn't just lose control of your bladder. No, my friend, what you've done is become a proud member of the...
Ejaculation Nation
Wait, but ejaculating is just something willies do! Y'know, when they shoot out spunk?
The stuff that came outta ME is clear-ish and slippery.
slidey slide
Ah! Actually, ejaculation is something that almost every body can do! It just works and looks a bit differently depending on which set of junk you have.
A bit (a LOT) less is known about vulvas that ejaculate than their phallic counterparts, but I'll tell ya what I know.

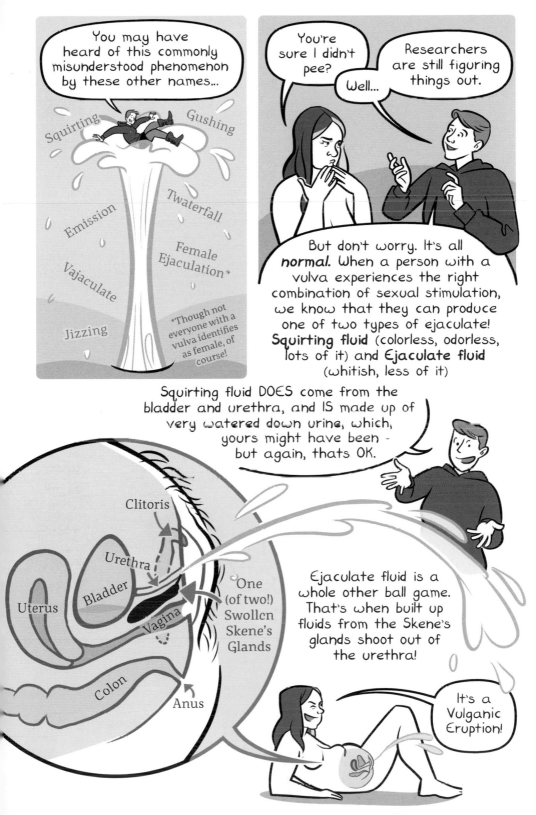

You may have heard of this commonly misunderstood phenomenon by these other names...

Squirting

Gushing

Emission

Twaterfall

Vajaculate

Female Ejaculation*

Jizzing

*Though not everyone with a vulva identifies as female, of course!

You're sure I didn't pee?

Well...

Researchers are still figuring things out.

But don't worry. It's all **normal**. When a person with a vulva experiences the right combination of sexual stimulation, we know that they can produce one of two types of ejaculate! **Squirting fluid** (colorless, odorless, lots of it) and **Ejaculate fluid** (whitish, less of it)

Squirting fluid DOES come from the bladder and urethra, and IS made up of very watered down urine, which, yours might have been - but again, that's OK.

Clitoris

Urethra

Bladder

Uterus

Vagina

°One (of two!) Swollen Skene's Glands

Colon

Anus

Ejaculate fluid is a whole other ball game. That's when built up fluids from the Skene's glands shoot out of the urethra!

It's a Vulganic Eruption!

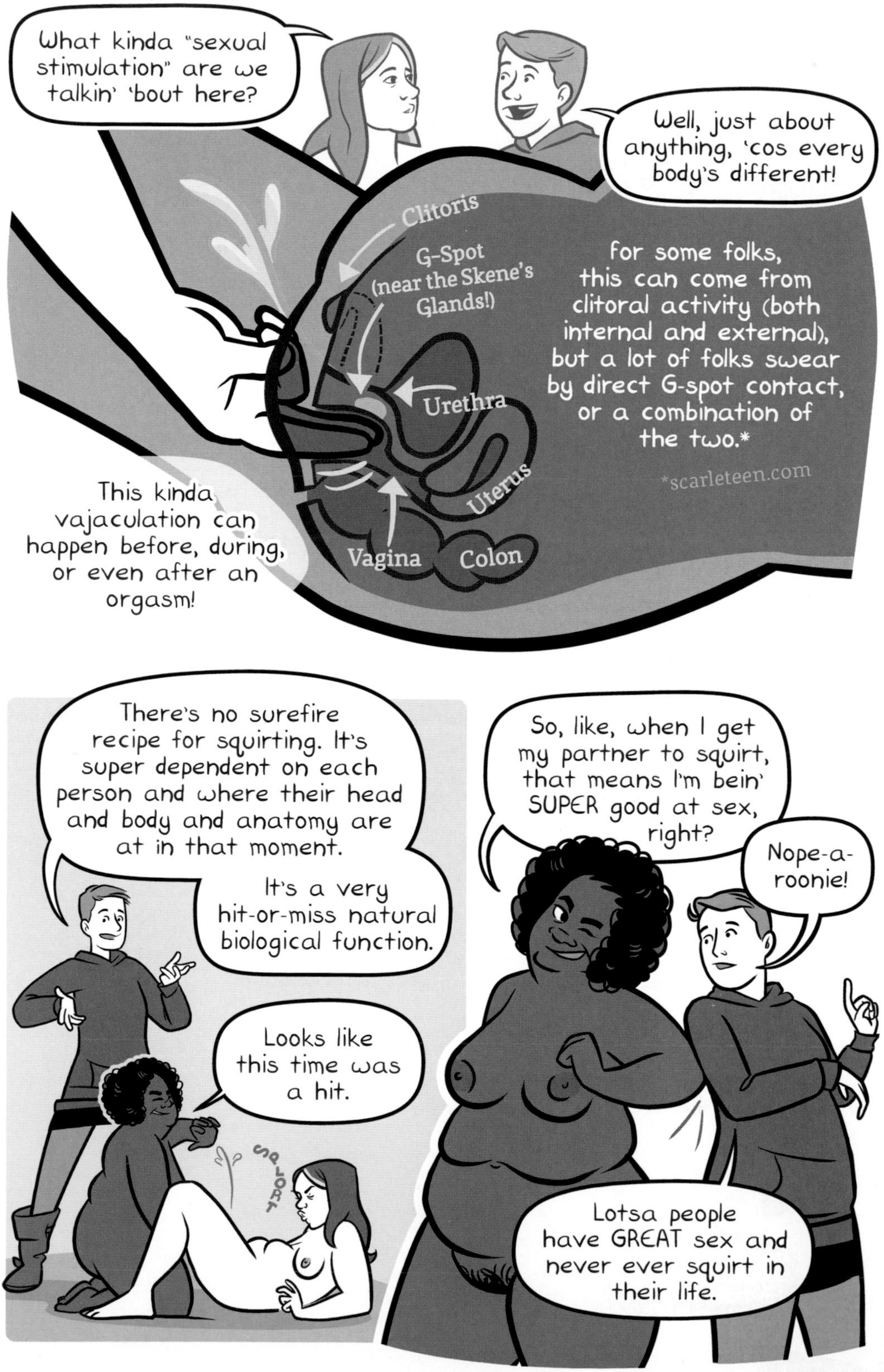
What kinda "sexual stimulation" are we talkin' 'bout here?
Well, just about anything, 'cos every body's different!
Clitoris
G-Spot (near the Skene's Glands!)
Urethra
Uterus
Vagina
Colon
For some folks, this can come from clitoral activity (both internal and external), but a lot of folks swear by direct G-spot contact, or a combination of the two.*
*scarleteen.com
This kinda vajaculation can happen before, during, or even after an orgasm!
There's no surefire recipe for squirting. It's super dependent on each person and where their head and body and anatomy are at in that moment.
It's a very hit-or-miss natural biological function.
Looks like this time was a hit.
SPLORT
So, like, when I get my partner to squirt, that means I'm bein' SUPER good at sex, right?
Nope-a-roonie!
Lotsa people have GREAT sex and never ever squirt in their life.

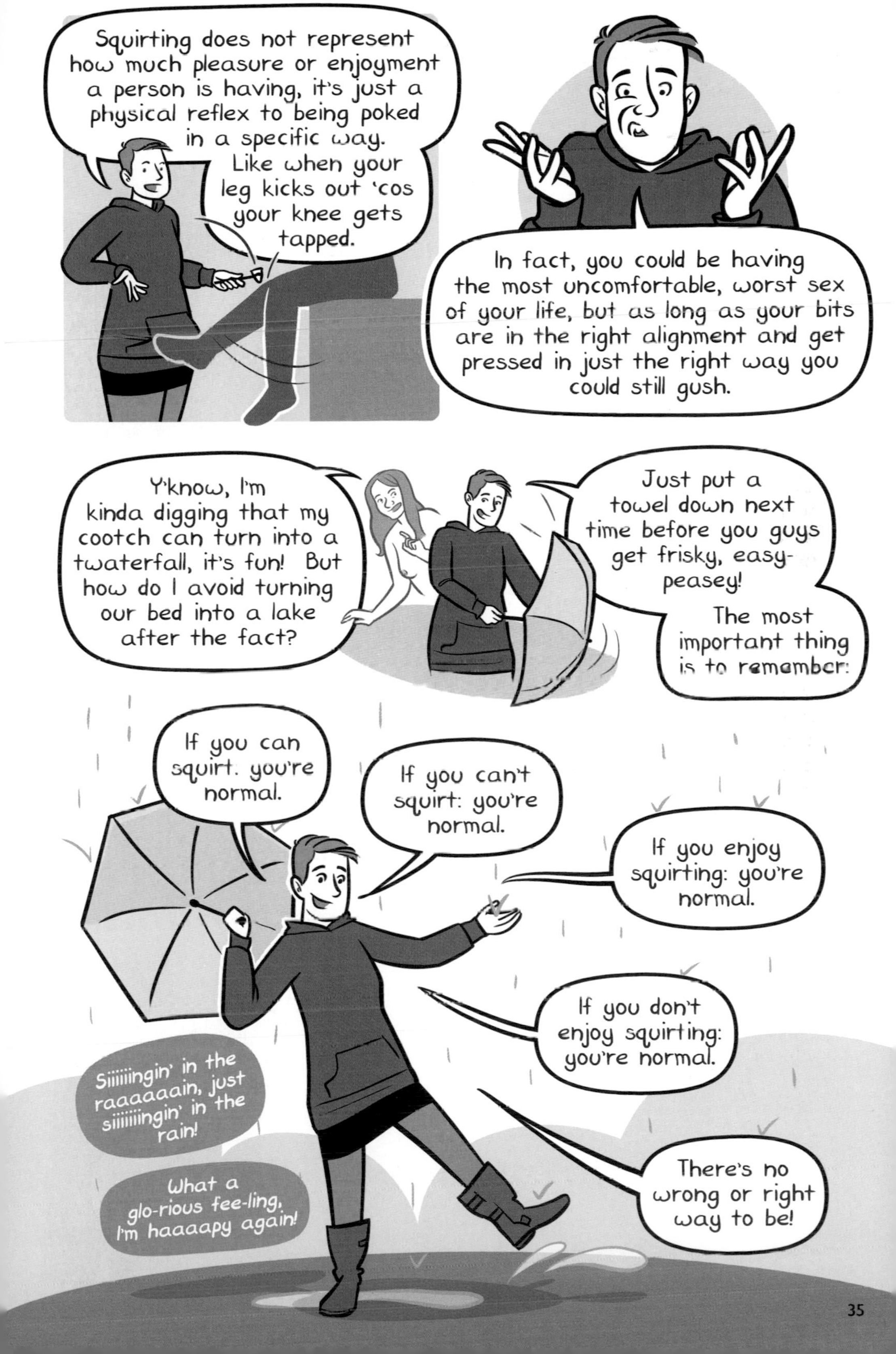
Squirting does not represent how much pleasure or enjoyment a person is having, it's just a physical reflex to being poked in a specific way.
Like when your leg kicks out 'cos your knee gets tapped.
In fact, you could be having the most uncomfortable, worst sex of your life, but as long as your bits are in the right alignment and get pressed in just the right way you could still gush.
Y'know, I'm kinda digging that my cootch can turn into a twaterfall, it's fun! But how do I avoid turning our bed into a lake after the fact?
Just put a towel down next time before you guys get frisky, easy-peasey!
The most important thing is to remember:
If you can squirt. you're normal.
If you can't squirt: you're normal.
If you enjoy squirting: you're normal.
If you don't enjoy squirting: you're normal.
There's no wrong or right way to be!
Siiiiiingin' in the raaaaaain, just siiiiiingin' in the rain!
What a glo-rious fee-ling, I'm haaaapy again!

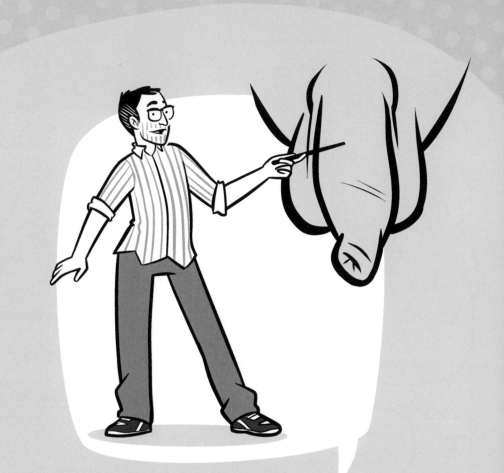

Foreskin

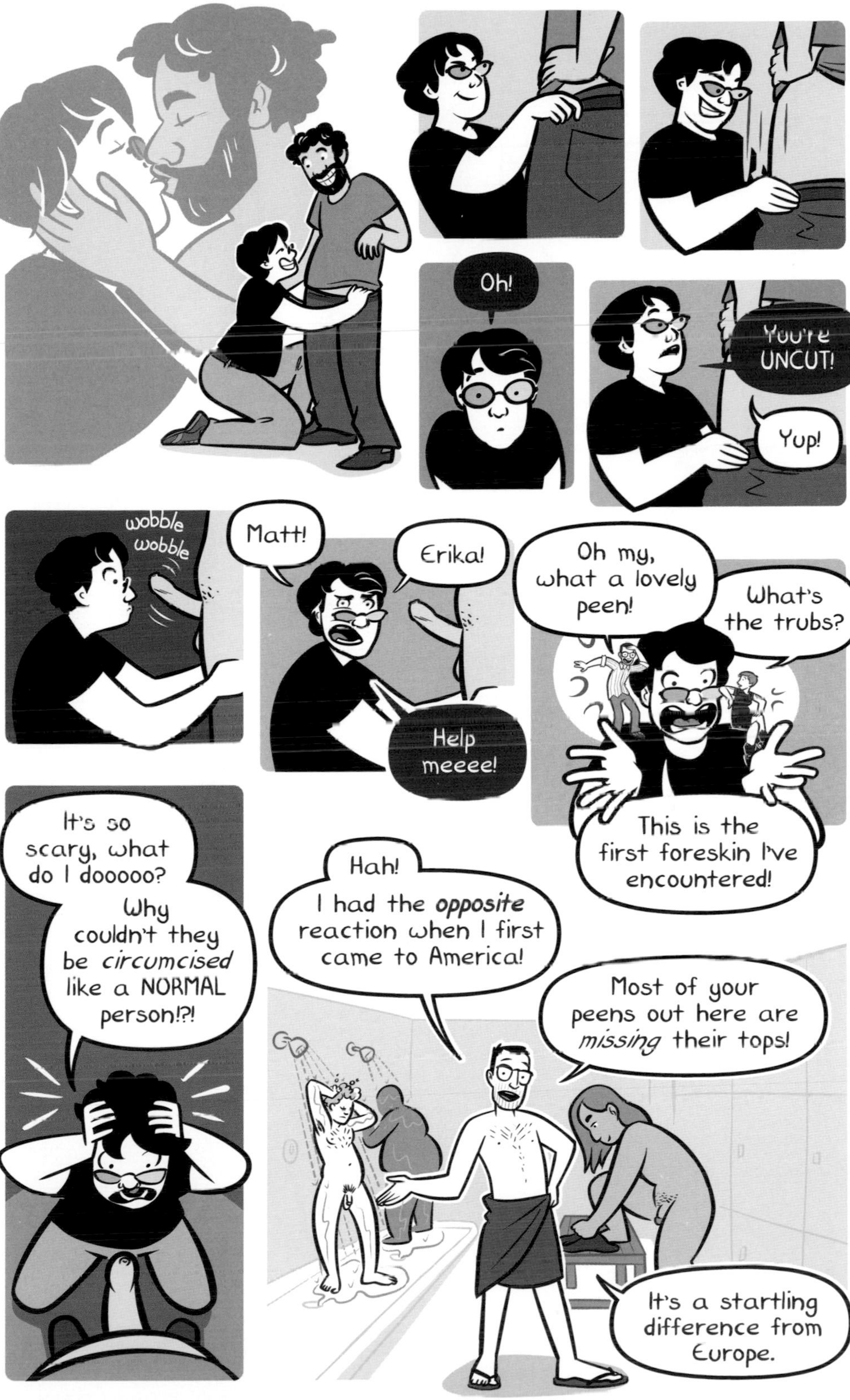
Oh!
You're UNCUT!
Yup!
wobble wobble
Matt!
Erika!
Help meeee!
Oh my, what a lovely peen!
What's the trubs?
This is the first foreskin I've encountered!
It's so scary, what do I dooooo?
Why couldn't they be *circumcised* like a NORMAL person!?!
Hah!
I had the ***opposite*** reaction when I first came to America!
Most of your peens out here are *missing* their tops!
It's a startling difference from Europe.

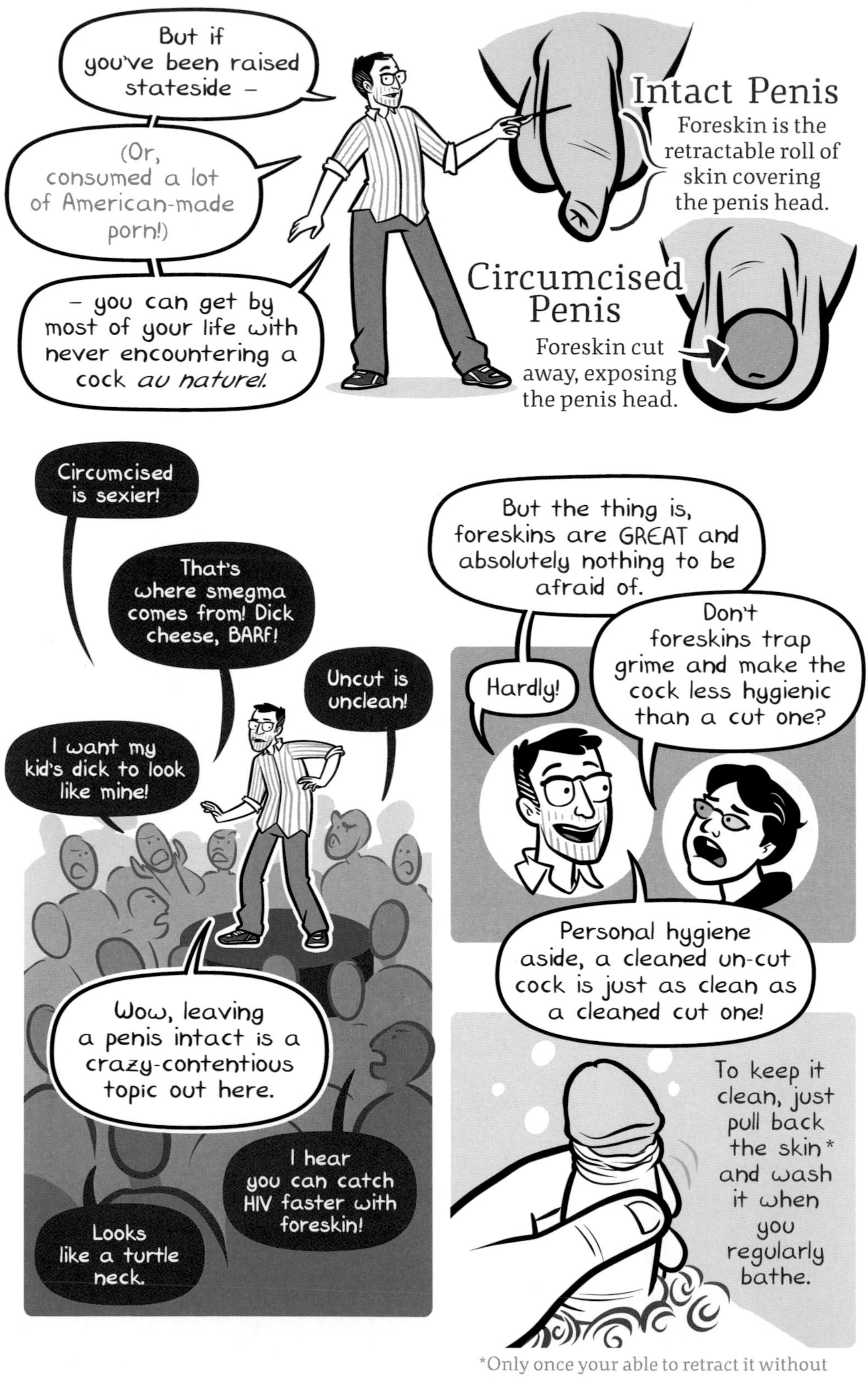

But if you've been raised stateside –
(Or, consumed a lot of American-made porn!)
– you can get by most of your life with never encountering a cock *au naturel.*
Intact Penis
Foreskin is the retractable roll of skin covering the penis head.
Circumcised Penis
Foreskin cut away, exposing the penis head.
Circumcised is sexier!
That's where smegma comes from! Dick cheese, BARF!
Uncut is unclean!
I want my kid's dick to look like mine!
Wow, leaving a penis intact is a crazy-contentious topic out here.
I hear you can catch HIV faster with foreskin!
Looks like a turtle neck.
But the thing is, foreskins are GREAT and absolutely nothing to be afraid of.
Hardly!
Don't foreskins trap grime and make the cock less hygienic than a cut one?
Personal hygiene aside, a cleaned un-cut cock is just as clean as a cleaned cut one!
To keep it clean, just pull back the skin* and wash it when you regularly bathe.

*Only once your able to retract it without force. Sometime between 5-16 years old.

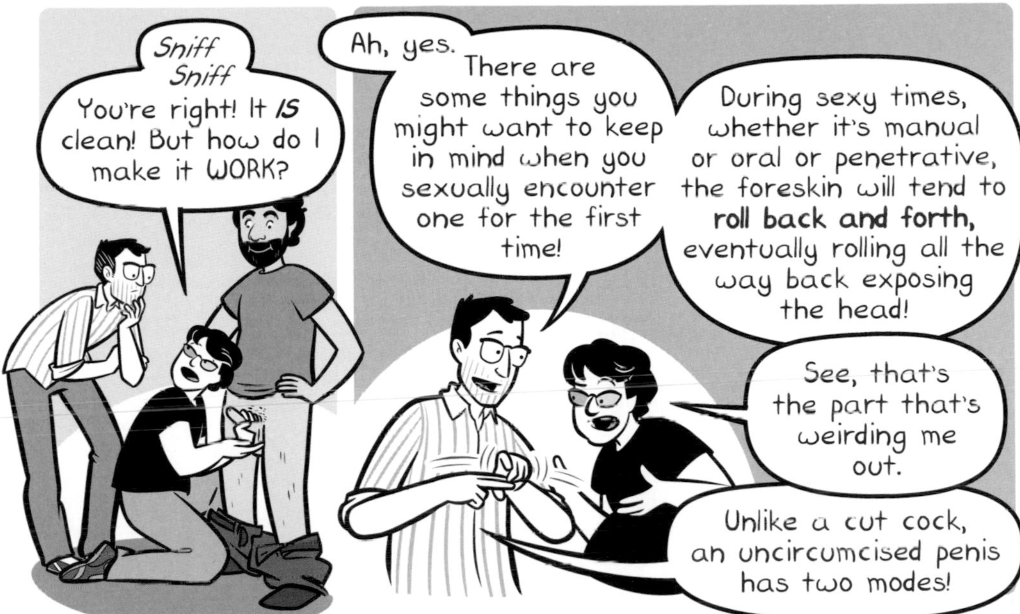
Sniff
Sniff
You're right! It *IS* clean! But how do I make it WORK?
Ah, yes.
There are some things you might want to keep in mind when you sexually encounter one for the first time!
During sexy times, whether it's manual or oral or penetrative, the foreskin will tend to **roll back and forth,** eventually rolling all the way back exposing the head!
See, that's the part that's weirding me out.
Unlike a cut cock, an uncircumcised penis has two modes!

Rolled Up!

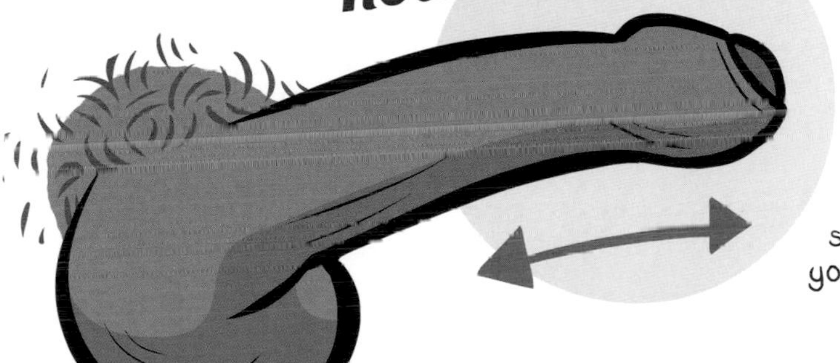

The foreskin will help protect the sensitive head and give it a different, more subdued sensation during sexy times.

That added skin surface area gives you more to play with during handjobs!

Pulled Back!*

*Don't fret if yours can't do this yet, some people's needs stretching that comes with age and some don't ever fully roll back.

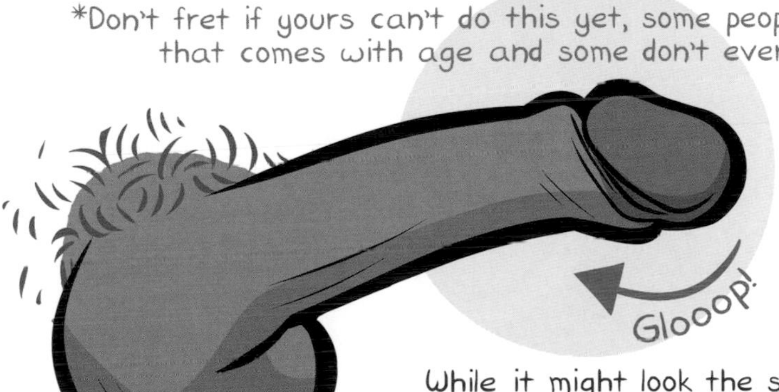
Glooop!

In this state an uncircumcised cock will resemble a circumcised one, but with an added roll of skin behind the head.

While it might look the same, it will probably react differently than a cut one: that head is a lot more sensitive!

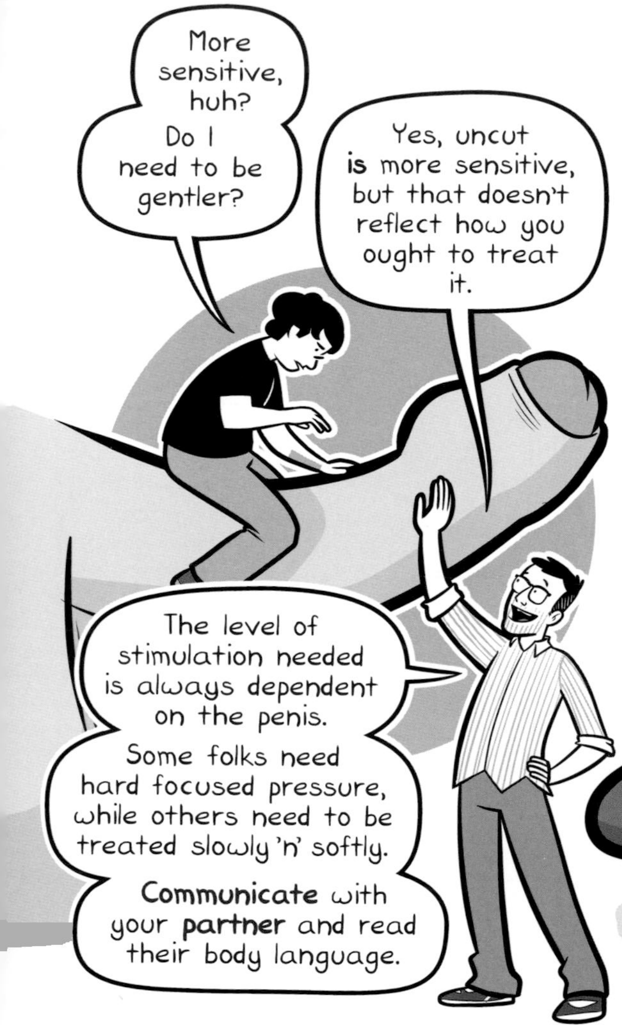
More sensitive, huh?
Do I need to be gentler?
Yes, uncut **is** more sensitive, but that doesn't reflect how you ought to treat it.
The level of stimulation needed is always dependent on the penis.
Some folks need hard focused pressure, while others need to be treated slowly 'n' softly.
Communicate with your **partner** and read their body language.

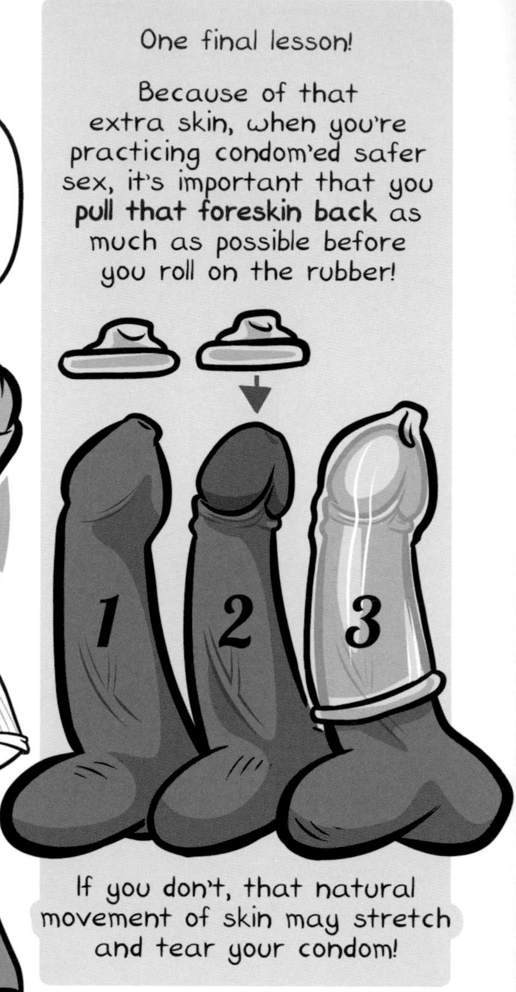
One final lesson!
Because of that extra skin, when you're practicing condom'ed safer sex, it's important that you **pull that foreskin back** as much as possible before you roll on the rubber!
1
2
3
If you don't, that natural movement of skin may stretch and tear your condom!

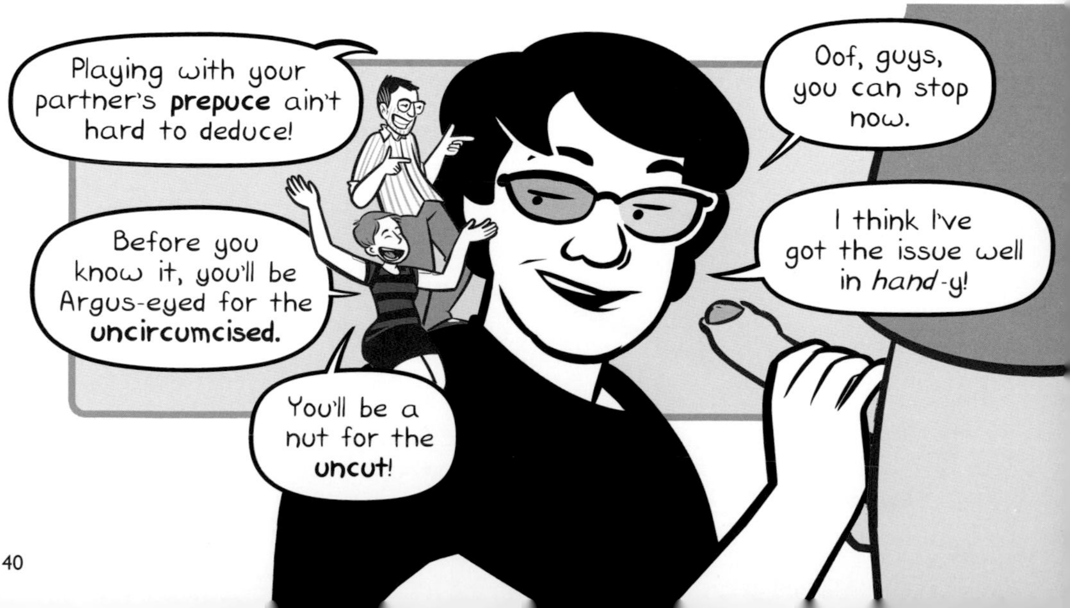
Playing with your partner's **prepuce** ain't hard to deduce!
Before you know it, you'll be Argus-eyed for the **uncircumcised.**
You'll be a nut for the **uncut**!
Oof, guys, you can stop now.
I think I've got the issue well in *hand*-y!

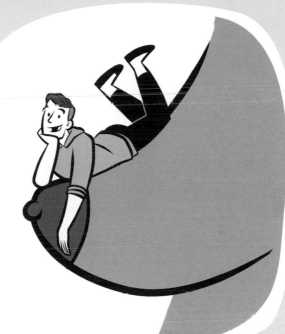

Breasts

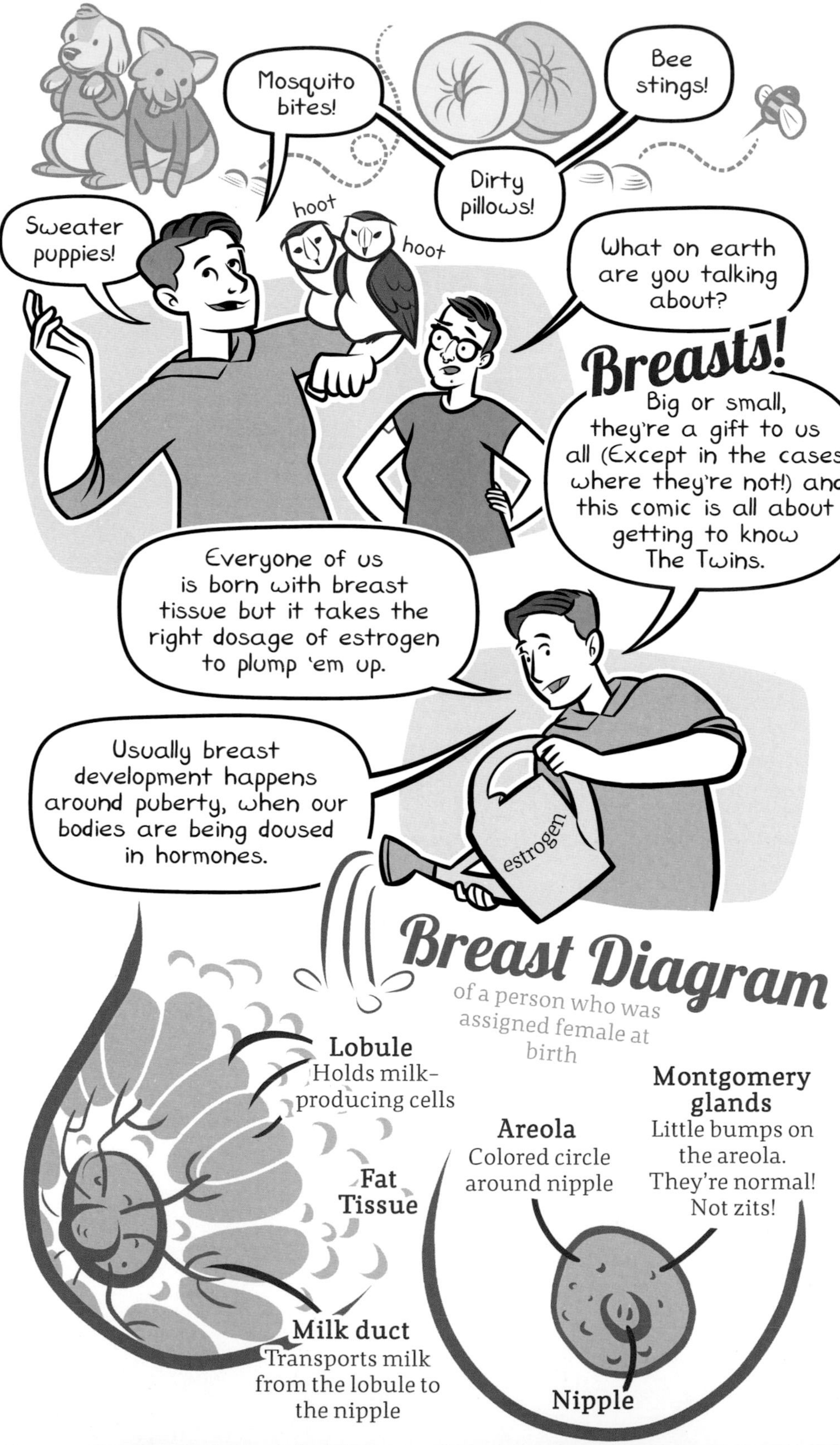

Sweater puppies!
Mosquito bites!
Dirty pillows!
Bee stings!
hoot
hoot
What on earth are you talking about?
Breasts!
Big or small, they're a gift to us all (Except in the cases where they're not!) and this comic is all about getting to know The Twins.
Everyone of us is born with breast tissue but it takes the right dosage of estrogen to plump 'em up.
Usually breast development happens around puberty, when our bodies are being doused in hormones.
estrogen
Breast Diagram
of a person who was assigned female at birth
Lobule
Holds milk-producing cells
Fat Tissue
Milk duct
Transports milk from the lobule to the nipple
Areola
Colored circle around nipple
Montgomery glands
Little bumps on the areola. They're normal! Not zits!
Nipple

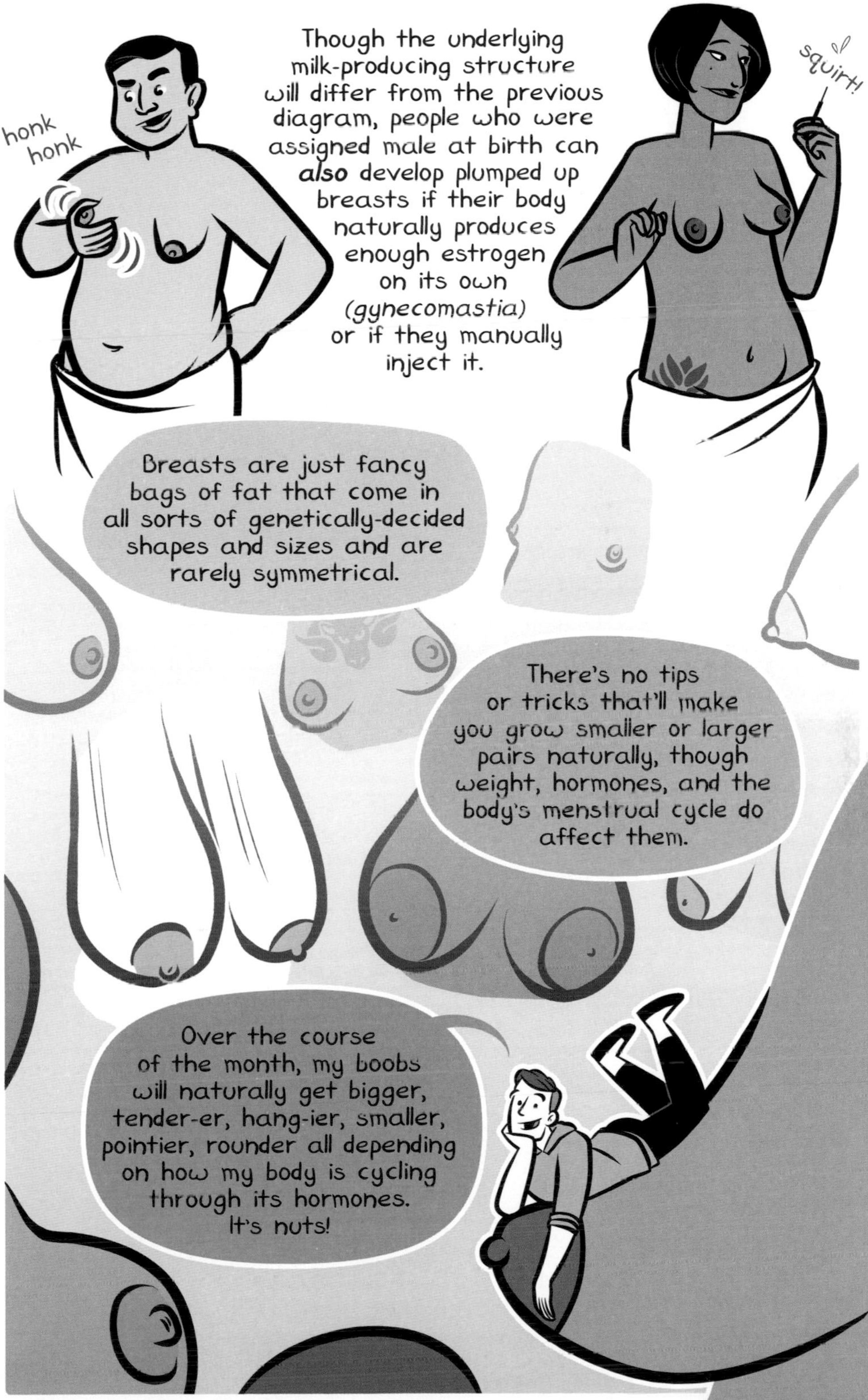
honk honk
Though the underlying milk-producing structure will differ from the previous diagram, people who were assigned male at birth can *also* develop plumped up breasts if their body naturally produces enough estrogen on its own (*gynecomastia*) or if they manually inject it.
squirt!
Breasts are just fancy bags of fat that come in all sorts of genetically-decided shapes and sizes and are rarely symmetrical.
There's no tips or tricks that'll make you grow smaller or larger pairs naturally, though weight, hormones, and the body's menstrual cycle do affect them.
Over the course of the month, my boobs will naturally get bigger, tender-er, hang-ier, smaller, pointier, rounder all depending on how my body is cycling through its hormones. It's nuts!

Over a lifetime, a person's breasts will change, especially from pregnancy and later in life as their natural hormone supply ages.

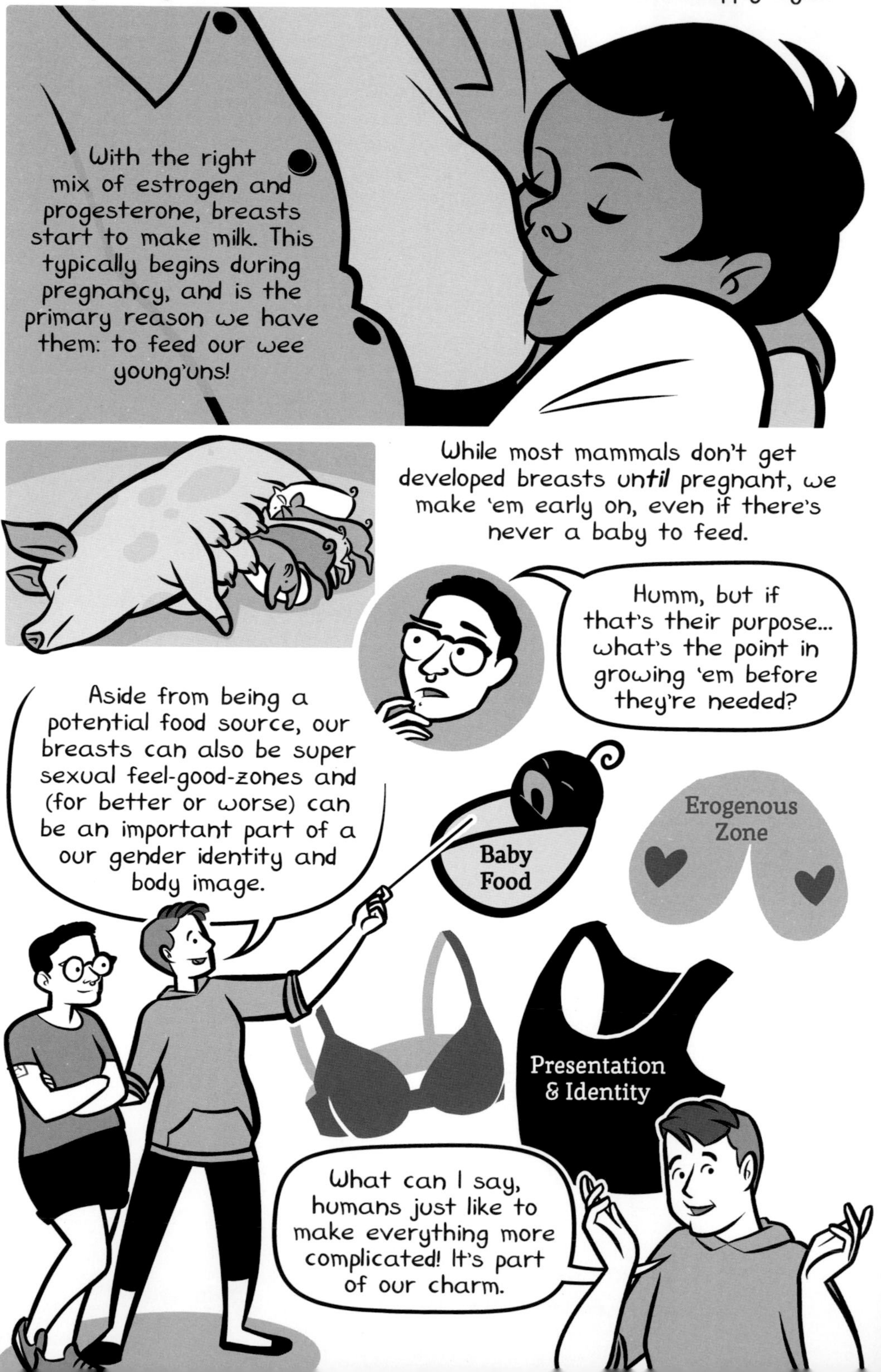
With the right mix of estrogen and progesterone, breasts start to make milk. This typically begins during pregnancy, and is the primary reason we have them: to feed our wee young'uns!
While most mammals don't get developed breasts *until* pregnant, we make 'em early on, even if there's never a baby to feed.
Humm, but if that's their purpose... what's the point in growing 'em before they're needed?
Aside from being a potential food source, our breasts can also be super sexual feel-good-zones and (for better or worse) can be an important part of a our gender identity and body image.
Baby Food
Erogenous Zone
Presentation & Identity
What can I say, humans just like to make everything more complicated! It's part of our charm.

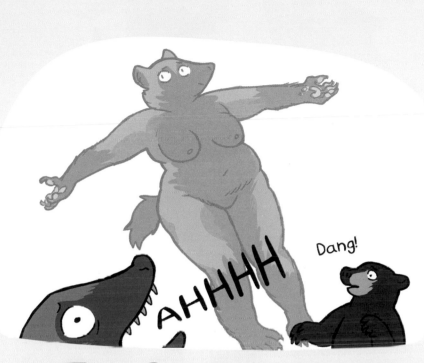

Body Image

By Abby Howard

Abbyhowardart.myportfolio.com

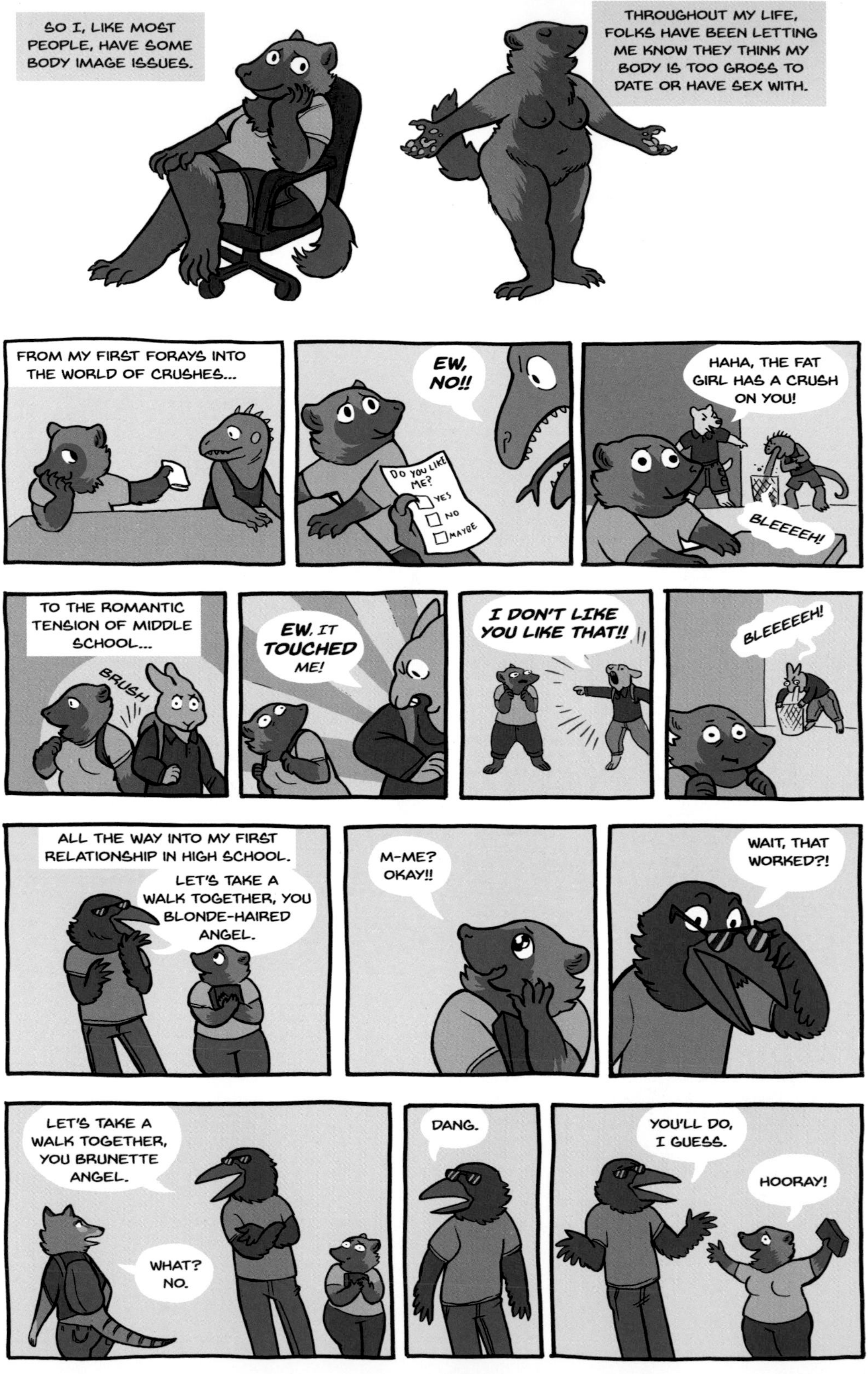
SO I, LIKE MOST PEOPLE, HAVE SOME BODY IMAGE ISSUES.
THROUGHOUT MY LIFE, FOLKS HAVE BEEN LETTING ME KNOW THEY THINK MY BODY IS TOO GROSS TO DATE OR HAVE SEX WITH.
FROM MY FIRST FORAYS INTO THE WORLD OF CRUSHES...
EW, NO!!
DO YOU LIKE ME?
YES
NO
MAYBE
HAHA, THE FAT GIRL HAS A CRUSH ON YOU!
BLEEEEH!
TO THE ROMANTIC TENSION OF MIDDLE SCHOOL...
BRUSH
EW, IT TOUCHED ME!
I DON'T LIKE YOU LIKE THAT!!
BLEEEEEH!
ALL THE WAY INTO MY FIRST RELATIONSHIP IN HIGH SCHOOL.
LET'S TAKE A WALK TOGETHER, YOU BLONDE-HAIRED ANGEL.
M-ME? OKAY!!
WAIT, THAT WORKED?!
LET'S TAKE A WALK TOGETHER, YOU BRUNETTE ANGEL.
WHAT? NO.
DANG.
YOU'LL DO, I GUESS.
HOORAY!

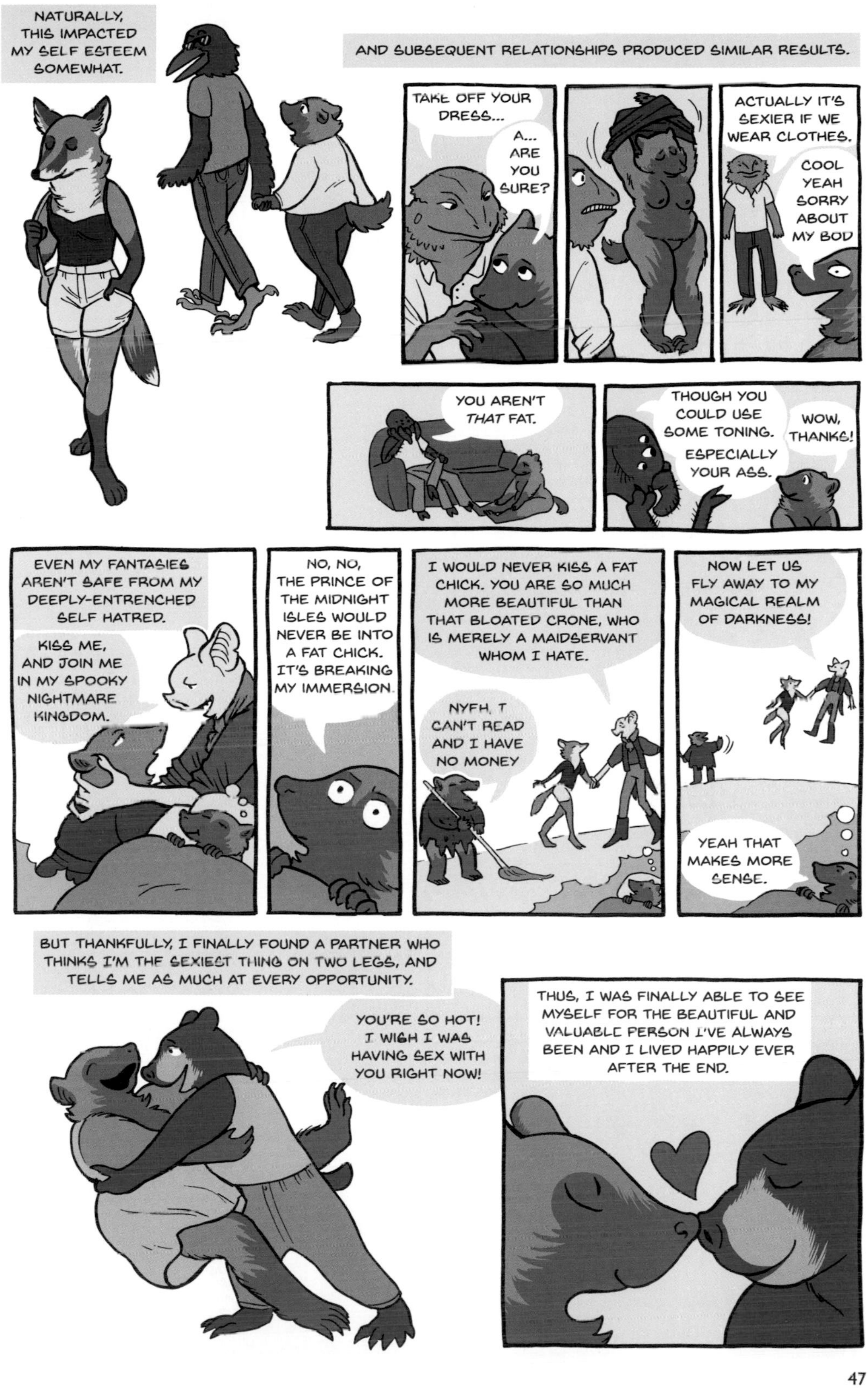
NATURALLY, THIS IMPACTED MY SELF ESTEEM SOMEWHAT.
AND SUBSEQUENT RELATIONSHIPS PRODUCED SIMILAR RESULTS.
TAKE OFF YOUR DRESS...
A... ARE YOU SURE?
ACTUALLY IT'S SEXIER IF WE WEAR CLOTHES.
COOL YEAH SORRY ABOUT MY BOD
YOU AREN'T *THAT* FAT.
THOUGH YOU COULD USE SOME TONING.
ESPECIALLY YOUR ASS.
WOW, THANKS!
EVEN MY FANTASIES AREN'T SAFE FROM MY DEEPLY-ENTRENCHED SELF HATRED.
KISS ME, AND JOIN ME IN MY SPOOKY NIGHTMARE KINGDOM.
NO, NO, THE PRINCE OF THE MIDNIGHT ISLES WOULD NEVER BE INTO A FAT CHICK. IT'S BREAKING MY IMMERSION.
I WOULD NEVER KISS A FAT CHICK. YOU ARE SO MUCH MORE BEAUTIFUL THAN THAT BLOATED CRONE, WHO IS MERELY A MAIDSERVANT WHOM I HATE.
NYFH, I CAN'T READ AND I HAVE NO MONEY
NOW LET US FLY AWAY TO MY MAGICAL REALM OF DARKNESS!
YEAH THAT MAKES MORE SENSE.
BUT THANKFULLY, I FINALLY FOUND A PARTNER WHO THINKS I'M THE SEXIEST THING ON TWO LEGS, AND TELLS ME AS MUCH AT EVERY OPPORTUNITY.
YOU'RE SO HOT! I WISH I WAS HAVING SEX WITH YOU RIGHT NOW!
THUS, I WAS FINALLY ABLE TO SEE MYSELF FOR THE BEAUTIFUL AND VALUABLE PERSON I'VE ALWAYS BEEN AND I LIVED HAPPILY EVER AFTER THE END.

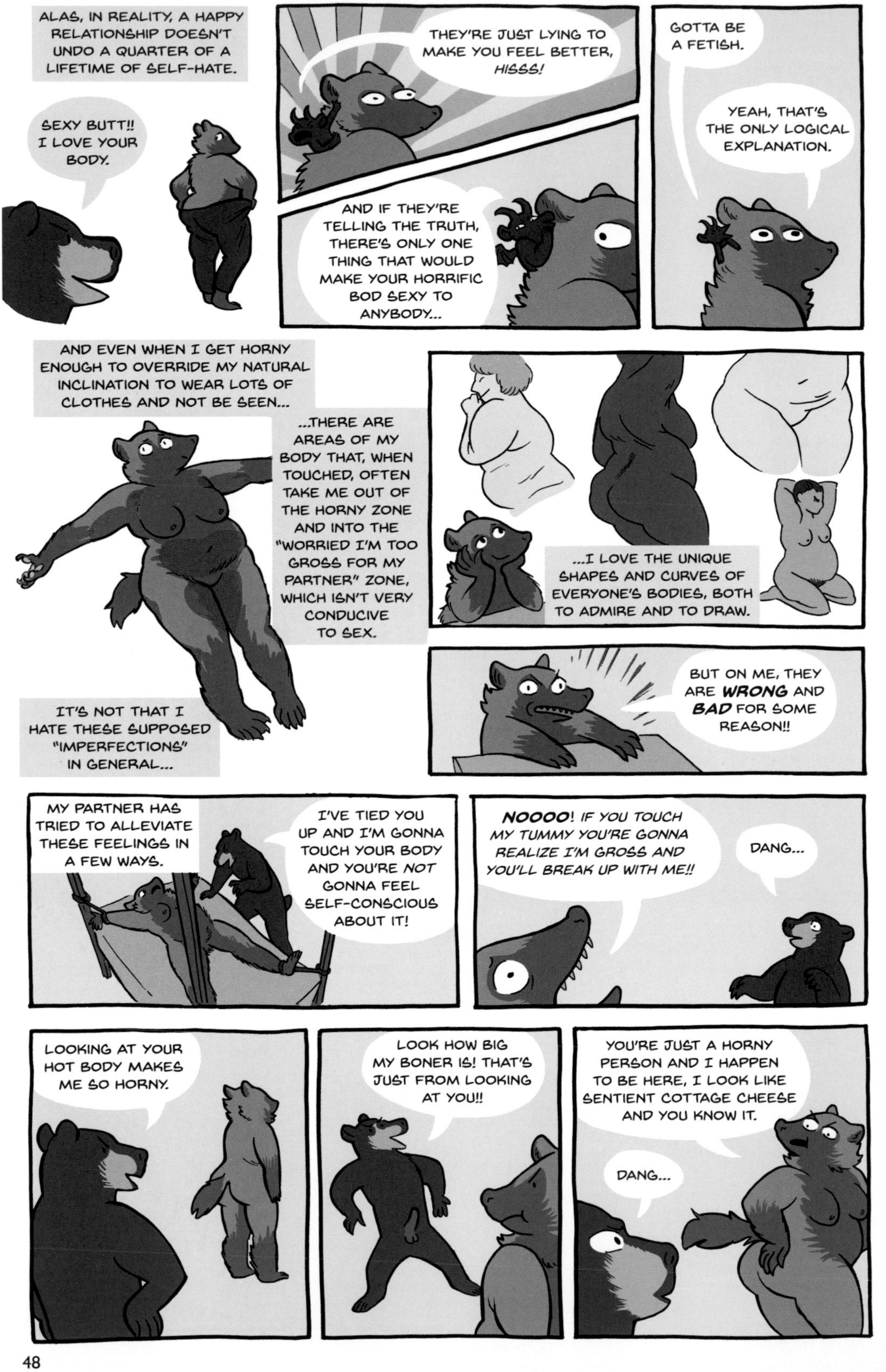
ALAS, IN REALITY, A HAPPY RELATIONSHIP DOESN'T UNDO A QUARTER OF A LIFETIME OF SELF-HATE.
SEXY BUTT!! I LOVE YOUR BODY.
THEY'RE JUST LYING TO MAKE YOU FEEL BETTER, HISSS!
AND IF THEY'RE TELLING THE TRUTH, THERE'S ONLY ONE THING THAT WOULD MAKE YOUR HORRIFIC BOD SEXY TO ANYBODY...
GOTTA BE A FETISH.
YEAH, THAT'S THE ONLY LOGICAL EXPLANATION.
AND EVEN WHEN I GET HORNY ENOUGH TO OVERRIDE MY NATURAL INCLINATION TO WEAR LOTS OF CLOTHES AND NOT BE SEEN...
...THERE ARE AREAS OF MY BODY THAT, WHEN TOUCHED, OFTEN TAKE ME OUT OF THE HORNY ZONE AND INTO THE "WORRIED I'M TOO GROSS FOR MY PARTNER" ZONE, WHICH ISN'T VERY CONDUCIVE TO SEX.
IT'S NOT THAT I HATE THESE SUPPOSED "IMPERFECTIONS" IN GENERAL...
...I LOVE THE UNIQUE SHAPES AND CURVES OF EVERYONE'S BODIES, BOTH TO ADMIRE AND TO DRAW.
BUT ON ME, THEY ARE WRONG AND BAD FOR SOME REASON!!
MY PARTNER HAS TRIED TO ALLEVIATE THESE FEELINGS IN A FEW WAYS.
I'VE TIED YOU UP AND I'M GONNA TOUCH YOUR BODY AND YOU'RE NOT GONNA FEEL SELF-CONSCIOUS ABOUT IT!
NOOOO! IF YOU TOUCH MY TUMMY YOU'RE GONNA REALIZE I'M GROSS AND YOU'LL BREAK UP WITH ME!!
DANG...
LOOKING AT YOUR HOT BODY MAKES ME SO HORNY.
LOOK HOW BIG MY BONER IS! THAT'S JUST FROM LOOKING AT YOU!!
YOU'RE JUST A HORNY PERSON AND I HAPPEN TO BE HERE, I LOOK LIKE SENTIENT COTTAGE CHEESE AND YOU KNOW IT.
DANG...

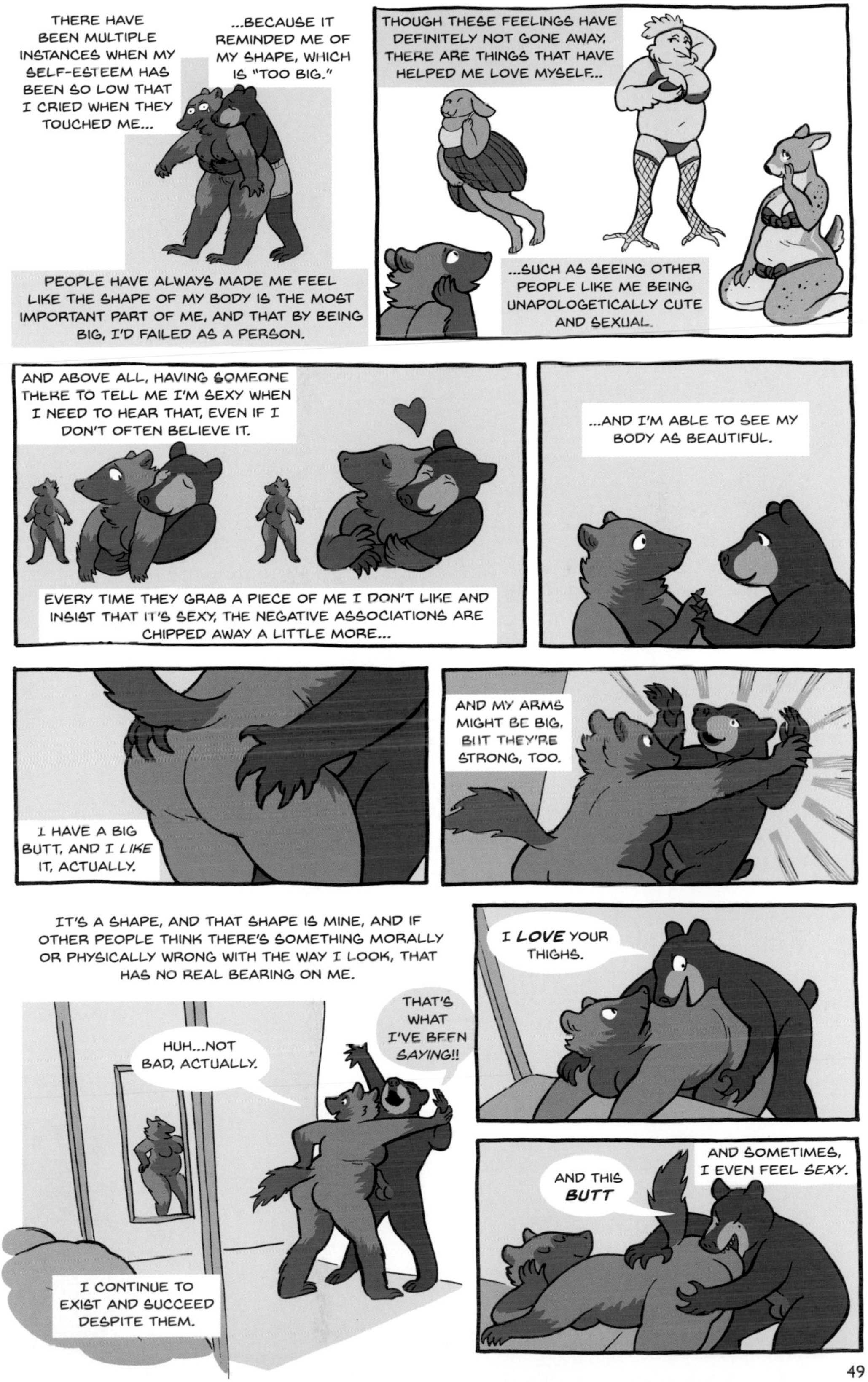

THERE HAVE BEEN MULTIPLE INSTANCES WHEN MY SELF-ESTEEM HAS BEEN SO LOW THAT I CRIED WHEN THEY TOUCHED ME...
...BECAUSE IT REMINDED ME OF MY SHAPE, WHICH IS "TOO BIG."
PEOPLE HAVE ALWAYS MADE ME FEEL LIKE THE SHAPE OF MY BODY IS THE MOST IMPORTANT PART OF ME, AND THAT BY BEING BIG, I'D FAILED AS A PERSON.
THOUGH THESE FEELINGS HAVE DEFINITELY NOT GONE AWAY, THERE ARE THINGS THAT HAVE HELPED ME LOVE MYSELF...
...SUCH AS SEEING OTHER PEOPLE LIKE ME BEING UNAPOLOGETICALLY CUTE AND SEXUAL.
AND ABOVE ALL, HAVING SOMEONE THERE TO TELL ME I'M SEXY WHEN I NEED TO HEAR THAT, EVEN IF I DON'T OFTEN BELIEVE IT.
EVERY TIME THEY GRAB A PIECE OF ME I DON'T LIKE AND INSIST THAT IT'S SEXY, THE NEGATIVE ASSOCIATIONS ARE CHIPPED AWAY A LITTLE MORE...
...AND I'M ABLE TO SEE MY BODY AS BEAUTIFUL.
I HAVE A BIG BUTT, AND I *LIKE* IT, ACTUALLY.
AND MY ARMS MIGHT BE BIG, BUT THEY'RE STRONG, TOO.
IT'S A SHAPE, AND THAT SHAPE IS MINE, AND IF OTHER PEOPLE THINK THERE'S SOMETHING MORALLY OR PHYSICALLY WRONG WITH THE WAY I LOOK, THAT HAS NO REAL BEARING ON ME.
HUH...NOT BAD, ACTUALLY.
THAT'S WHAT I'VE BEEN *SAYING*!!
I CONTINUE TO EXIST AND SUCCEED DESPITE THEM.
I ***LOVE*** YOUR THIGHS.
AND THIS ***BUTT***
AND SOMETIMES, I EVEN FEEL *SEXY*.

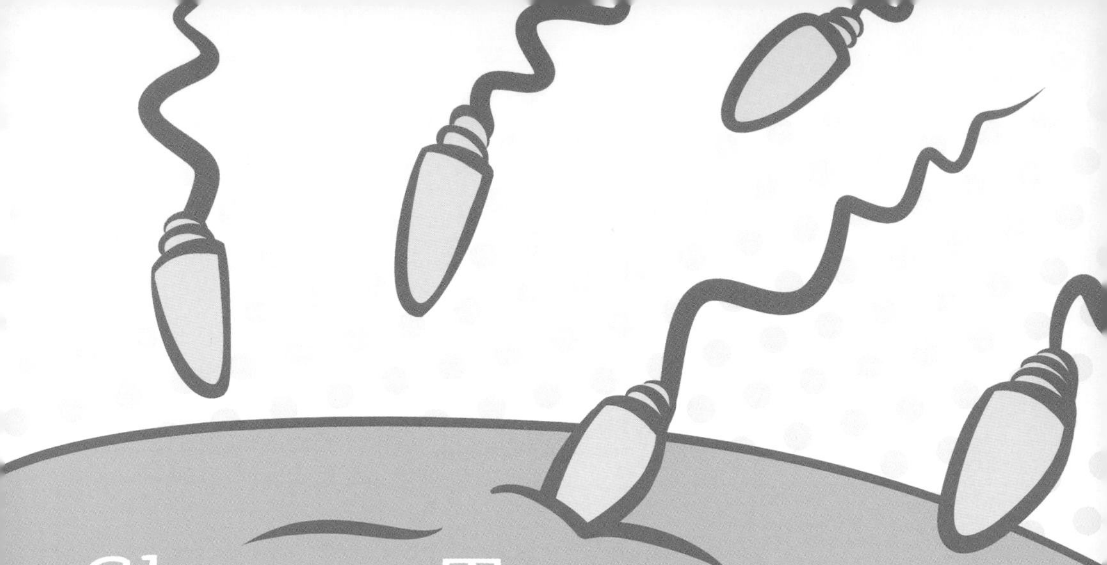

Chapter Two

Pregnancy & Abortion

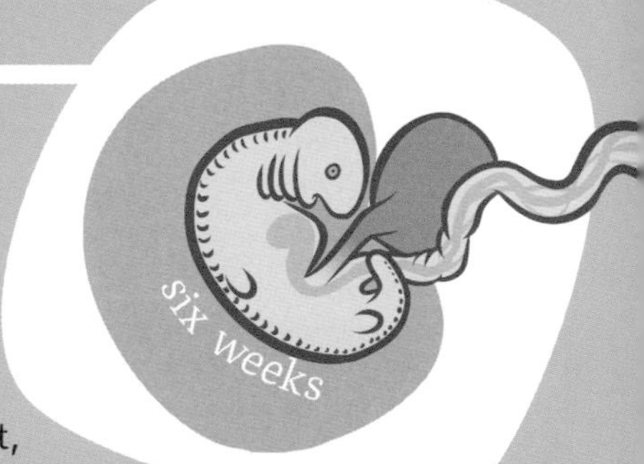
six weeks

If there's one thing us human beings are good at, it's reproducing! In this chapter, we'll talk about the mechanics of how our bodies can turn a few DNA-thick cells into a fully-formed baby nine months later.

We all know that a baby is made from sperm and egg combining inside a body, but... like... what *really* goes on in there? Turns out, lots of fascinating steps and transformations are happening out of sight. Do you know the difference between a fertilized egg, an embryo, and a fetus? You will be when you're done with this chapter! At the same time, we'll take a look at abortion and discuss the process to end a pregnancy early.

Our previous book covered contraceptives people can use to regulate their fertility, but some people want a more permanent solution. Lucky for them, sterilization exists! And, lucky for you, we've got a couple of comics to explain a few of those options too!

It is so common for pregnancies to end before they come to term, yet it's not widely discussed or understood in our society. Whether a miscarriage or an abortion, any person with a terminated pregnancy experiences a huge physical transition and deserves lots of understanding and support from their community. Educate yourself on these processes so you have the knowledge for yourself and to share with all your baby-making loved ones!

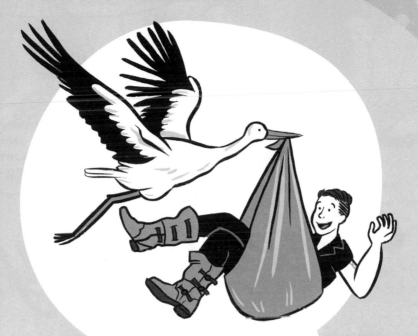

Conception &
Pregnancy

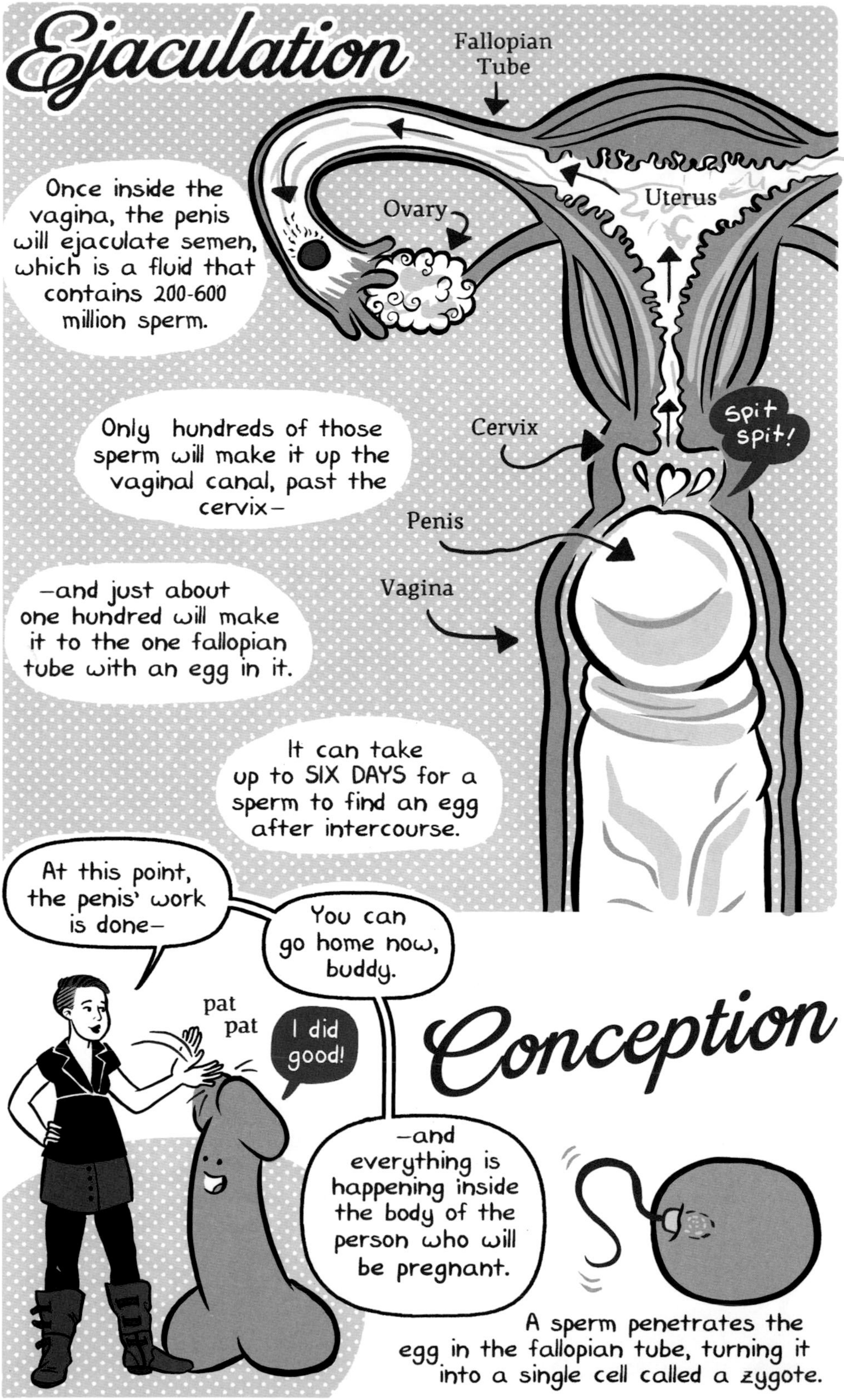
Ejaculation
Fallopian Tube
Once inside the vagina, the penis will ejaculate semen, which is a fluid that contains 200-600 million sperm.
Ovary
Uterus
Only hundreds of those sperm will make it up the vaginal canal, past the cervix–
Cervix
Spit spit!
Penis
–and just about one hundred will make it to the one fallopian tube with an egg in it.
Vagina
It can take up to SIX DAYS for a sperm to find an egg after intercourse.
At this point, the penis' work is done–
You can go home now, buddy.
pat pat
I did good!
Conception
–and everything is happening inside the body of the person who will be pregnant.
A sperm penetrates the egg in the fallopian tube, turning it into a single cell called a zygote.

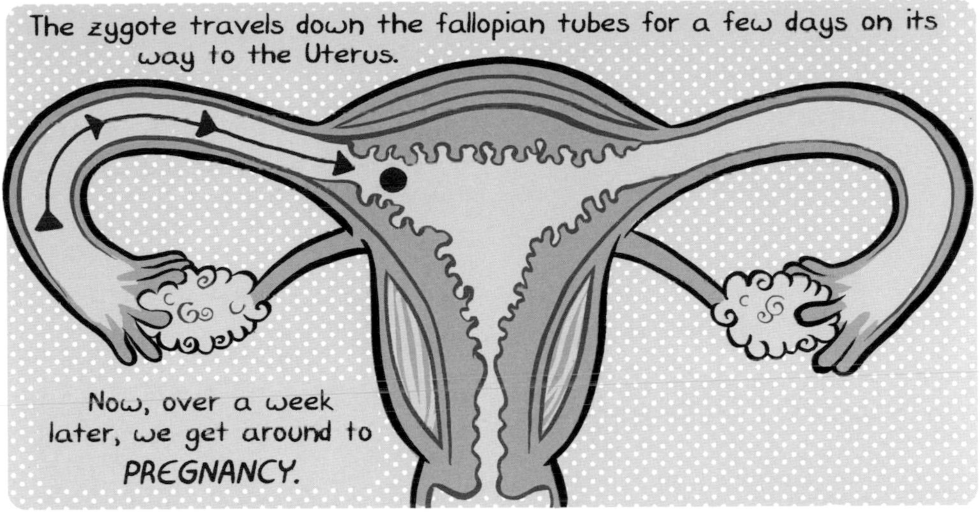

The zygote travels down the fallopian tubes for a few days on its way to the Uterus.
Now, over a week later, we get around to PREGNANCY.

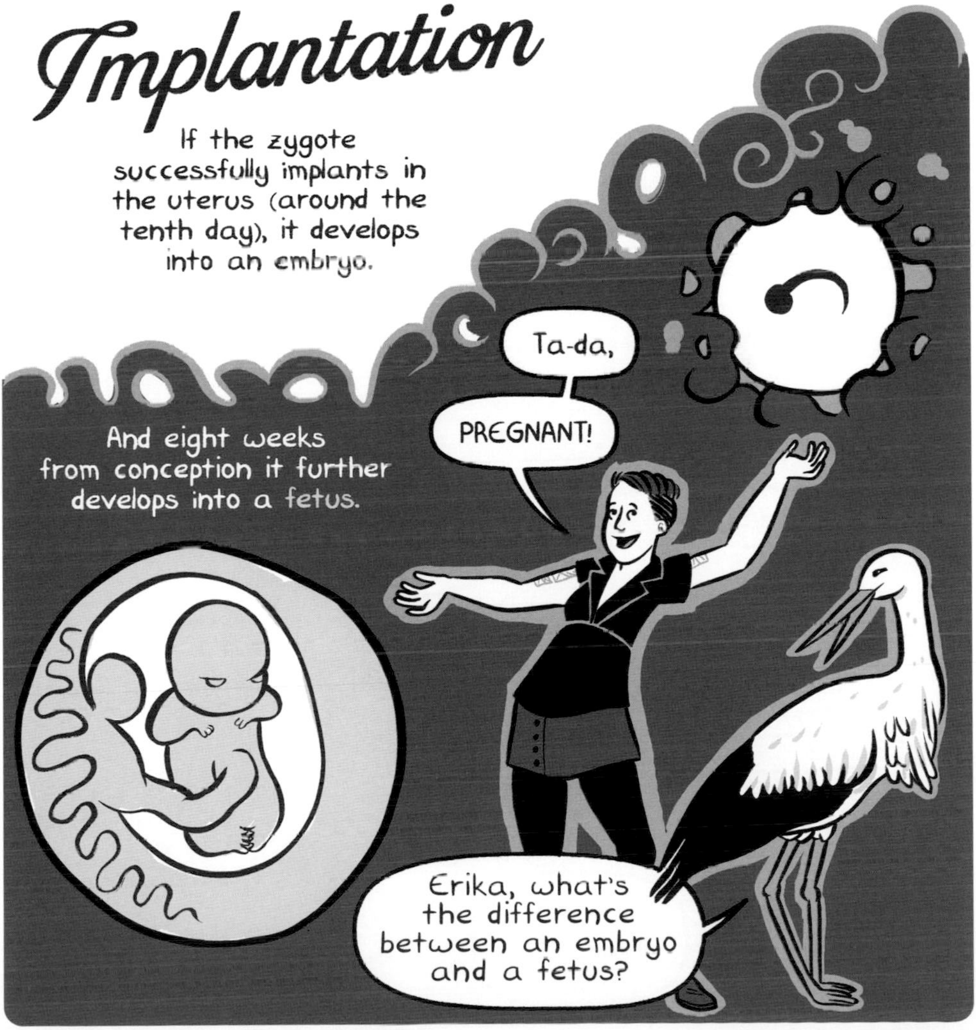

Implantation
If the zygote successfully implants in the uterus (around the tenth day), it develops into an embryo.
Ta-da,
PREGNANT!
And eight weeks from conception it further develops into a fetus.
Erika, what's the difference between an embryo and a fetus?

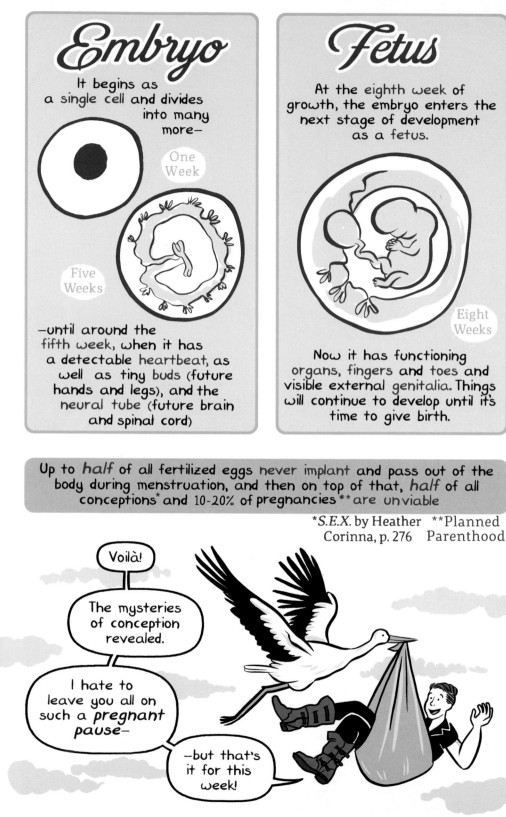

Embryo

It begins as a single cell and divides into many more—

One Week

Five Weeks

—until around the fifth week, when it has a detectable heartbeat, as well as tiny buds (future hands and legs), and the neural tube (future brain and spinal cord)

Fetus

At the eighth week of growth, the embryo enters the next stage of development as a fetus.

Eight Weeks

Now it has functioning organs, fingers and toes and visible external genitalia. Things will continue to develop until it's time to give birth.

Up to *half* of all fertilized eggs never implant and pass out of the body during menstruation, and then on top of that, *half* of all conceptions* and 10-20% of pregnancies** are unviable

*S.E.X. by Heather Corinna, p. 276   **Planned Parenthood

Voilà!

The mysteries of conception revealed.

I hate to leave you all on such a *pregnant pause*—

—but that's it for this week!

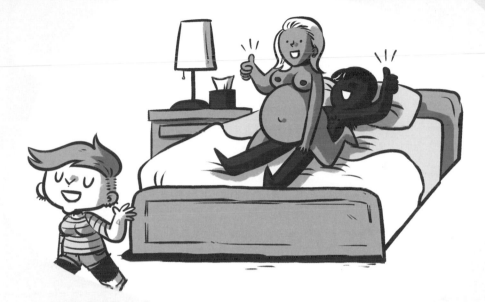

Pregnancy Sex
By Boum
Boumfolio.com

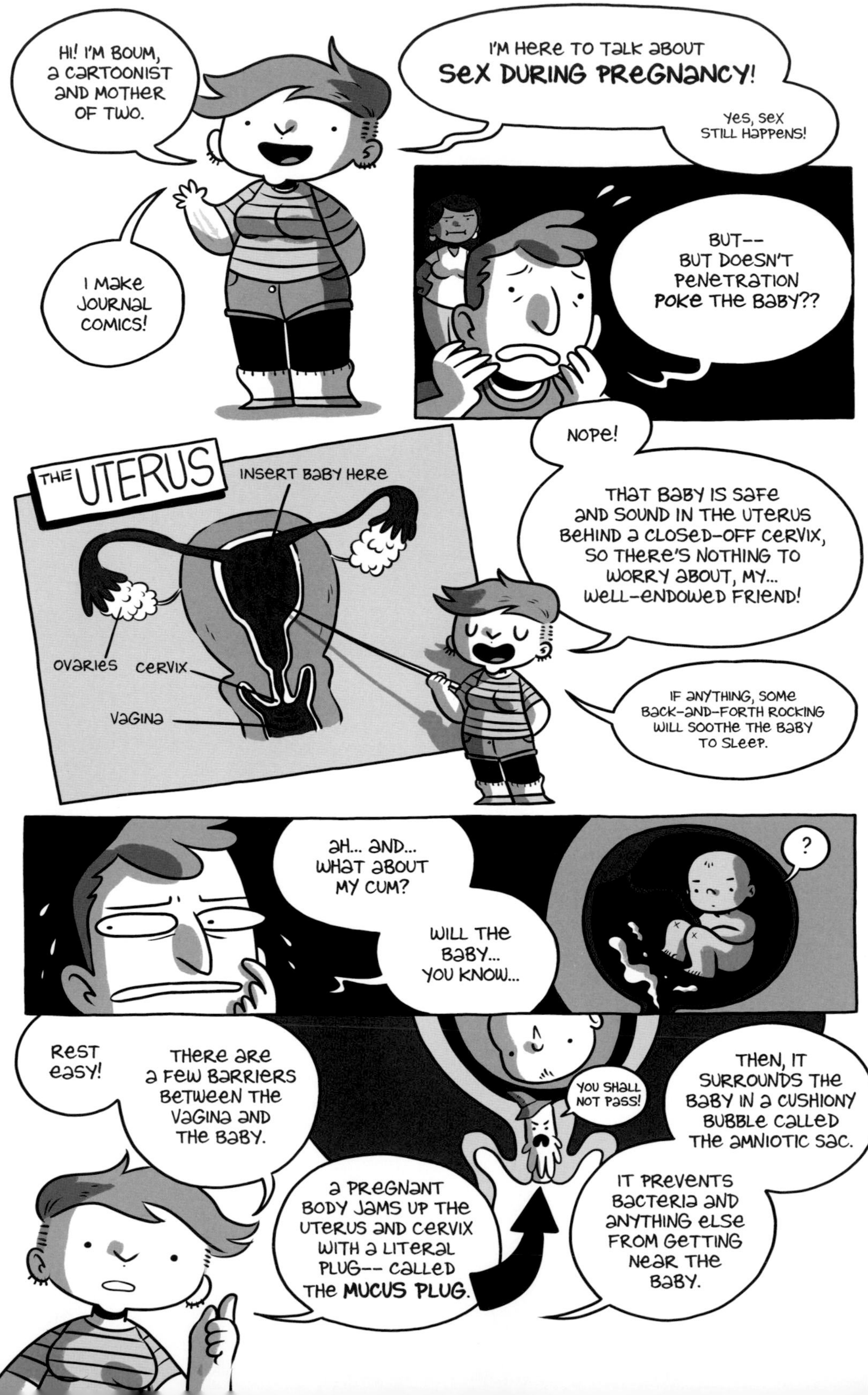
HI! I'M BOUM, A CARTOONIST AND MOTHER OF TWO.
I'M HERE TO TALK ABOUT SEX DURING PREGNANCY!
YES, SEX STILL HAPPENS!
I MAKE JOURNAL COMICS!
BUT-- BUT DOESN'T PENETRATION POKE THE BABY??
THE UTERUS
INSERT BABY HERE
OVARIES
CERVIX
VAGINA
NOPE!
THAT BABY IS SAFE AND SOUND IN THE UTERUS BEHIND A CLOSED-OFF CERVIX, SO THERE'S NOTHING TO WORRY ABOUT, MY... WELL-ENDOWED FRIEND!
IF ANYTHING, SOME BACK-AND-FORTH ROCKING WILL SOOTHE THE BABY TO SLEEP.
AH... AND... WHAT ABOUT MY CUM?
WILL THE BABY... YOU KNOW...
?
REST EASY!
THERE ARE A FEW BARRIERS BETWEEN THE VAGINA AND THE BABY.
A PREGNANT BODY JAMS UP THE UTERUS AND CERVIX WITH A LITERAL PLUG-- CALLED THE MUCUS PLUG.
YOU SHALL NOT PASS!
THEN, IT SURROUNDS THE BABY IN A CUSHIONY BUBBLE CALLED THE AMNIOTIC SAC.
IT PREVENTS BACTERIA AND ANYTHING ELSE FROM GETTING NEAR THE BABY.

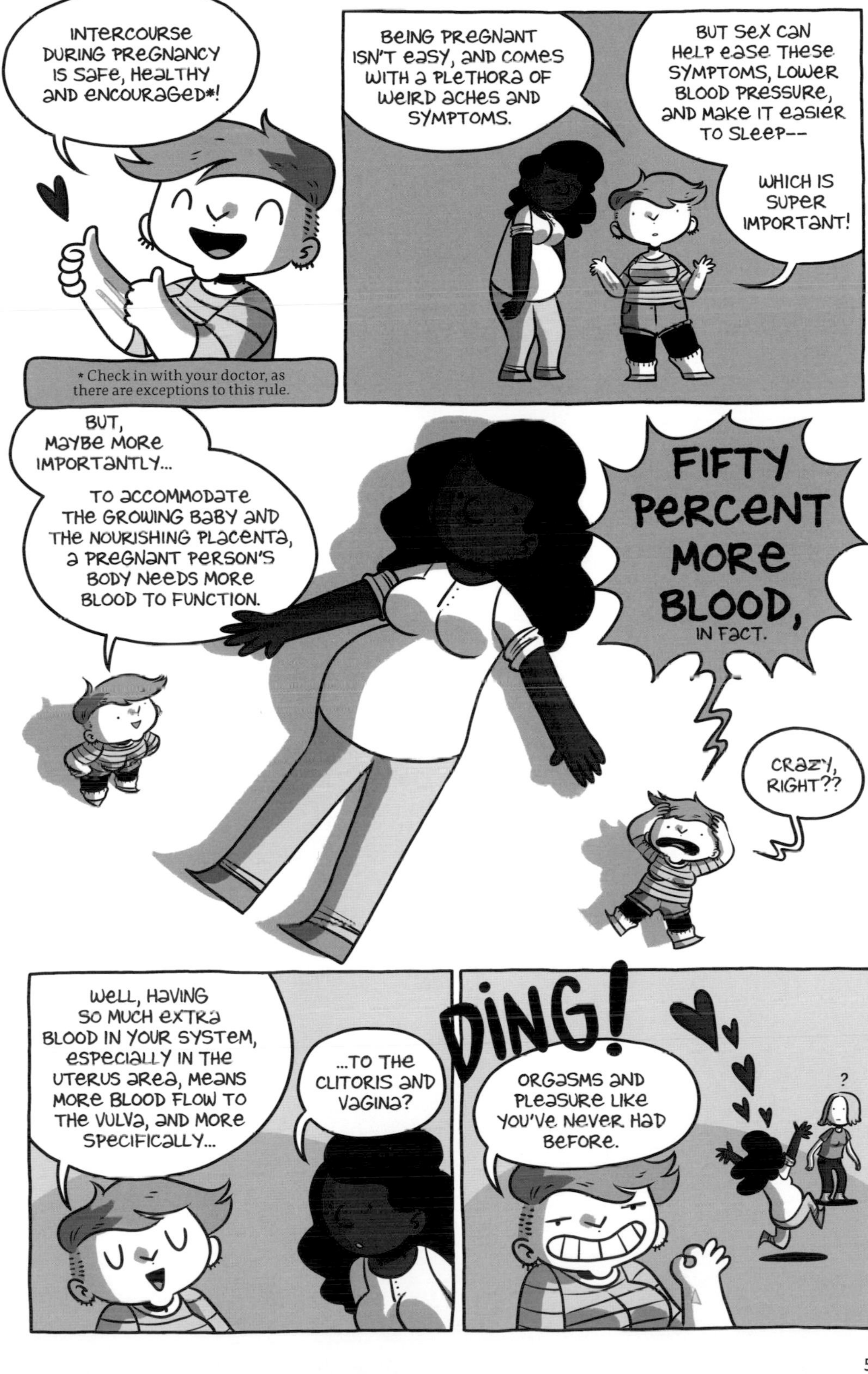
INTERCOURSE DURING PREGNANCY IS SAFE, HEALTHY AND ENCOURAGED*!
* Check in with your doctor, as there are exceptions to this rule.
BEING PREGNANT ISN'T EASY, AND COMES WITH A PLETHORA OF WEIRD ACHES AND SYMPTOMS.
BUT SEX CAN HELP EASE THESE SYMPTOMS, LOWER BLOOD PRESSURE, AND MAKE IT EASIER TO SLEEP--
WHICH IS SUPER IMPORTANT!
BUT, MAYBE MORE IMPORTANTLY...
TO ACCOMMODATE THE GROWING BABY AND THE NOURISHING PLACENTA, A PREGNANT PERSON'S BODY NEEDS MORE BLOOD TO FUNCTION.
FIFTY PERCENT MORE BLOOD, IN FACT.
CRAZY, RIGHT??
WELL, HAVING SO MUCH EXTRA BLOOD IN YOUR SYSTEM, ESPECIALLY IN THE UTERUS AREA, MEANS MORE BLOOD FLOW TO THE VULVA, AND MORE SPECIFICALLY...
...TO THE CLITORIS AND VAGINA?
DING!
ORGASMS AND PLEASURE LIKE YOU'VE NEVER HAD BEFORE.
?

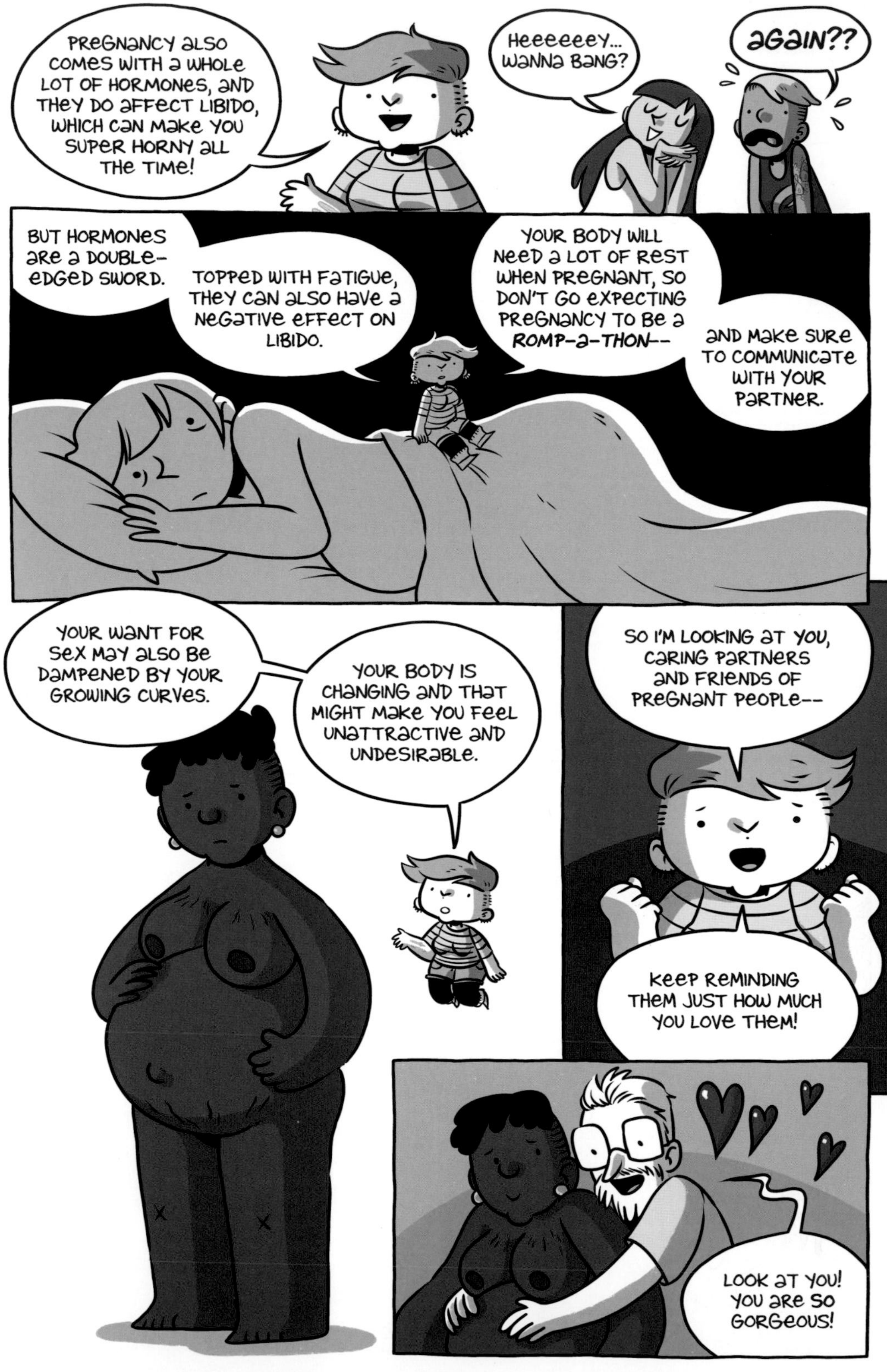
PREGNANCY ALSO COMES WITH A WHOLE LOT OF HORMONES, AND THEY DO AFFECT LIBIDO, WHICH CAN MAKE YOU SUPER HORNY ALL THE TIME!
HEEEEEEY... WANNA BANG?
AGAIN??
BUT HORMONES ARE A DOUBLE-EDGED SWORD.
TOPPED WITH FATIGUE, THEY CAN ALSO HAVE A NEGATIVE EFFECT ON LIBIDO.
YOUR BODY WILL NEED A LOT OF REST WHEN PREGNANT, SO DON'T GO EXPECTING PREGNANCY TO BE A ROMP-A-THON--
AND MAKE SURE TO COMMUNICATE WITH YOUR PARTNER.
YOUR WANT FOR SEX MAY ALSO BE DAMPENED BY YOUR GROWING CURVES.
YOUR BODY IS CHANGING AND THAT MIGHT MAKE YOU FEEL UNATTRACTIVE AND UNDESIRABLE.
SO I'M LOOKING AT YOU, CARING PARTNERS AND FRIENDS OF PREGNANT PEOPLE--
KEEP REMINDING THEM JUST HOW MUCH YOU LOVE THEM!
LOOK AT YOU! YOU ARE SO GORGEOUS!

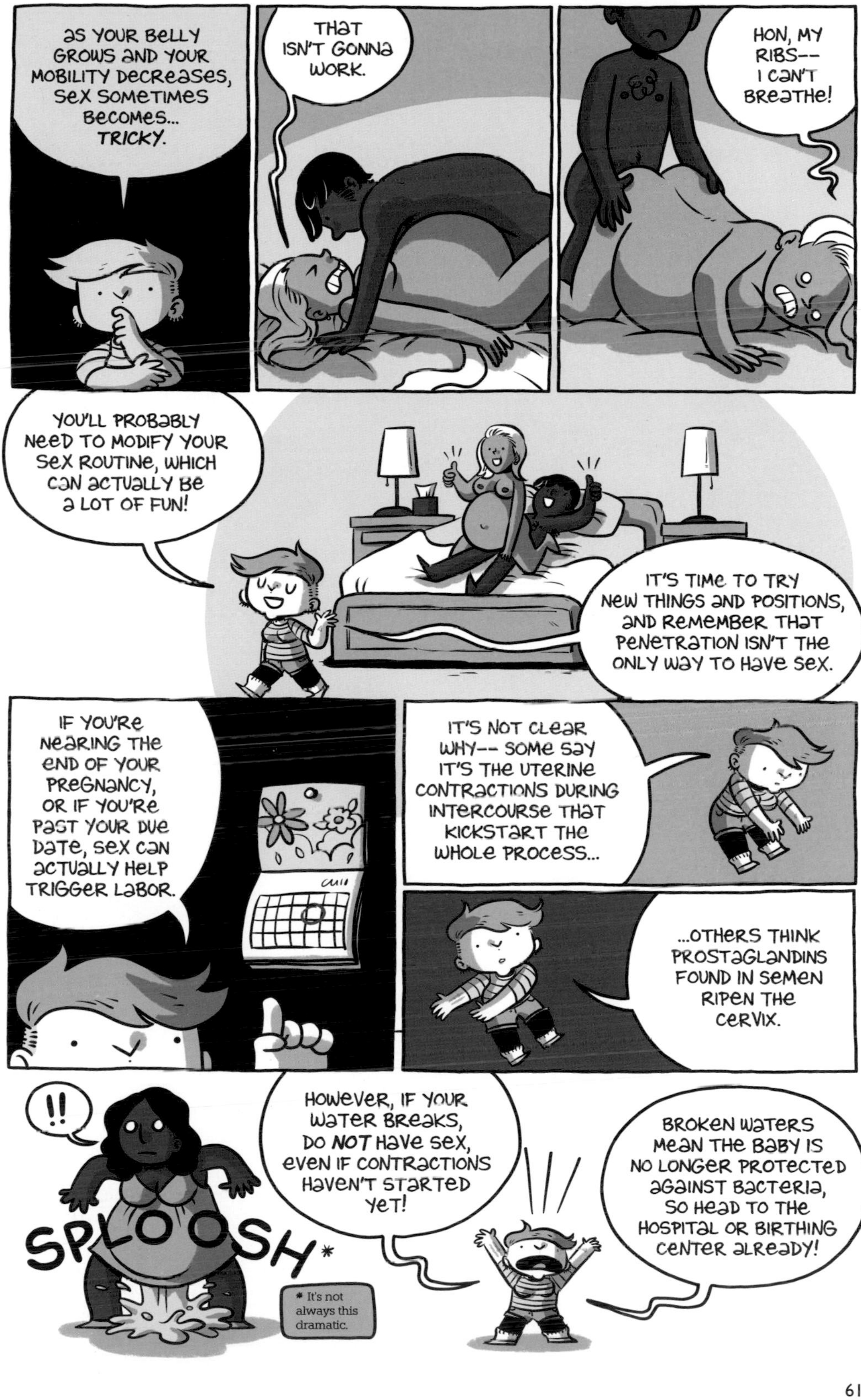
AS YOUR BELLY GROWS AND YOUR MOBILITY DECREASES, SEX SOMETIMES BECOMES... TRICKY.
THAT ISN'T GONNA WORK.
HON, MY RIBS-- I CAN'T BREATHE!
YOU'LL PROBABLY NEED TO MODIFY YOUR SEX ROUTINE, WHICH CAN ACTUALLY BE A LOT OF FUN!
IT'S TIME TO TRY NEW THINGS AND POSITIONS, AND REMEMBER THAT PENETRATION ISN'T THE ONLY WAY TO HAVE SEX.
IF YOU'RE NEARING THE END OF YOUR PREGNANCY, OR IF YOU'RE PAST YOUR DUE DATE, SEX CAN ACTUALLY HELP TRIGGER LABOR.
IT'S NOT CLEAR WHY-- SOME SAY IT'S THE UTERINE CONTRACTIONS DURING INTERCOURSE THAT KICKSTART THE WHOLE PROCESS...
...OTHERS THINK PROSTAGLANDINS FOUND IN SEMEN RIPEN THE CERVIX.
!!
SPLOOSH*
* It's not always this dramatic.
HOWEVER, IF YOUR WATER BREAKS, DO NOT HAVE SEX, EVEN IF CONTRACTIONS HAVEN'T STARTED YET!
BROKEN WATERS MEAN THE BABY IS NO LONGER PROTECTED AGAINST BACTERIA, SO HEAD TO THE HOSPITAL OR BIRTHING CENTER ALREADY!

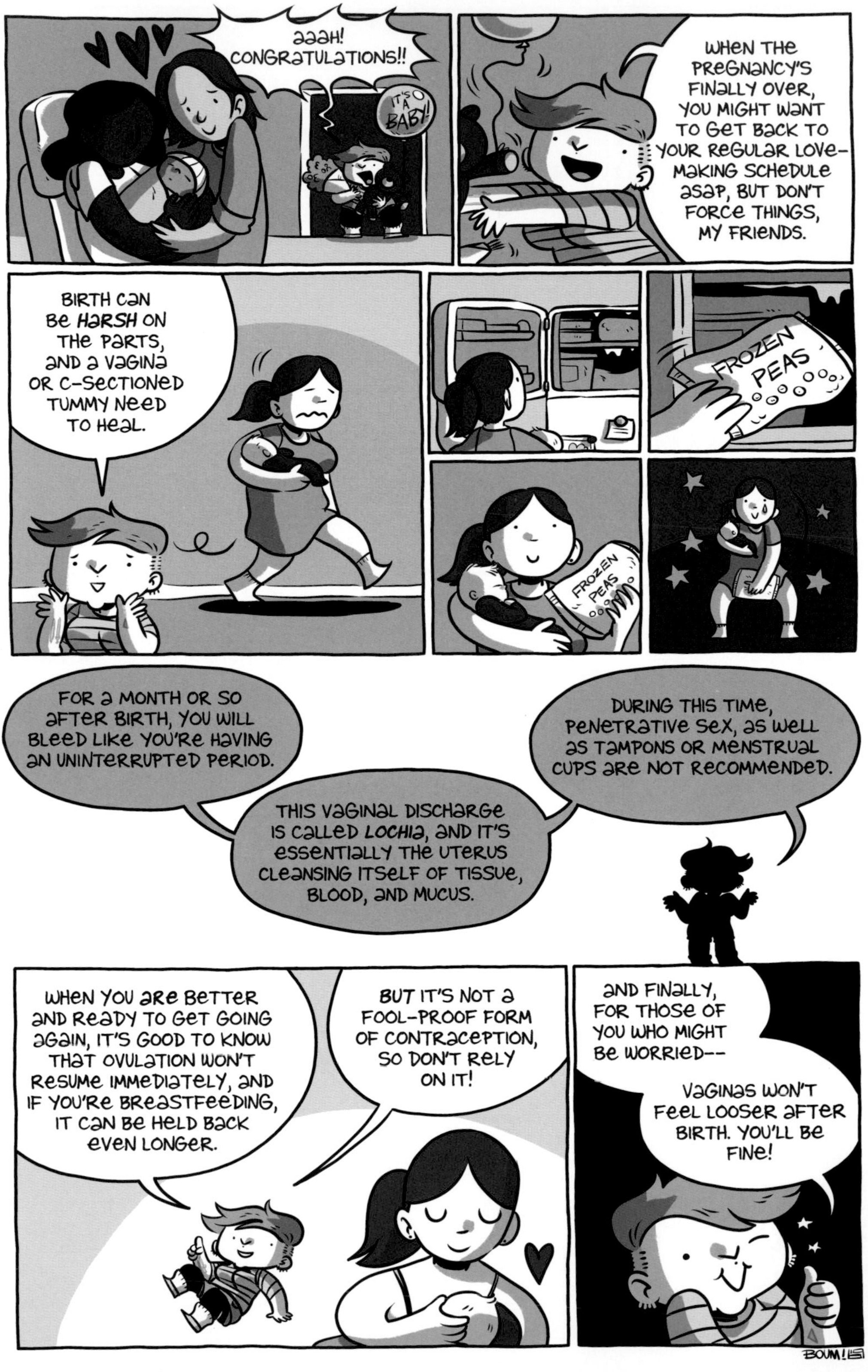
AAAH! CONGRATULATIONS!!
IT'S A BABY!
WHEN THE PREGNANCY'S FINALLY OVER, YOU MIGHT WANT TO GET BACK TO YOUR REGULAR LOVE-MAKING SCHEDULE ASAP, BUT DON'T FORCE THINGS, MY FRIENDS.
BIRTH CAN BE *HARSH* ON THE PARTS, AND A VAGINA OR C-SECTIONED TUMMY NEED TO HEAL.
FROZEN PEAS
FROZEN PEAS
FOR A MONTH OR SO AFTER BIRTH, YOU WILL BLEED LIKE YOU'RE HAVING AN UNINTERRUPTED PERIOD.
THIS VAGINAL DISCHARGE IS CALLED *LOCHIA*, AND IT'S ESSENTIALLY THE UTERUS CLEANSING ITSELF OF TISSUE, BLOOD, AND MUCUS.
DURING THIS TIME, PENETRATIVE SEX, AS WELL AS TAMPONS OR MENSTRUAL CUPS ARE NOT RECOMMENDED.
WHEN YOU ARE BETTER AND READY TO GET GOING AGAIN, IT'S GOOD TO KNOW THAT OVULATION WON'T RESUME IMMEDIATELY, AND IF YOU'RE BREASTFEEDING, IT CAN BE HELD BACK EVEN LONGER.
BUT IT'S NOT A FOOL-PROOF FORM OF CONTRACEPTION, SO DON'T RELY ON IT!
AND FINALLY, FOR THOSE OF YOU WHO MIGHT BE WORRIED--
VAGINAS WON'T FEEL LOOSER AFTER BIRTH. YOU'LL BE FINE!
BOUM!

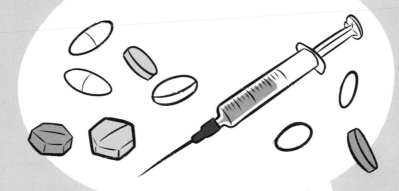

Medication Abortion
& Stages of Pregnancy

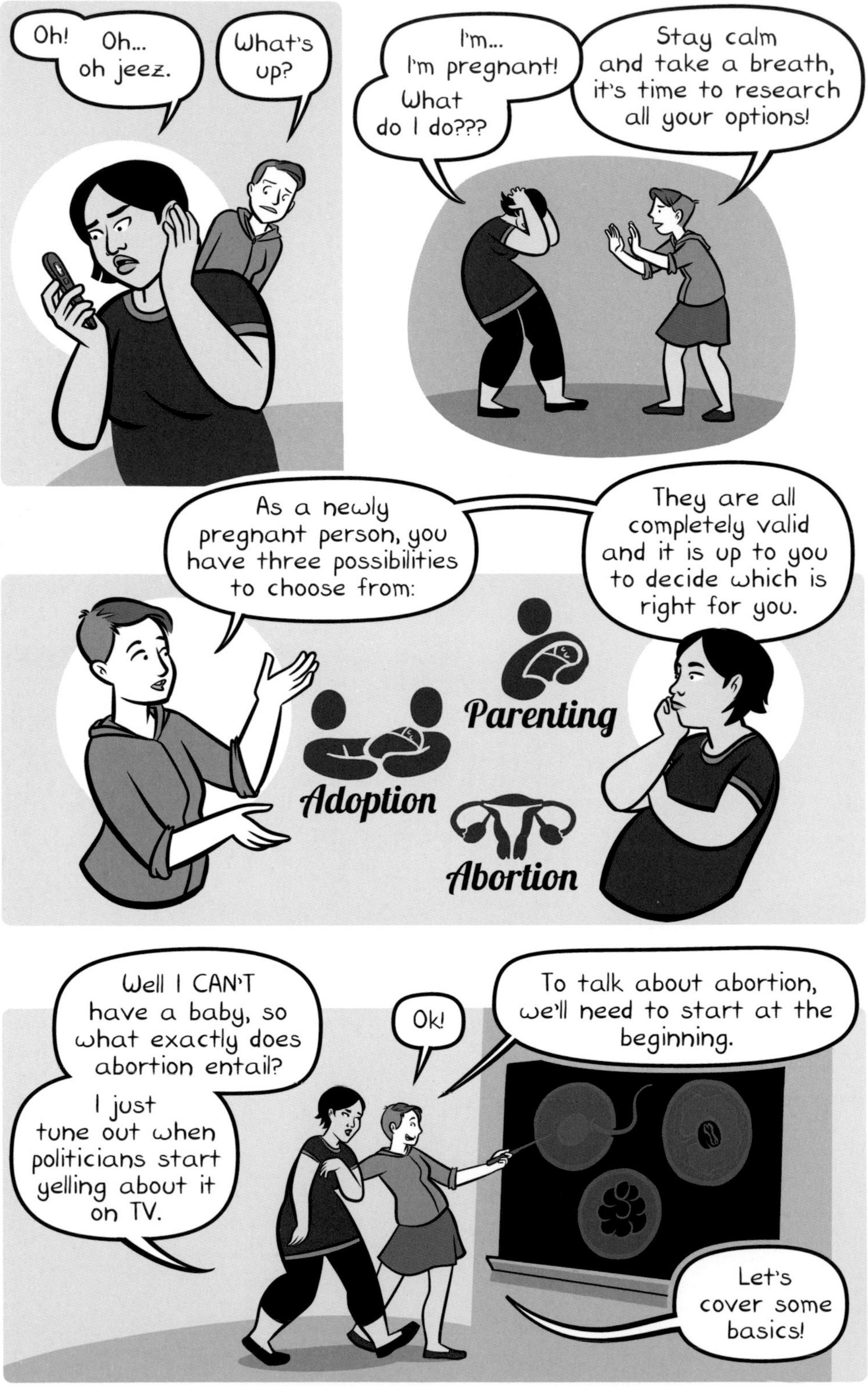
Oh! Oh... oh jeez.
What's up?
I'm... I'm pregnant! What do I do???
Stay calm and take a breath, it's time to research all your options!
As a newly pregnant person, you have three possibilities to choose from:
They are all completely valid and it is up to you to decide which is right for you.
Parenting
Adoption
Abortion
Well I CAN'T have a baby, so what exactly does abortion entail?
I just tune out when politicians start yelling about it on TV.
Ok!
To talk about abortion, we'll need to start at the beginning.
Let's cover some basics!

Stages of Pregnancy

Conception

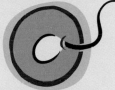

When your egg meets sperm in one of your fallopian tubes, we have conception!

Implantation & Embryo Development (1–5 weeks)

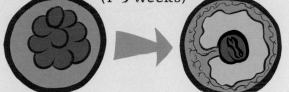

That fertilized egg (the *blastocyst*) will slowly travel to your uterus and implant itself, becoming an *embryo* and making you officially pregnant!

Around the 5 - 7 weeks mark, there's enough there for the embryo to have a detectable heartbeat, tiny buds (future hands and legs), and the beginning of a neural tube (future brain and spinal cord)

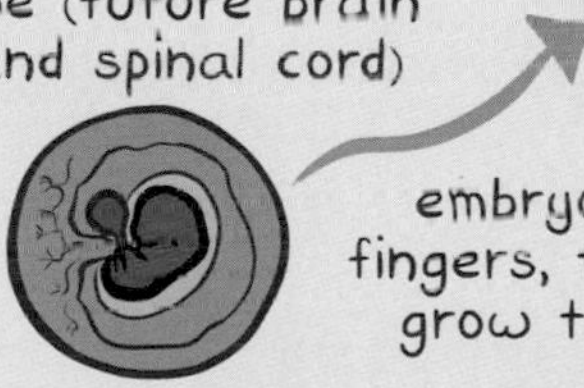

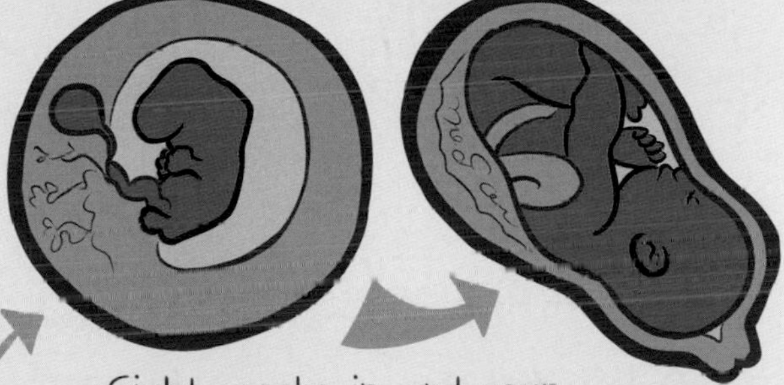

Fetus (8 weeks – 40 ish weeks)

Eight weeks in and your embryo will develop into a fetus with organs, fingers, toes, and genitalia that will continue to grow through all the next stages until birth.

The timeline of a pregnancy is tracked through 'Trimesters':

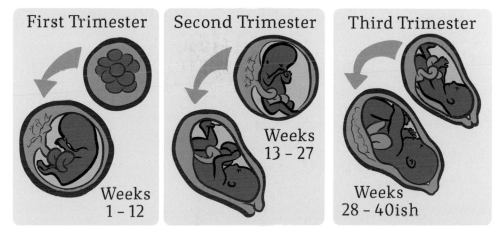

First Trimester
Weeks 1 – 12

Second Trimester
Weeks 13 – 27

Third Trimester
Weeks 28 – 40ish

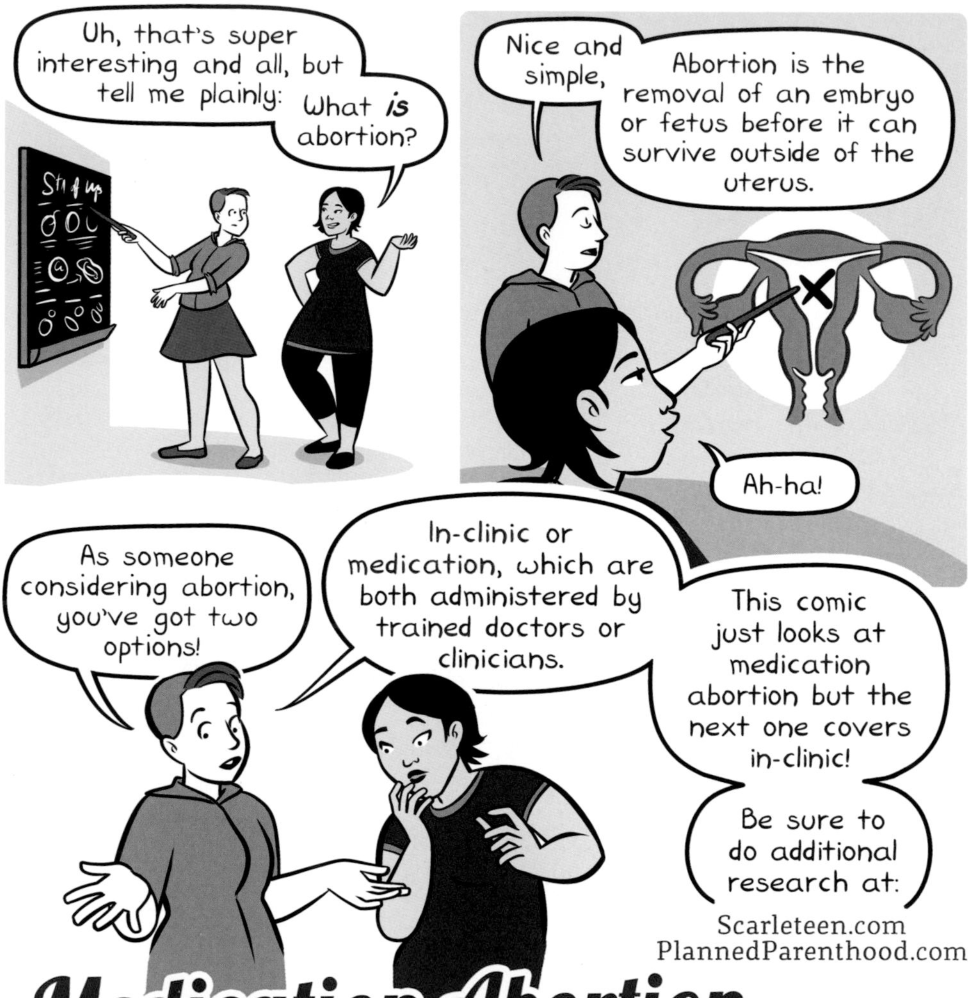

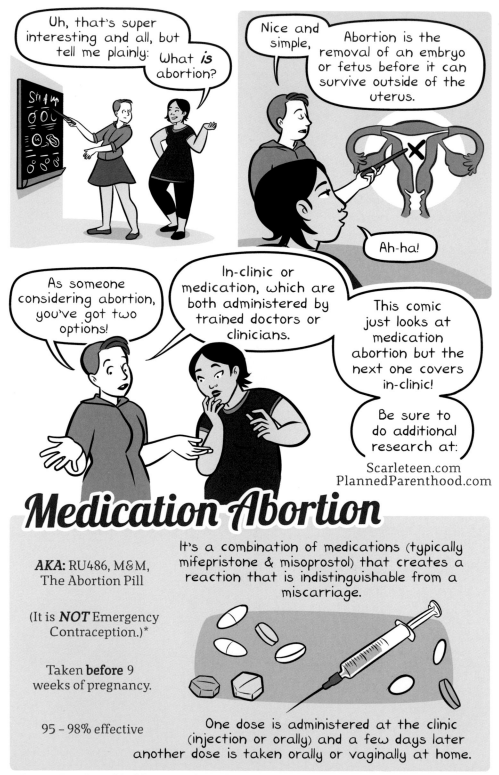

Uh, that's super interesting and all, but tell me plainly:
What *is* abortion?
Nice and simple,
Abortion is the removal of an embryo or fetus before it can survive outside of the uterus.
Ah-ha!
As someone considering abortion, you've got two options!
In-clinic or medication, which are both administered by trained doctors or clinicians.
This comic just looks at medication abortion but the next one covers in-clinic!
Be sure to do additional research at:
Scarleteen.com
PlannedParenthood.com

Medication Abortion

AKA: RU486, M&M, The Abortion Pill

It's a combination of medications (typically mifepristone & misoprostol) that creates a reaction that is indistinguishable from a miscarriage.

(It is ***NOT*** Emergency Contraception.)*

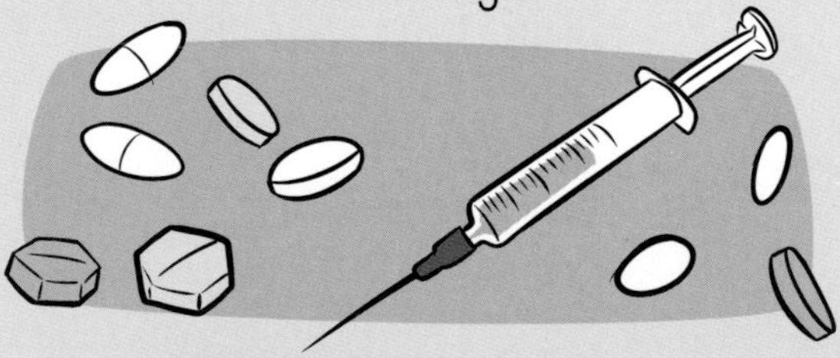

Taken **before** 9 weeks of pregnancy.

95 – 98% effective

One dose is administered at the clinic (injection or orally) and a few days later another dose is taken orally or vaginally at home.

* Covered on Page 66 of *Drawn to Sex: The Basics*

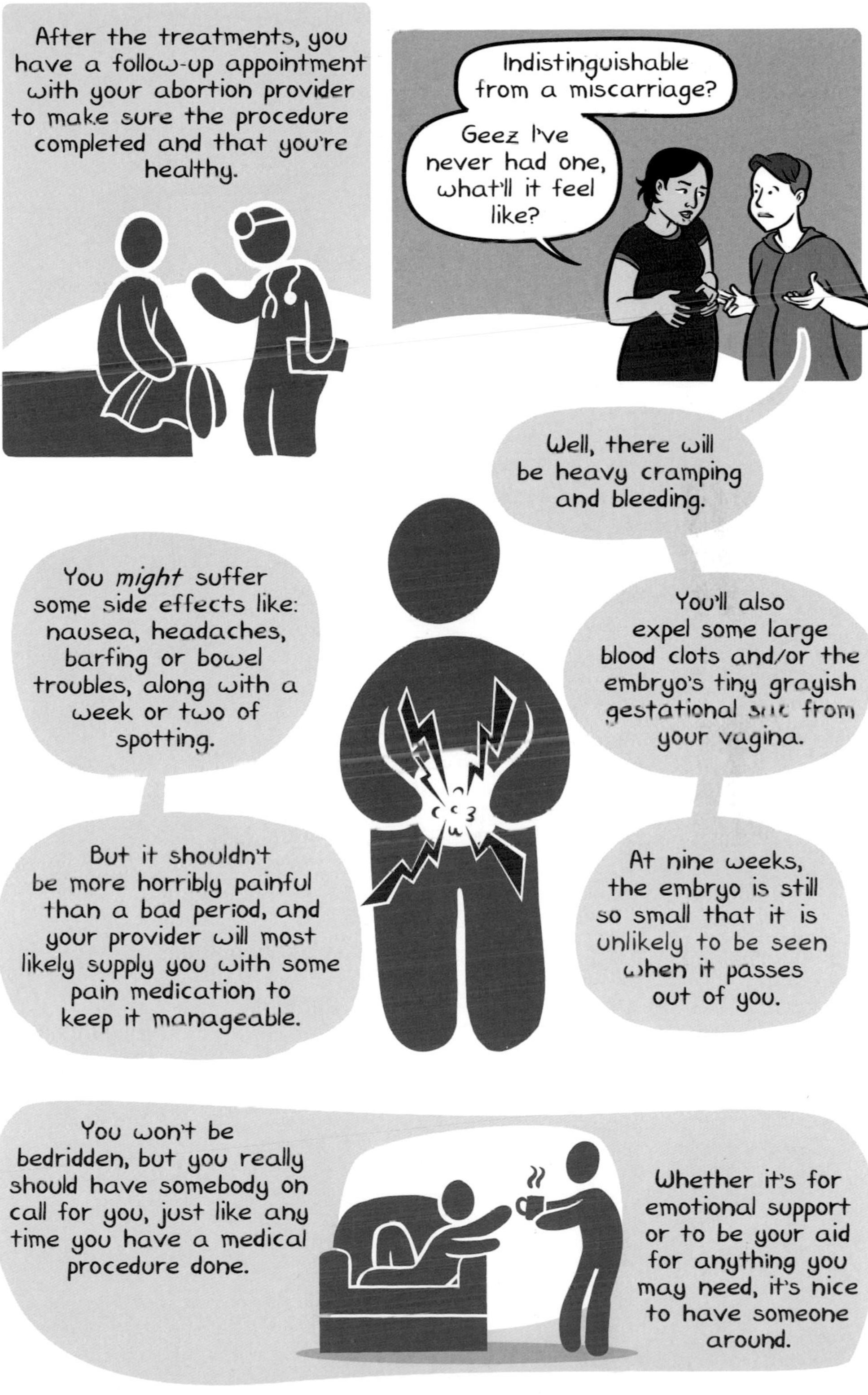

After the treatments, you have a follow-up appointment with your abortion provider to make sure the procedure completed and that you're healthy.
Indistinguishable from a miscarriage?
Geez I've never had one, what'll it feel like?
Well, there will be heavy cramping and bleeding.
You'll also expel some large blood clots and/or the embryo's tiny grayish gestational sac from your vagina.
At nine weeks, the embryo is still so small that it is unlikely to be seen when it passes out of you.
You *might* suffer some side effects like: nausea, headaches, barfing or bowel troubles, along with a week or two of spotting.
But it shouldn't be more horribly painful than a bad period, and your provider will most likely supply you with some pain medication to keep it manageable.
You won't be bedridden, but you really should have somebody on call for you, just like any time you have a medical procedure done.
Whether it's for emotional support or to be your aid for anything you may need, it's nice to have someone around.

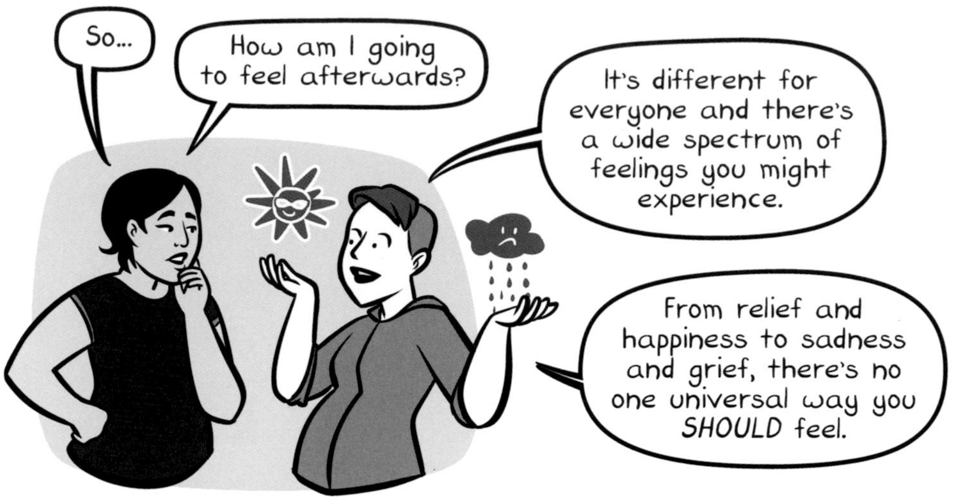
So...
How am I going to feel afterwards?
It's different for everyone and there's a wide spectrum of feelings you might experience.
From relief and happiness to sadness and grief, there's no one universal way you *SHOULD* feel.

Pregnancy hormones not only cause big changes in your body but can also create **giant mood swings**, and it's normal to feel some depression or intense emotions when you're no longer pregnant–

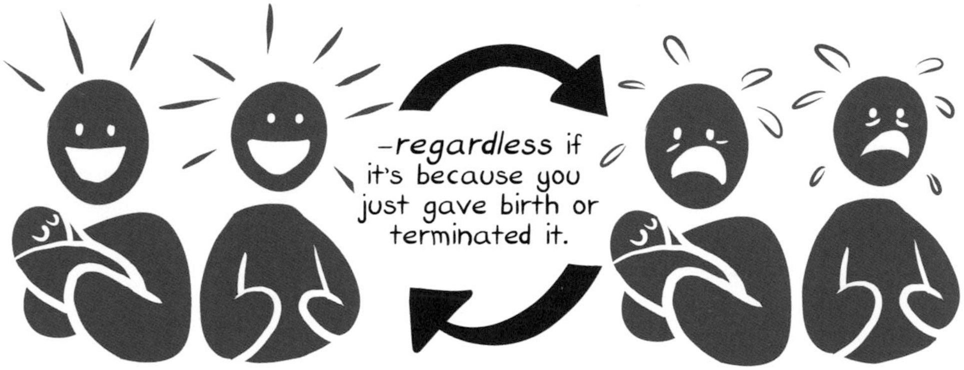
–*regardless* if it's because you just gave birth or terminated it.

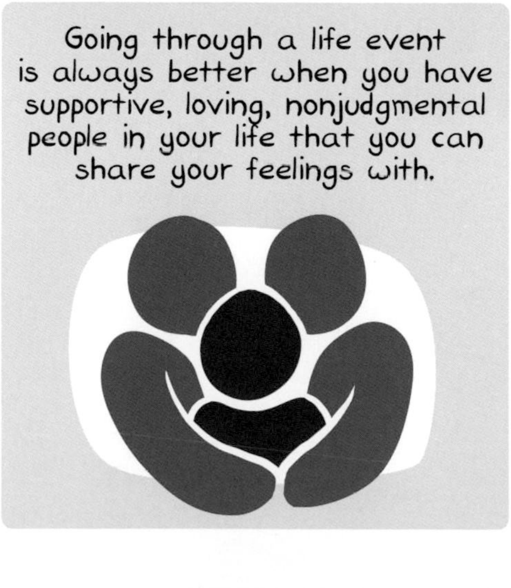
Going through a life event is always better when you have supportive, loving, nonjudgmental people in your life that you can share your feelings with.

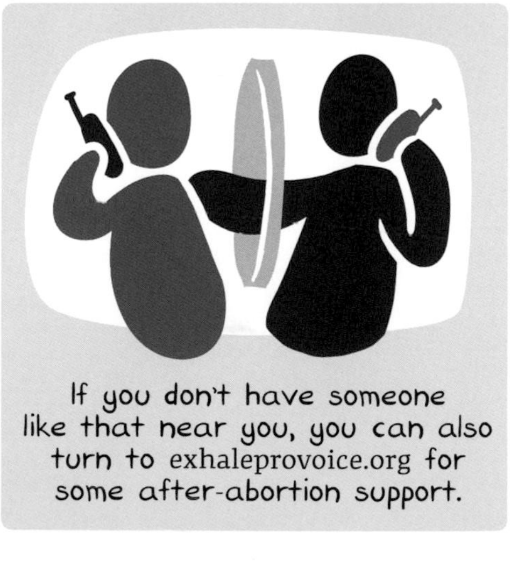
If you don't have someone like that near you, you can also turn to exhaleprovoice.org for some after-abortion support.

Take care of yourself physically and emotionally by doing things you enjoy afterwards, like spending time with friends, sleeping, eating, going to the movies, or whatever!

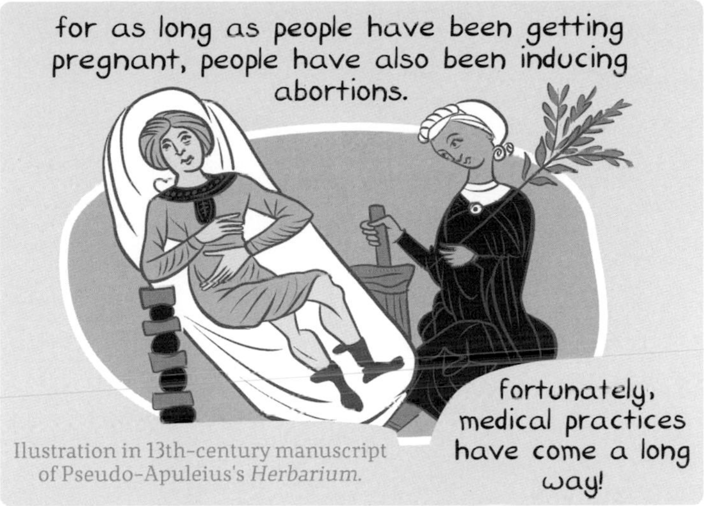
for as long as people have been getting pregnant, people have also been inducing abortions.
fortunately, medical practices have come a long way!
Illustration in 13th-century manuscript of Pseudo-Apuleius's *Herbarium*.

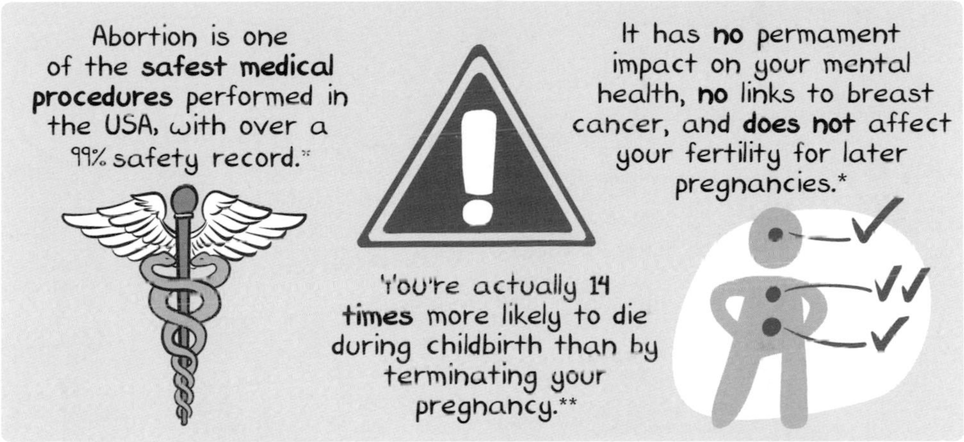
Abortion is one of the **safest medical procedures** performed in the USA, with over a 99% safety record.*
It has **no** permament impact on your mental health, **no** links to breast cancer, and **does not** affect your fertility for later pregnancies.*
You're actually 14 **times** more likely to die during childbirth than by terminating your pregnancy.**

*plannedparenthood.org

**pubmed.ncbi.nlm.nih.gov
PMID: 22270271

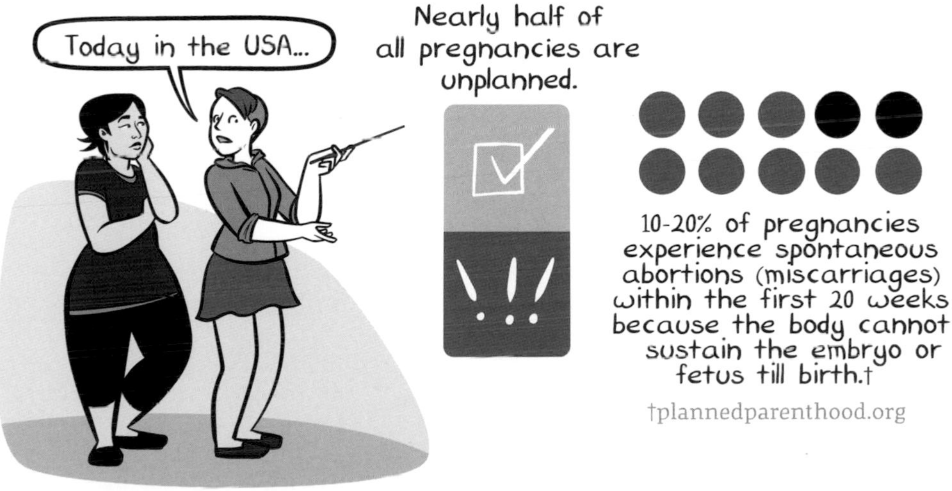
Today in the USA...
Nearly half of all pregnancies are unplanned.
10-20% of pregnancies experience spontaneous abortions (miscarriages) within the first 20 weeks because the body cannot sustain the embryo or fetus till birth.†

†plannedparenthood.org

In the United States...

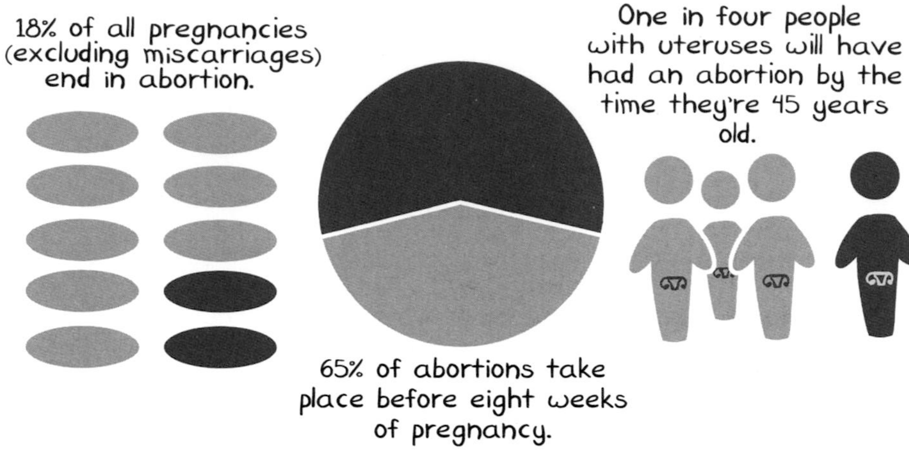
18% of all pregnancies (excluding miscarriages) end in abortion.
65% of abortions take place before eight weeks of pregnancy.
One in four people with uteruses will have had an abortion by the time they're 45 years old.

Satistics from Guttmacher.org

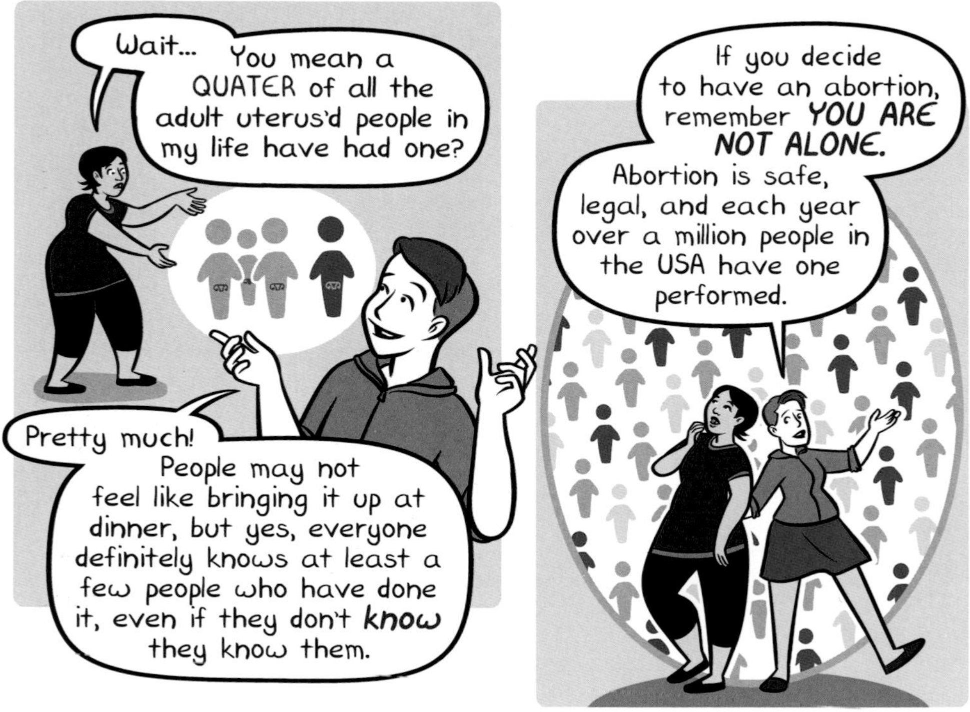
Wait... You mean a QUATER of all the adult uterus'd people in my life have had one?
Pretty much! People may not feel like bringing it up at dinner, but yes, everyone definitely knows at least a few people who have done it, even if they don't **know** they know them.
If you decide to have an abortion, remember ***YOU ARE NOT ALONE.*** Abortion is safe, legal, and each year over a million people in the USA have one performed.

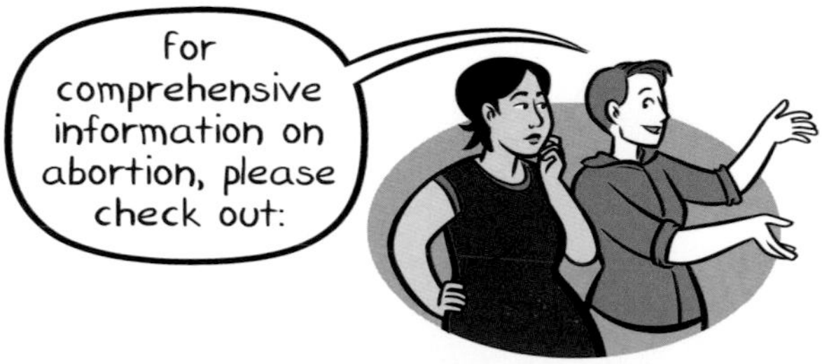
For comprehensive information on abortion, please check out:

scarleteen.com

exhaleprovoice.org

plannedparenthood.org

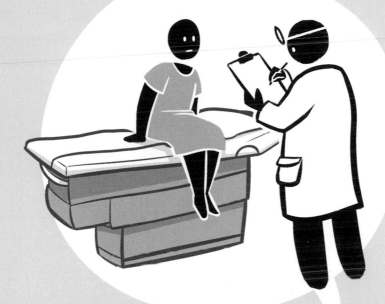

In-Clinic Abortion

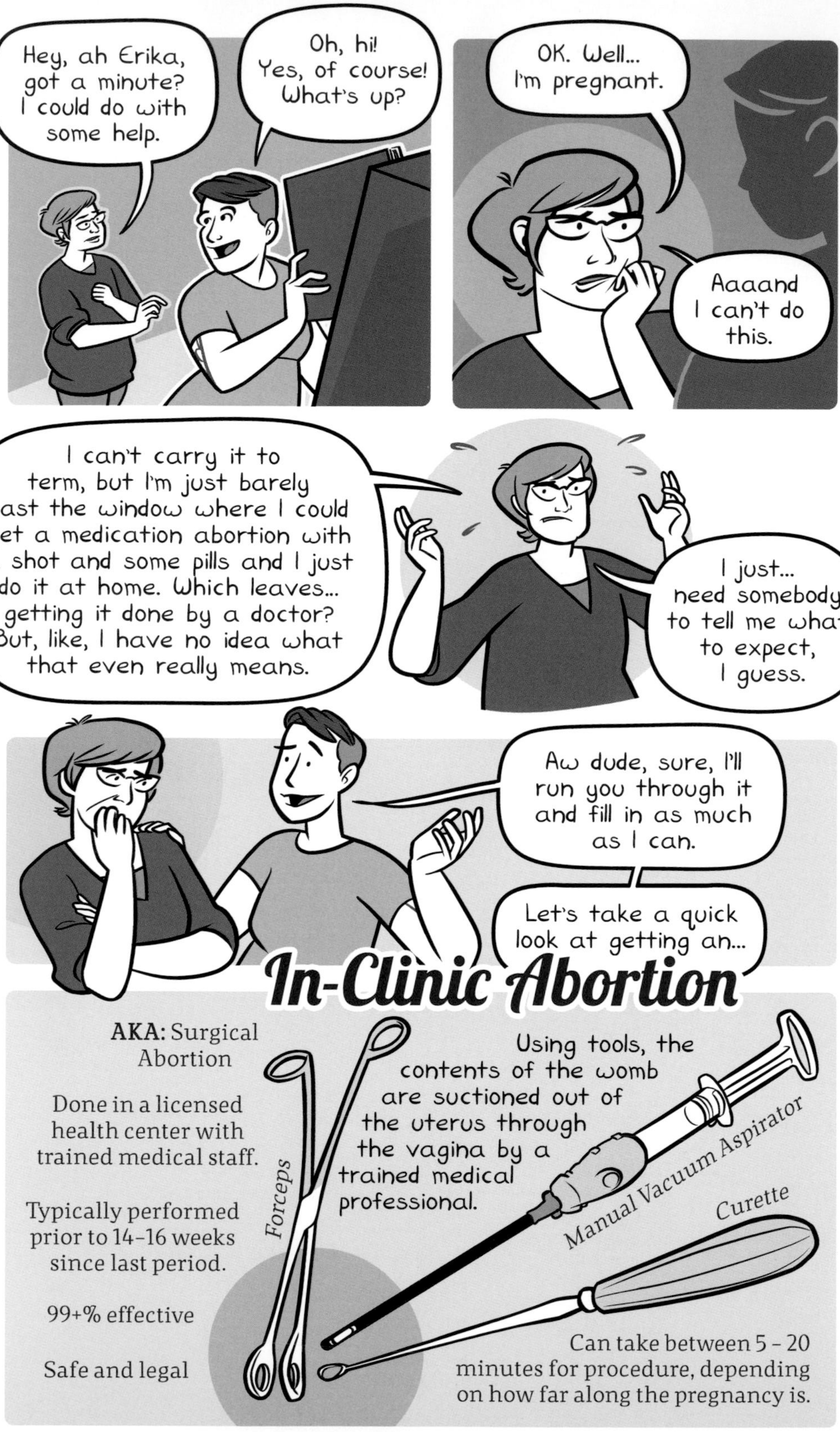
Hey, ah Erika, got a minute? I could do with some help.
Oh, hi! Yes, of course! What's up?
OK. Well... I'm pregnant.
Aaaand I can't do this.
I can't carry it to term, but I'm just barely past the window where I could get a medication abortion with a shot and some pills and I just do it at home. Which leaves... getting it done by a doctor? But, like, I have no idea what that even really means.
I just... need somebody to tell me what to expect, I guess.
Aw dude, sure, I'll run you through it and fill in as much as I can.
Let's take a quick look at getting an...
In-Clinic Abortion
AKA: Surgical Abortion
Done in a licensed health center with trained medical staff.
Typically performed prior to 14-16 weeks since last period.
99+% effective
Safe and legal
Using tools, the contents of the womb are suctioned out of the uterus through the vagina by a trained medical professional.
Forceps
Manual Vacuum Aspirator
Curette
Can take between 5 - 20 minutes for procedure, depending on how far along the pregnancy is.

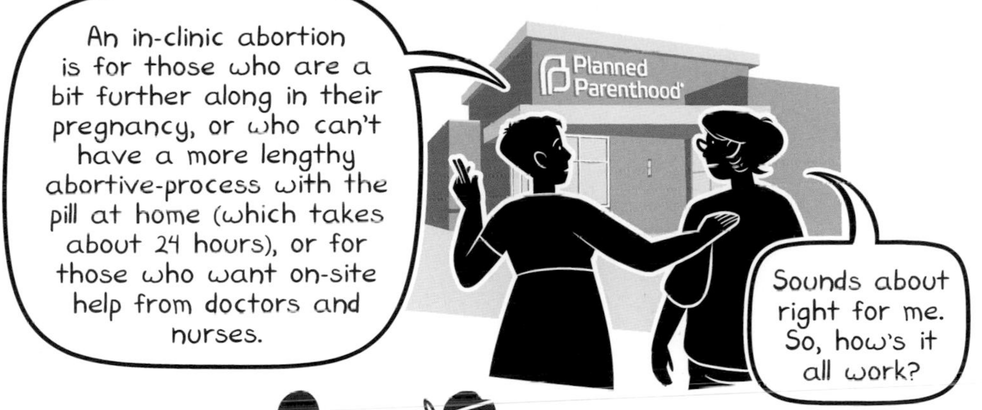

An in-clinic abortion is for those who are a bit further along in their pregnancy, or who can't have a more lengthy abortive-process with the pill at home (which takes about 24 hours), or for those who want on-site help from doctors and nurses.

Sounds about right for me. So, how's it all work?

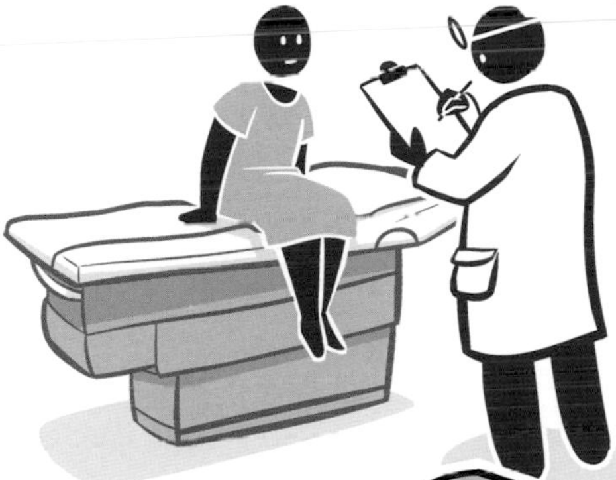

Well, before any kind of procedure, there's a lot of talking and tests! You'll meet with a medical worker and talk over your options. Then there will be an exam, blood work and maybe an ultrasound to see how far along you might be.

When it comes to the actual procedure, you'll be given some pain killers, antibiotics, and something to dilate your cervix (so the suction tube will be able to fit through and into your uterus).

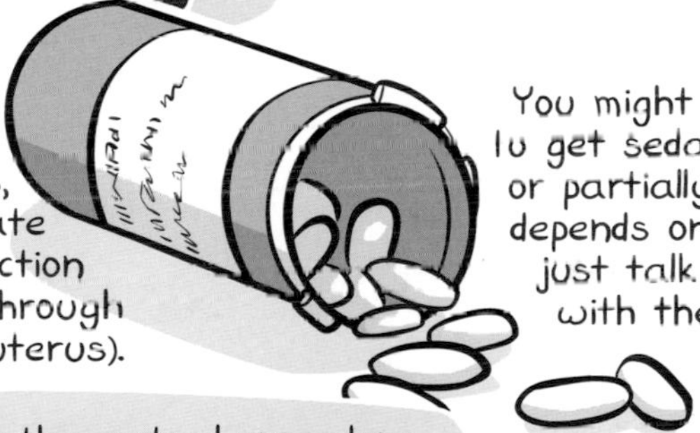

You might be able to get sedated (fully or partially), but it depends on a lot—just talk it out with the doc.

For the actual procedure, there are two methods:

Suction Abortion & Dilation and Evacuation

AKA: Vacuum Aspiration

5-10 minutes

Usually for abortions prior to 14–16 weeks after last period.

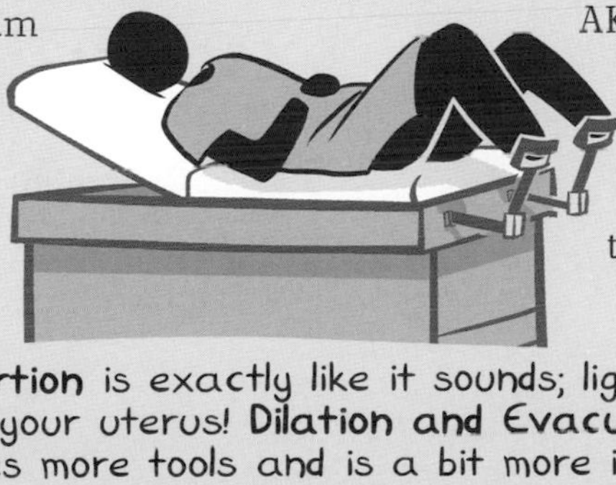

AKA: D&E

10-20 minutes

Usually for abortions later than 16 weeks after last period.

Suction Abortion is exactly like it sounds; light suction is used to empty your uterus! **Dilation and Evacuation** is similar but utilizes more tools and is a bit more involved.

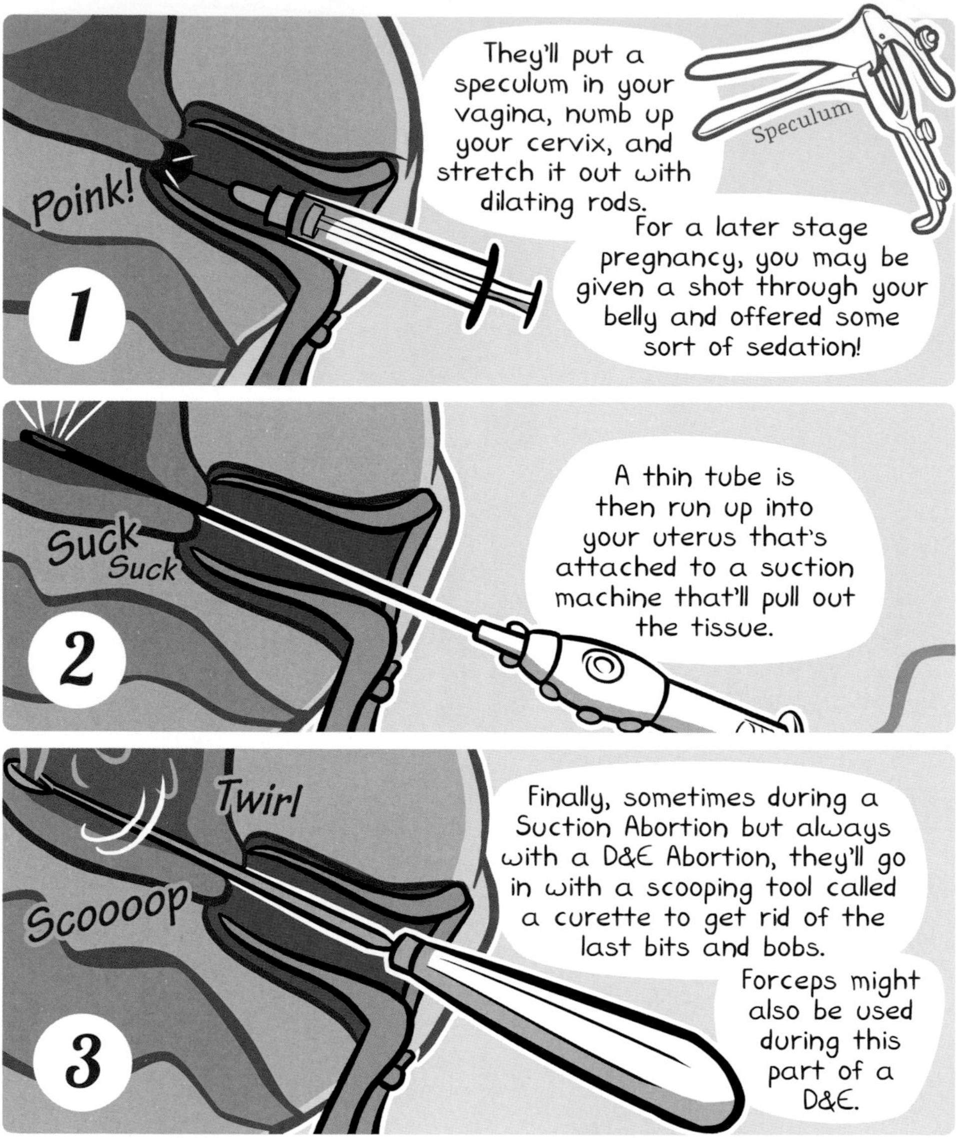
Poink!
1
They'll put a speculum in your vagina, numb up your cervix, and stretch it out with dilating rods.
Speculum
For a later stage pregnancy, you may be given a shot through your belly and offered some sort of sedation!
Suck
Suck
2
A thin tube is then run up into your uterus that's attached to a suction machine that'll pull out the tissue.
Twirl
Scoooop
3
Finally, sometimes during a Suction Abortion but always with a D&E Abortion, they'll go in with a scooping tool called a curette to get rid of the last bits and bobs.
Forceps might also be used during this part of a D&E.

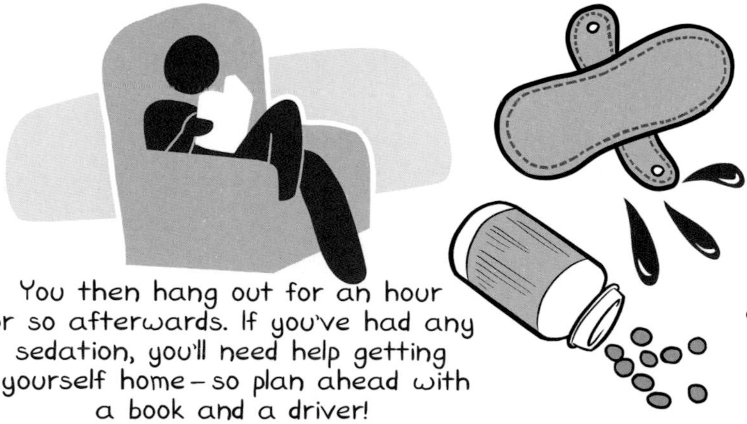

You then hang out for an hour or so afterwards. If you've had any sedation, you'll need help getting yourself home – so plan ahead with a book and a driver!

You'll probably experience some bleeding and cramping too, so bring some pads, give yourself the day off, and keep that ibuprofen within hands' reach.

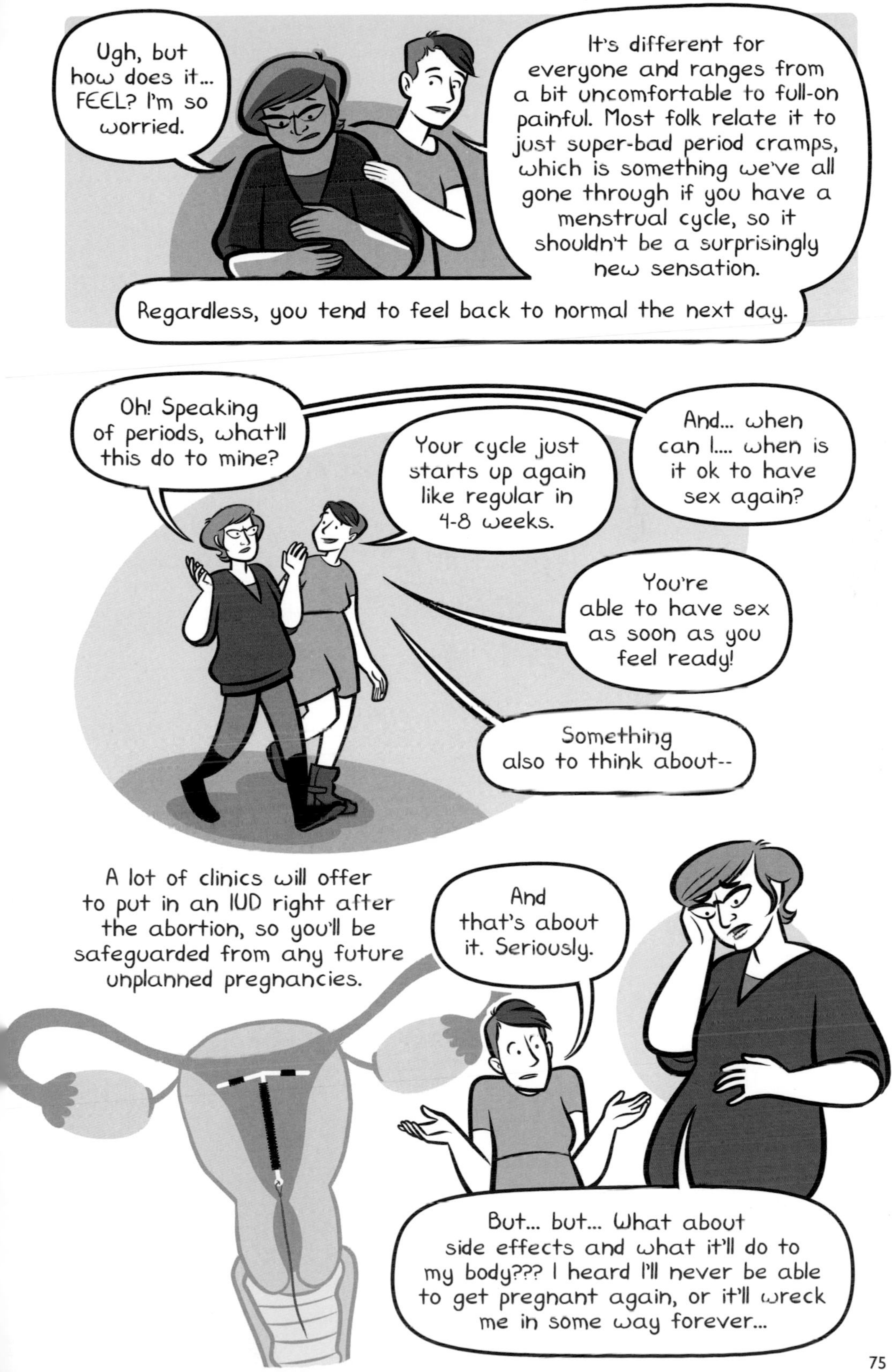
Ugh, but how does it... FEEL? I'm so worried.
It's different for everyone and ranges from a bit uncomfortable to full-on painful. Most folk relate it to just super-bad period cramps, which is something we've all gone through if you have a menstrual cycle, so it shouldn't be a surprisingly new sensation.
Regardless, you tend to feel back to normal the next day.
Oh! Speaking of periods, what'll this do to mine?
Your cycle just starts up again like regular in 4-8 weeks.
And... when can I.... when is it ok to have sex again?
You're able to have sex as soon as you feel ready!
Something also to think about--
A lot of clinics will offer to put in an IUD right after the abortion, so you'll be safeguarded from any future unplanned pregnancies.
And that's about it. Seriously.
But... but... What about side effects and what it'll do to my body??? I heard I'll never be able to get pregnant again, or it'll wreck me in some way forever...

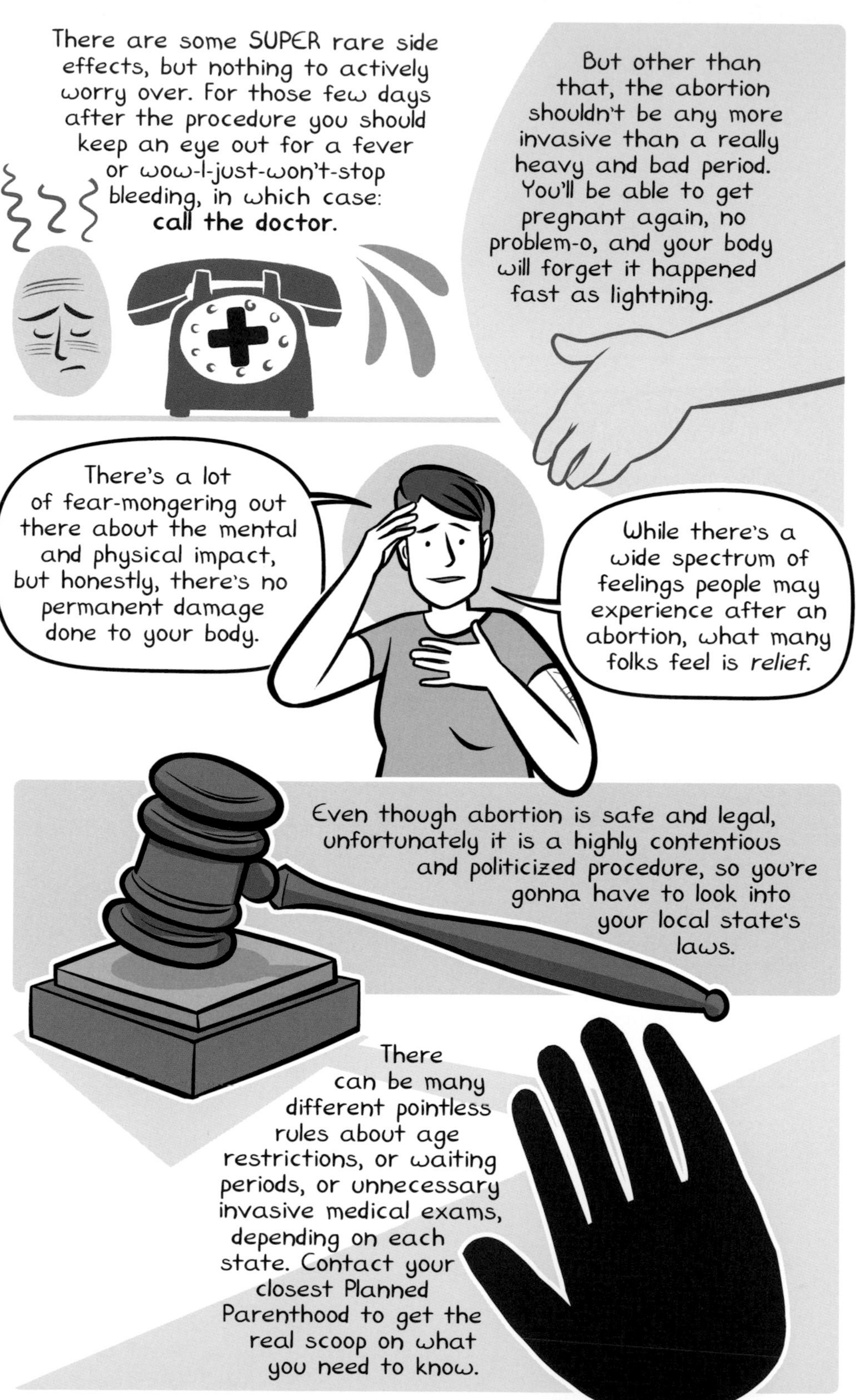
There are some SUPER rare side effects, but nothing to actively worry over. For those few days after the procedure you should keep an eye out for a fever or wow-I-just-won't-stop bleeding, in which case: **call the doctor**.
But other than that, the abortion shouldn't be any more invasive than a really heavy and bad period. You'll be able to get pregnant again, no problem-o, and your body will forget it happened fast as lightning.
There's a lot of fear-mongering out there about the mental and physical impact, but honestly, there's no permanent damage done to your body.
While there's a wide spectrum of feelings people may experience after an abortion, what many folks feel is *relief*.
Even though abortion is safe and legal, unfortunately it is a highly contentious and politicized procedure, so you're gonna have to look into your local state's laws.
There can be many different pointless rules about age restrictions, or waiting periods, or unnecessary invasive medical exams, depending on each state. Contact your closest Planned Parenthood to get the real scoop on what you need to know.

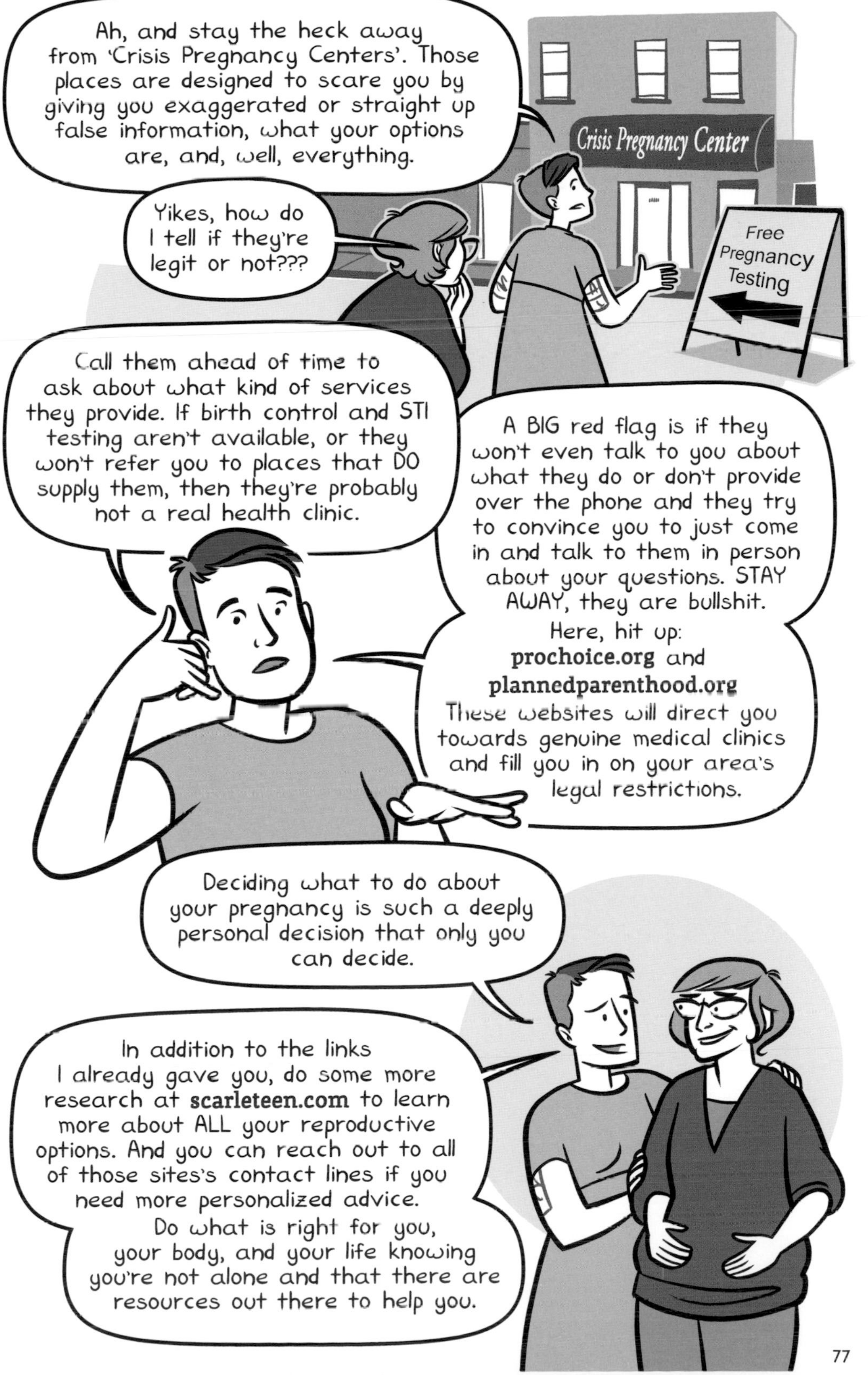
Ah, and stay the heck away from 'Crisis Pregnancy Centers'. Those places are designed to scare you by giving you exaggerated or straight up false information, what your options are, and, well, everything.
Crisis Pregnancy Center
Yikes, how do I tell if they're legit or not???
Free Pregnancy Testing
Call them ahead of time to ask about what kind of services they provide. If birth control and STI testing aren't available, or they won't refer you to places that DO supply them, then they're probably not a real health clinic.
A BIG red flag is if they won't even talk to you about what they do or don't provide over the phone and they try to convince you to just come in and talk to them in person about your questions. STAY AWAY, they are bullshit.
Here, hit up: **prochoice.org** and **plannedparenthood.org** These websites will direct you towards genuine medical clinics and fill you in on your area's legal restrictions.
Deciding what to do about your pregnancy is such a deeply personal decision that only you can decide.
In addition to the links I already gave you, do some more research at **scarleteen.com** to learn more about ALL your reproductive options. And you can reach out to all of those sites's contact lines if you need more personalized advice.
Do what is right for you, your body, and your life knowing you're not alone and that there are resources out there to help you.

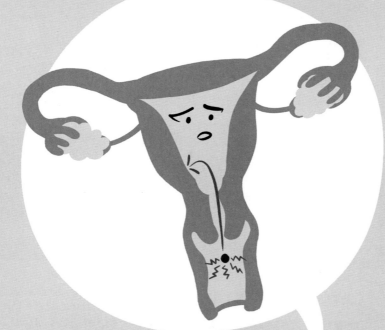

Miscarriage

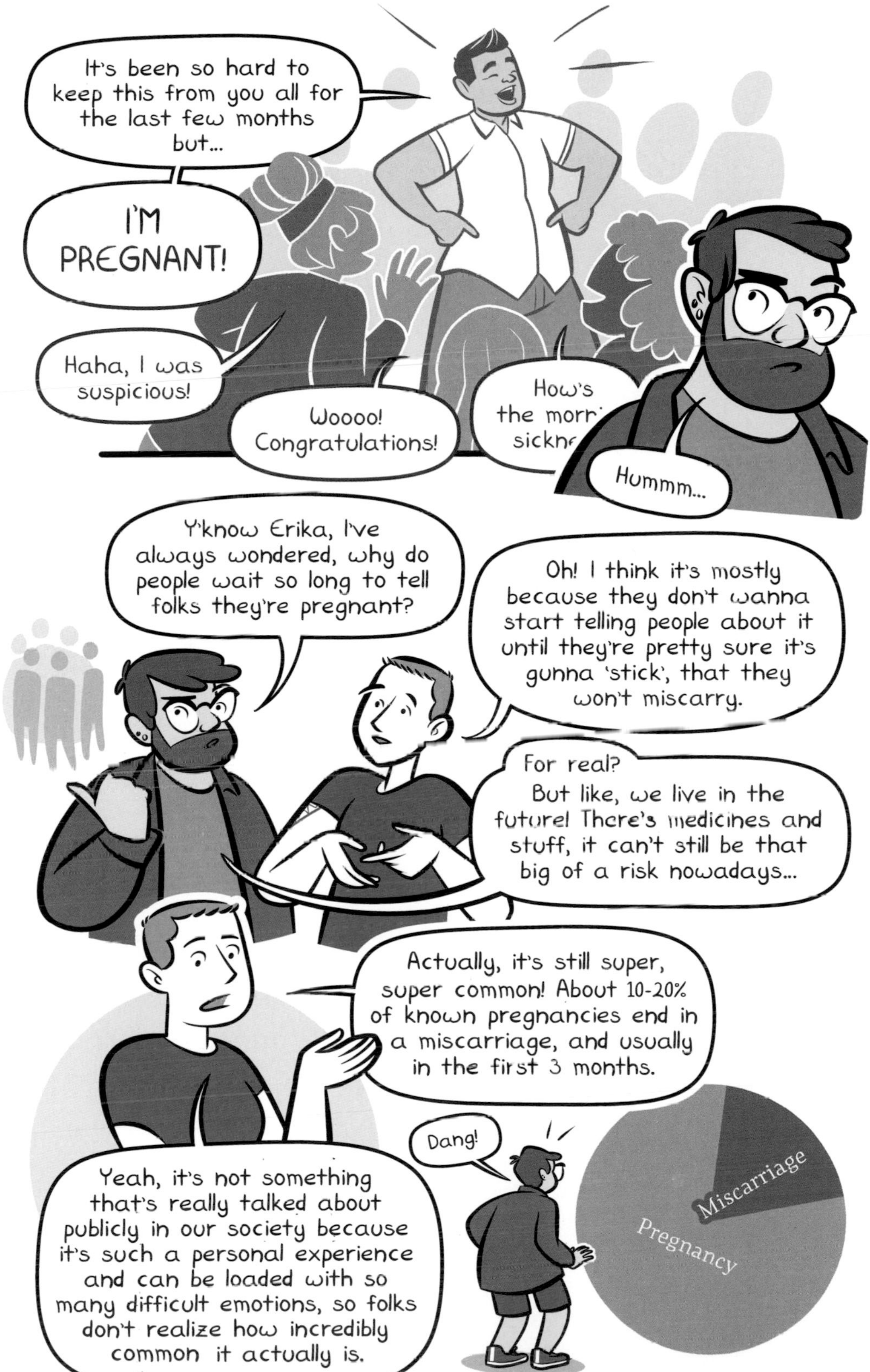
It's been so hard to keep this from you all for the last few months but...
I'M PREGNANT!
Haha, I was suspicious!
Woooo! Congratulations!
How's the morn sickn
Hummm...
Y'know Erika, I've always wondered, why do people wait so long to tell folks they're pregnant?
Oh! I think it's mostly because they don't wanna start telling people about it until they're pretty sure it's gunna 'stick', that they won't miscarry.
For real?
But like, we live in the future! There's medicines and stuff, it can't still be that big of a risk nowadays...
Actually, it's still super, super common! About 10-20% of known pregnancies end in a miscarriage, and usually in the first 3 months.
Dang!
Miscarriage
Pregnancy
Yeah, it's not something that's really talked about publicly in our society because it's such a personal experience and can be loaded with so many difficult emotions, so folks don't realize how incredibly common it actually is.

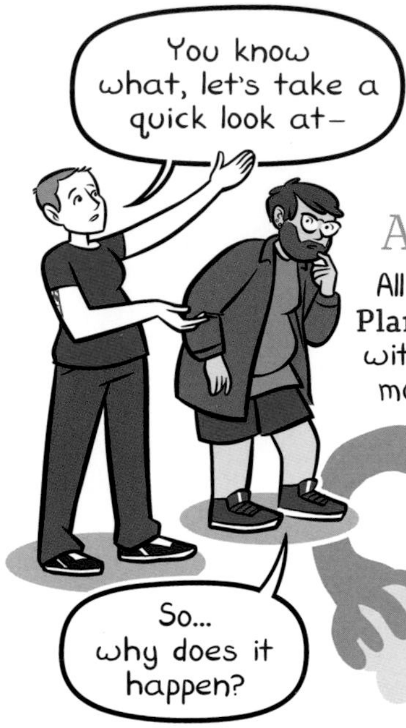
You know what, let's take a quick look at–
So... why does it happen?

Miscarriage

AKA: *Spontaneous Abortion*

All the information here was sourced from PlannedParenthood.org and Scarleteen.org. As with everything we cover, there is so much more information available on this subject than we can include in this comic, so we encourage you to dive into more research!

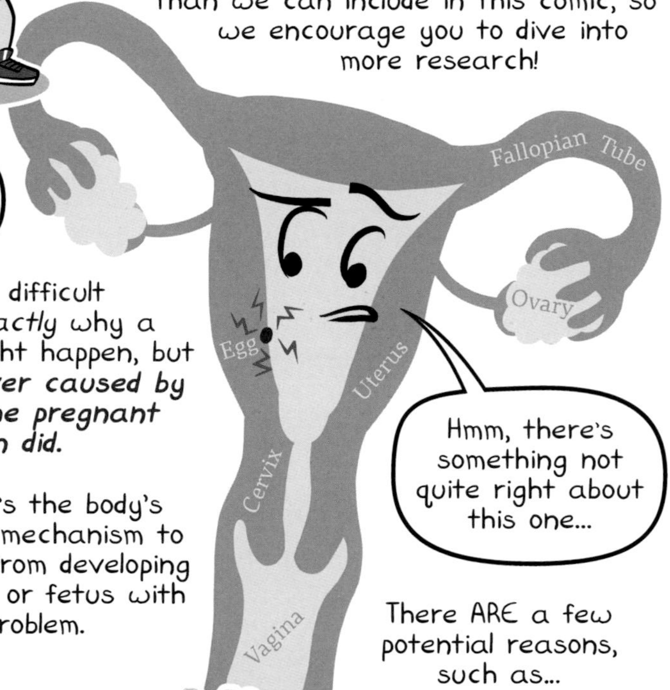
Fallopian Tube
Ovary
Egg
Uterus
Cervix
Vagina
Hmm, there's something not quite right about this one...

It's really difficult to know *exactly* why a miscarriage might happen, but it's ***almost never caused by something the pregnant person did.***

Usually, it's the body's protective mechanism to protect it from developing an embryo or fetus with a problem.

There ARE a few potential reasons, such as...

What Causes a Miscarriage?

When the fertilized egg randomly has the wrong number of chromosomes or the fetus develops a congenital defect.

- Serious injury or major infection.
- Some illnesses like severe diabetes can increase the odds of miscarriage.
- Abnormalities in the uterus can cause a late miscarriage (after 3 months)
- Having had more than 2 miscarriages in a row ups the odds too.

What DOESN'T Cause a Miscarriage?

- Minor injuries (like falling)
- Most medications
- Working
- Exercise
- Sex

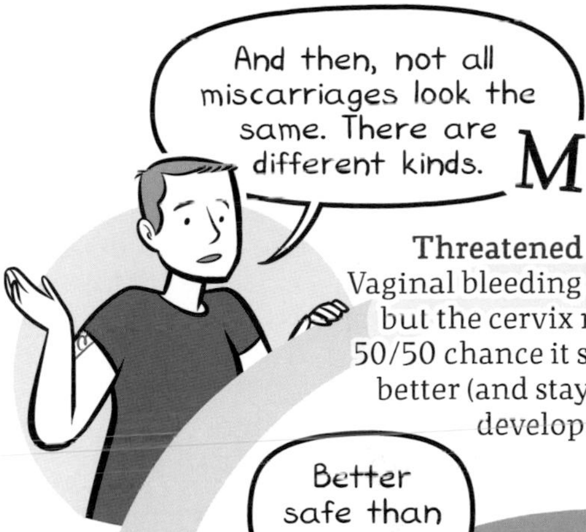

And then, not all miscarriages look the same. There are different kinds.

Types of Miscarriage

Threatened Miscarriage
Vaginal bleeding and mild cramps, but the cervix remains closed. 50/50 chance it stops and they get better (and stay pregnant), or it develops into a...

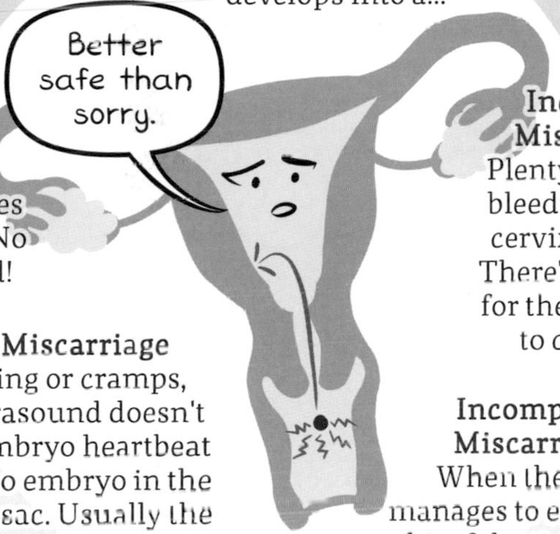

Better safe than sorry.

Complete Miscarriage
All the tissue comes out of the uterus. No treatment needed!

Inevitable Miscarriage
Plenty of vaginal bleeding and the cervix opens up. There's no chance for the pregnancy to continue.

Missed Miscarriage
No bleeding or cramps, but an ultrasound doesn't show an embryo heartbeat or there's no embryo in the pregnancy sac. Usually the tissue passes on its own, but sometimes they'll need treatment to remove the leftover tissue.

Incomplete Miscarriage
When the body manages to evacuate a bit of the tissue, but not all of it. The person may need treatment to remove what's left.

Treatment after a miscarriage is pretty much the same as the treatments for an abortion. Either medication is used to help the body evacuate what's left, or you go in for aspiration, where a small suction tube is used to remove the left over tissue.

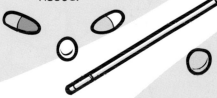

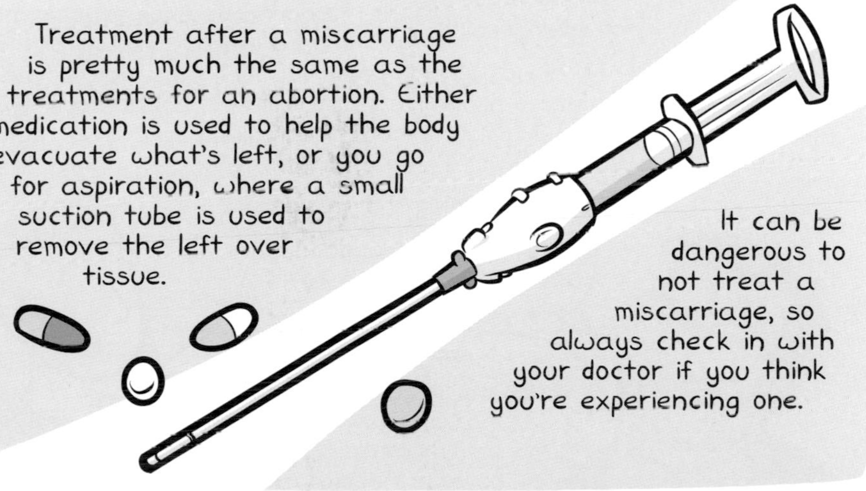

It can be dangerous to not treat a miscarriage, so always check in with your doctor if you think you're experiencing one.

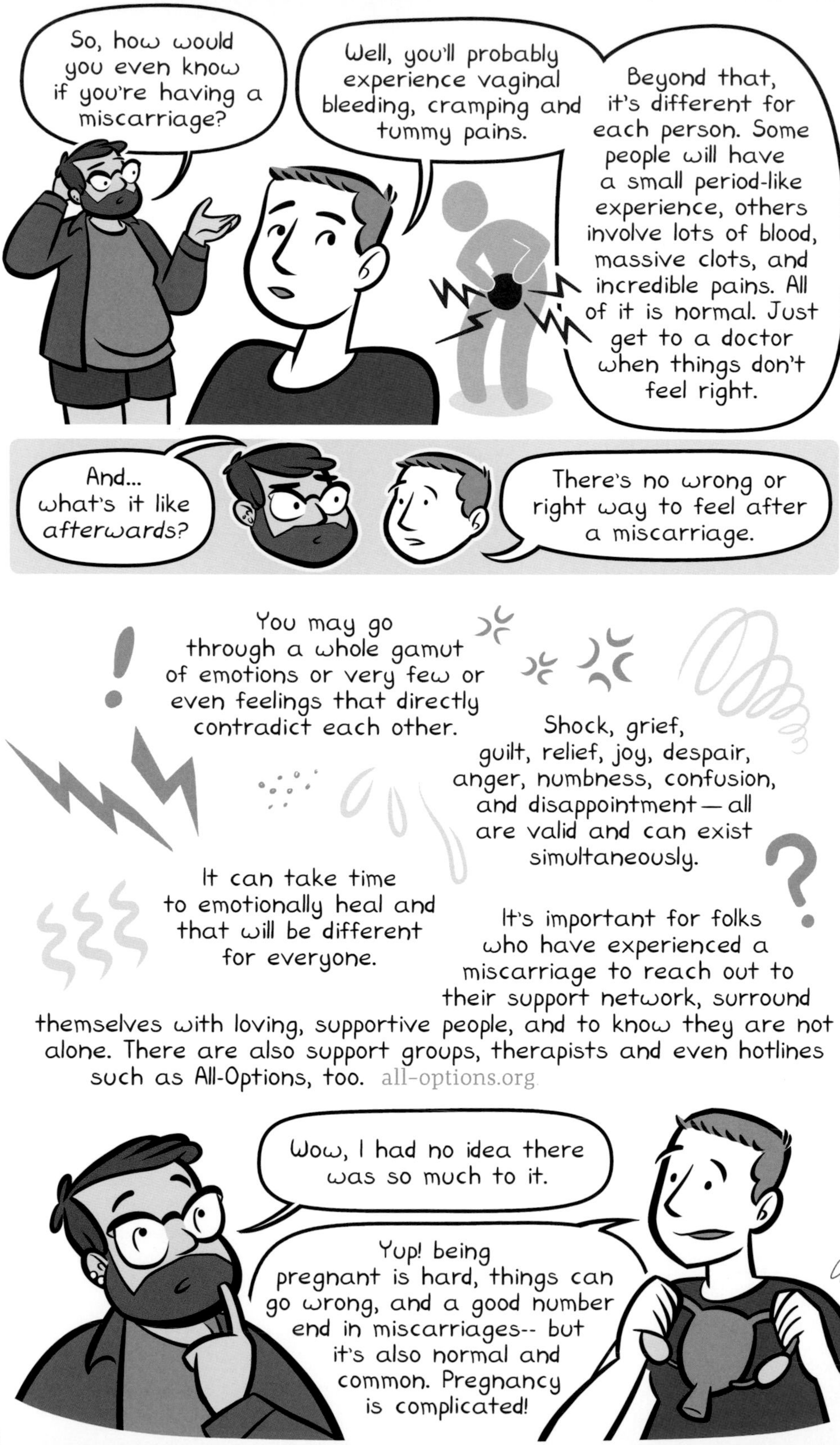

So, how would you even know if you're having a miscarriage?
Well, you'll probably experience vaginal bleeding, cramping and tummy pains.
Beyond that, it's different for each person. Some people will have a small period-like experience, others involve lots of blood, massive clots, and incredible pains. All of it is normal. Just get to a doctor when things don't feel right.
And... what's it like afterwards?
There's no wrong or right way to feel after a miscarriage.
You may go through a whole gamut of emotions or very few or even feelings that directly contradict each other.
Shock, grief, guilt, relief, joy, despair, anger, numbness, confusion, and disappointment— all are valid and can exist simultaneously.
It can take time to emotionally heal and that will be different for everyone.
It's important for folks who have experienced a miscarriage to reach out to their support network, surround themselves with loving, supportive people, and to know they are not alone. There are also support groups, therapists and even hotlines such as All-Options, too. all-options.org
Wow, I had no idea there was so much to it.
Yup! being pregnant is hard, things can go wrong, and a good number end in miscarriages-- but it's also normal and common. Pregnancy is complicated!

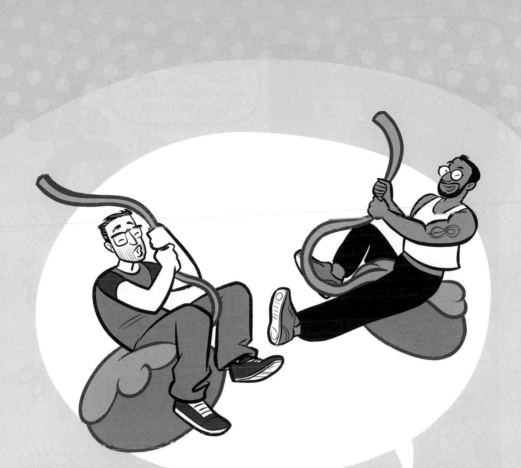

Vasectomy

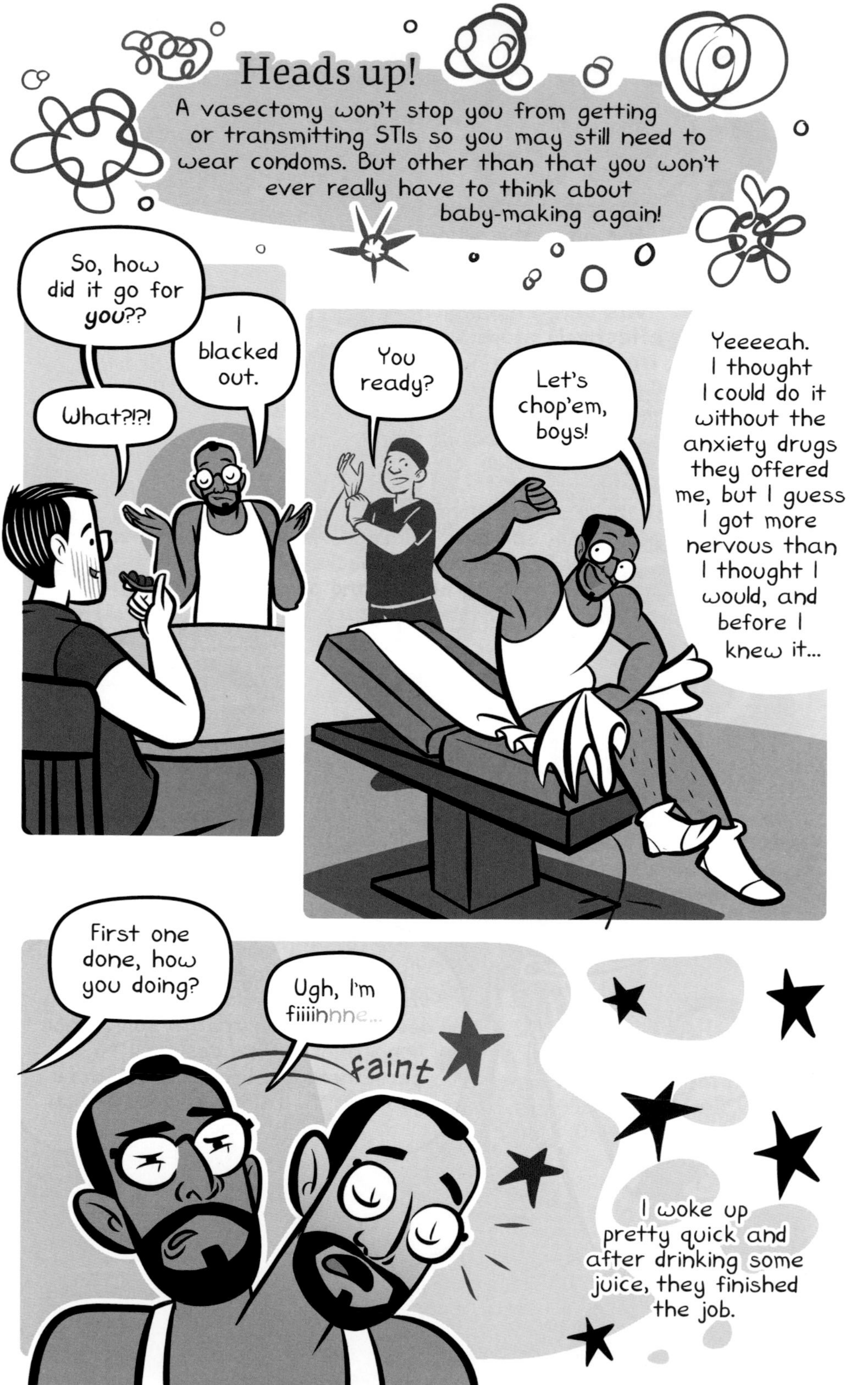
Heads up!
A vasectomy won't stop you from getting or transmitting STIs so you may still need to wear condoms. But other than that you won't ever really have to think about baby-making again!
So, how did it go for *you*??
I blacked out.
What?!?!
You ready?
Let's chop'em, boys!
Yeeeeah. I thought I could do it without the anxiety drugs they offered me, but I guess I got more nervous than I thought I would, and before I knew it...
First one done, how you doing?
Ugh, I'm fiiiinnne...
faint
I woke up pretty quick and after drinking some juice, they finished the job.

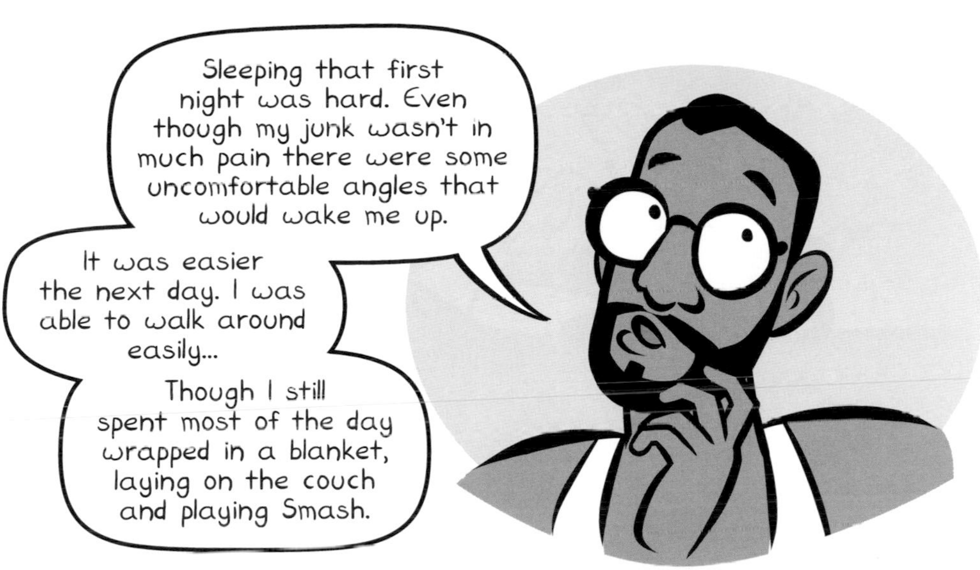
Sleeping that first night was hard. Even though my junk wasn't in much pain there were some uncomfortable angles that would wake me up.
It was easier the next day. I was able to walk around easily...
Though I still spent most of the day wrapped in a blanket, laying on the couch and playing Smash.

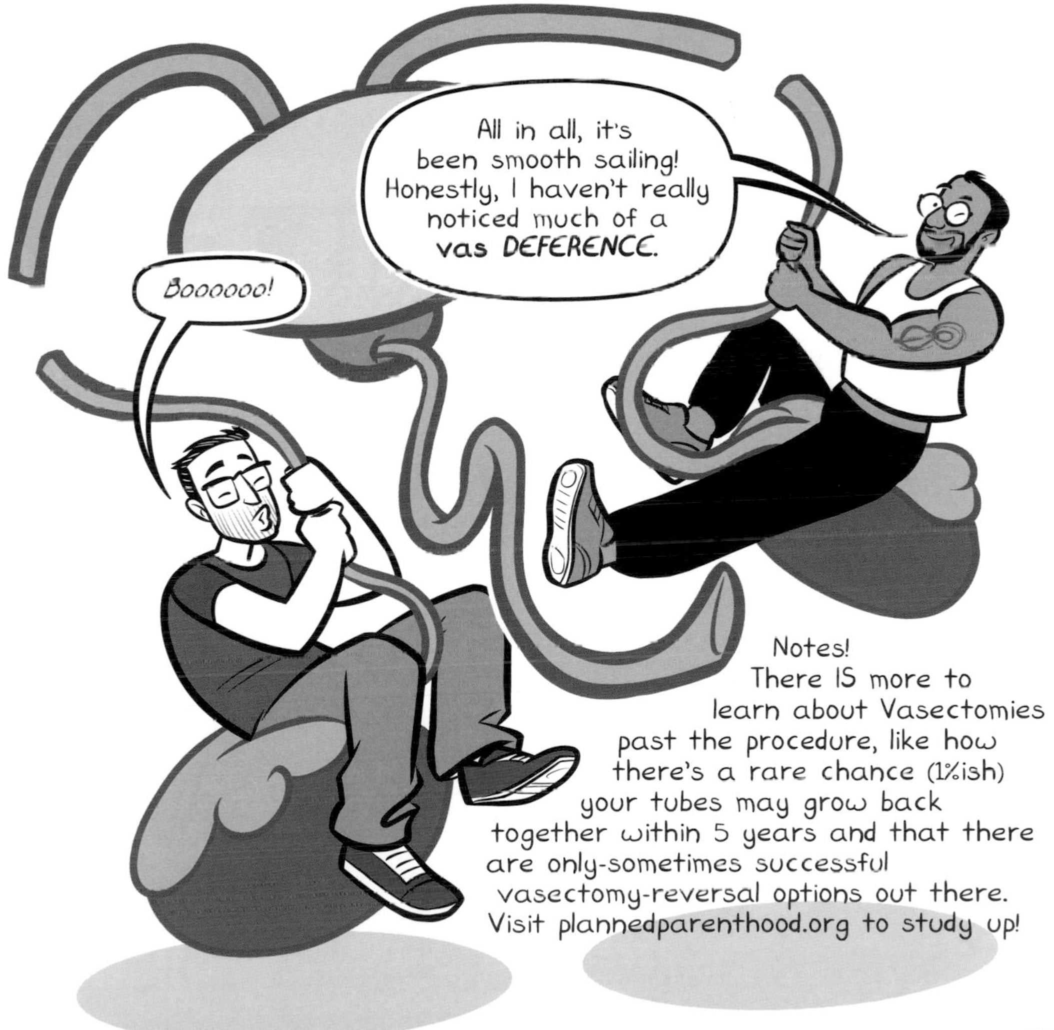
All in all, it's been smooth sailing! Honestly, I haven't really noticed much of a vas DEFERENCE.
Boooooo!
Notes!
There IS more to learn about Vasectomies past the procedure, like how there's a rare chance (1%ish) your tubes may grow back together within 5 years and that there are only-sometimes successful vasectomy-reversal options out there. Visit plannedparenthood.org to study up!

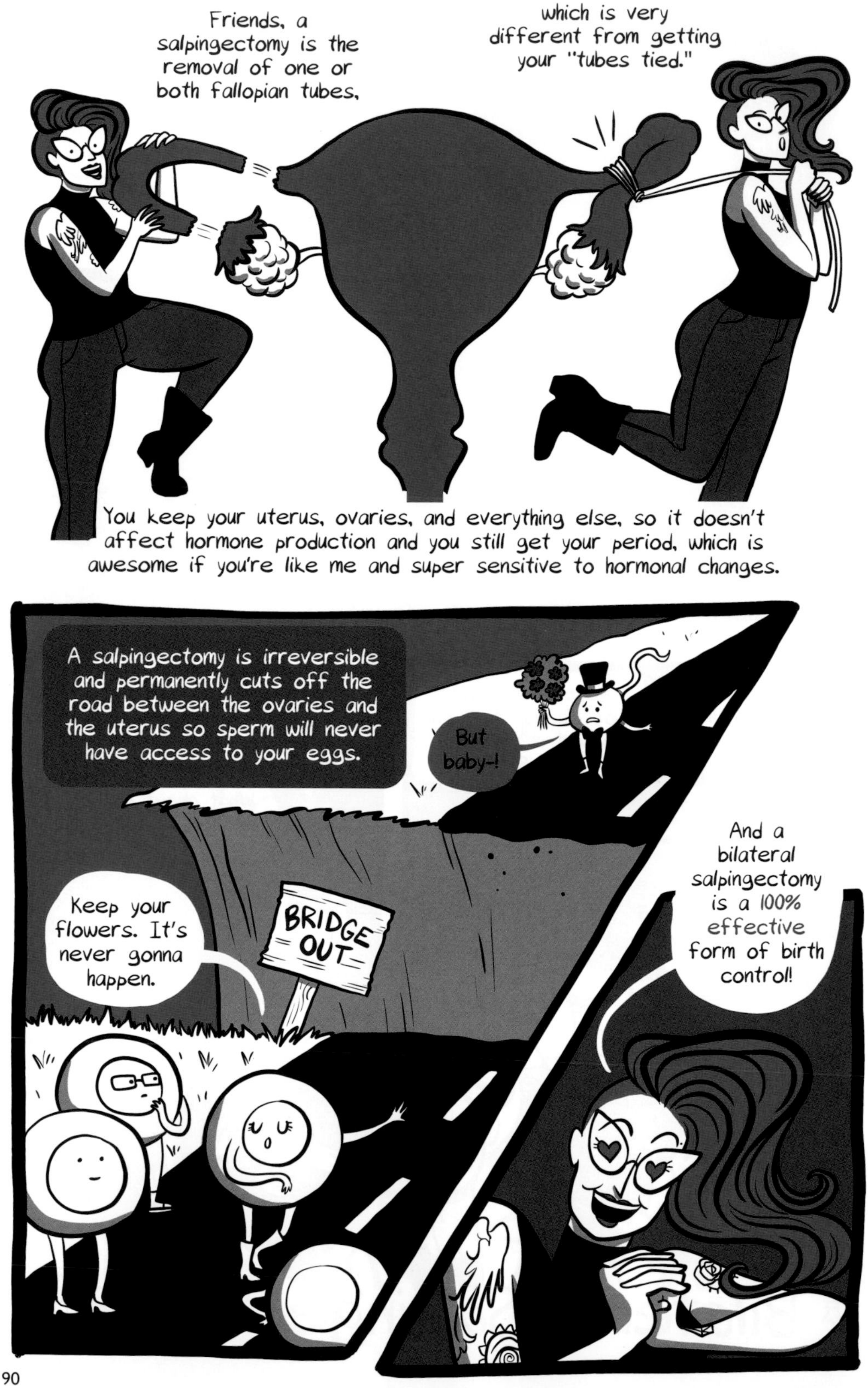
Friends, a salpingectomy is the removal of one or both fallopian tubes,
which is very different from getting your "tubes tied."
You keep your uterus, ovaries, and everything else, so it doesn't affect hormone production and you still get your period, which is awesome if you're like me and super sensitive to hormonal changes.
A salpingectomy is irreversible and permanently cuts off the road between the ovaries and the uterus so sperm will never have access to your eggs.
But baby-!
Keep your flowers. It's never gonna happen.
BRIDGE OUT
And a bilateral salpingectomy is a 100% effective form of birth control!

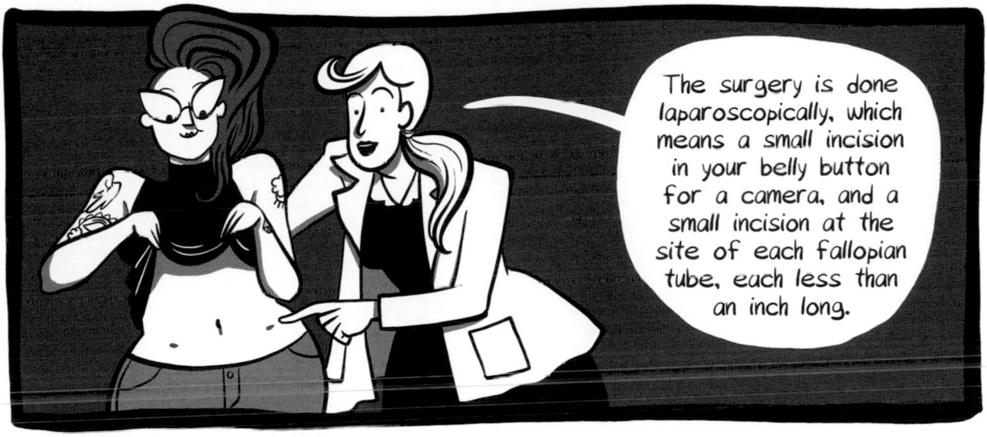
The surgery is done laparoscopically, which means a small incision in your belly button for a camera, and a small incision at the site of each fallopian tube, each less than an inch long.

It's a fairly quick outpatient procedure, but it is still a surgery with all the risks that occur anytime someone goes cutting into your body, including:

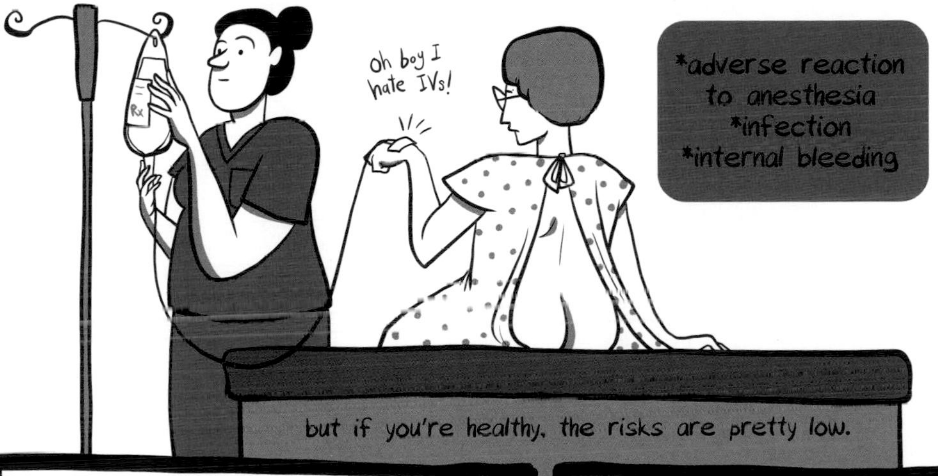
Oh boy I hate IVs!
Rx
*adverse reaction to anesthesia
*infection
*internal bleeding
but if you're healthy, the risks are pretty low.

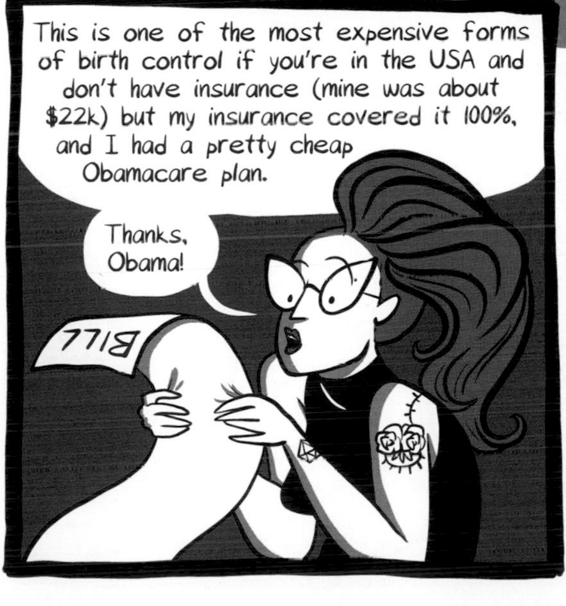
This is one of the most expensive forms of birth control if you're in the USA and don't have insurance (mine was about $22k) but my insurance covered it 100%, and I had a pretty cheap Obamacare plan.
Thanks, Obama!
BILL

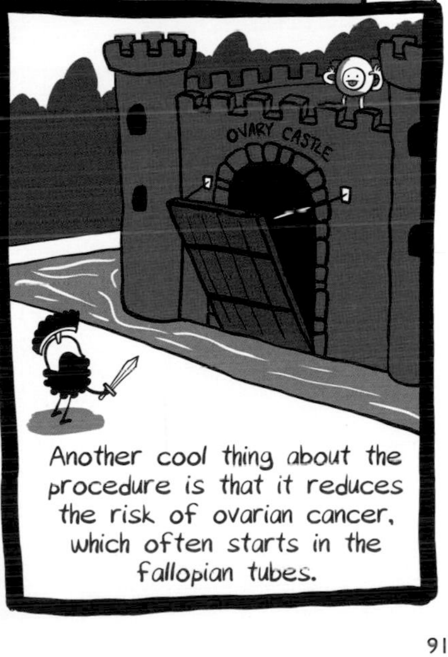
OVARY CASTLE
Another cool thing about the procedure is that it reduces the risk of ovarian cancer, which often starts in the fallopian tubes.

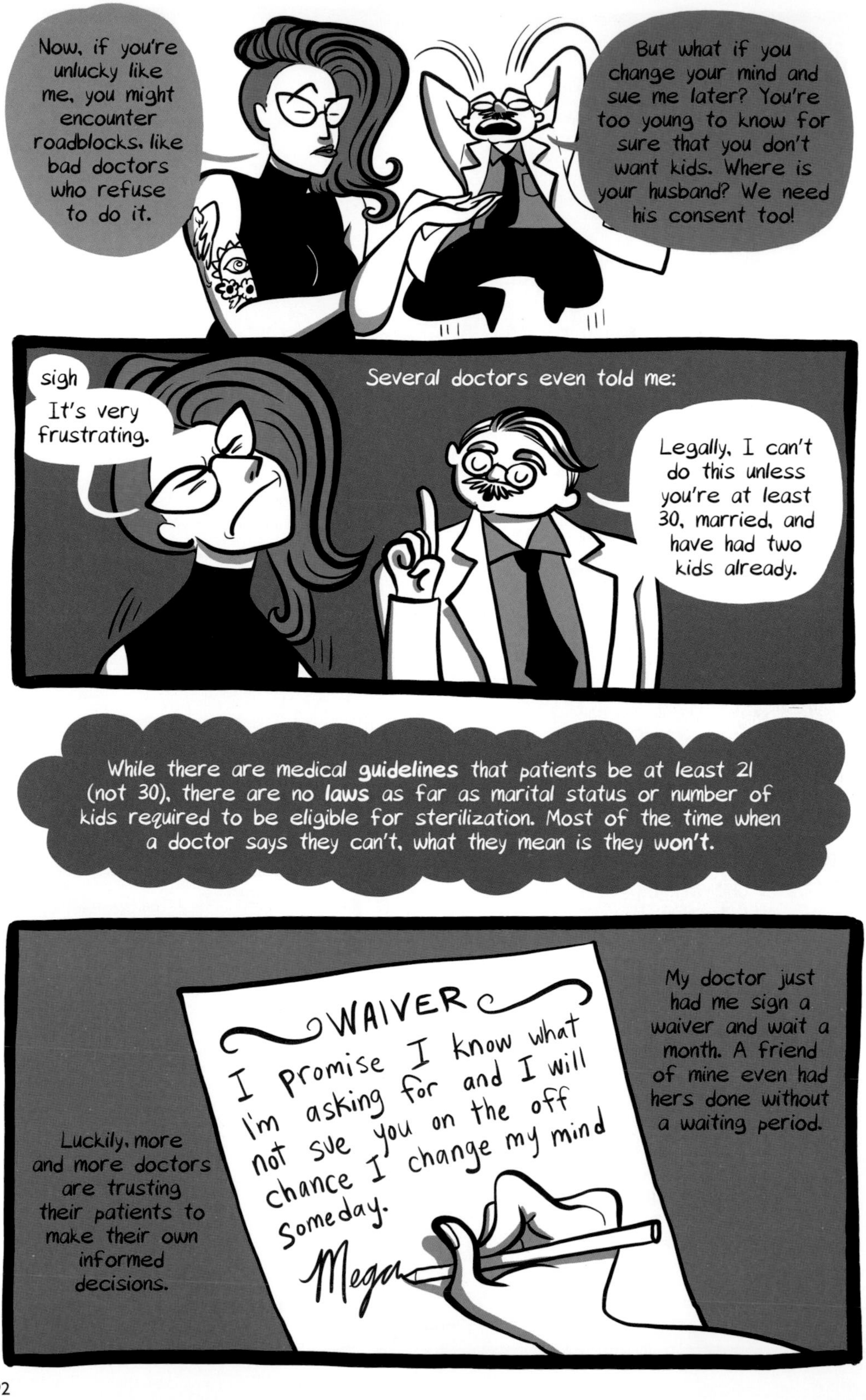
Now, if you're unlucky like me, you might encounter roadblocks, like bad doctors who refuse to do it.
But what if you change your mind and sue me later? You're too young to know for sure that you don't want kids. Where is your husband? We need his consent too!
sigh
It's very frustrating.
Several doctors even told me:
Legally, I can't do this unless you're at least 30, married, and have had two kids already.
While there are medical **guidelines** that patients be at least 21 (not 30), there are no **laws** as far as marital status or number of kids required to be eligible for sterilization. Most of the time when a doctor says they can't, what they mean is they **won't**.
Luckily, more and more doctors are trusting their patients to make their own informed decisions.
WAIVER
I promise I know what I'm asking for and I will not sue you on the off chance I change my mind someday.
Megan
My doctor just had me sign a waiver and wait a month. A friend of mine even had hers done without a waiting period.

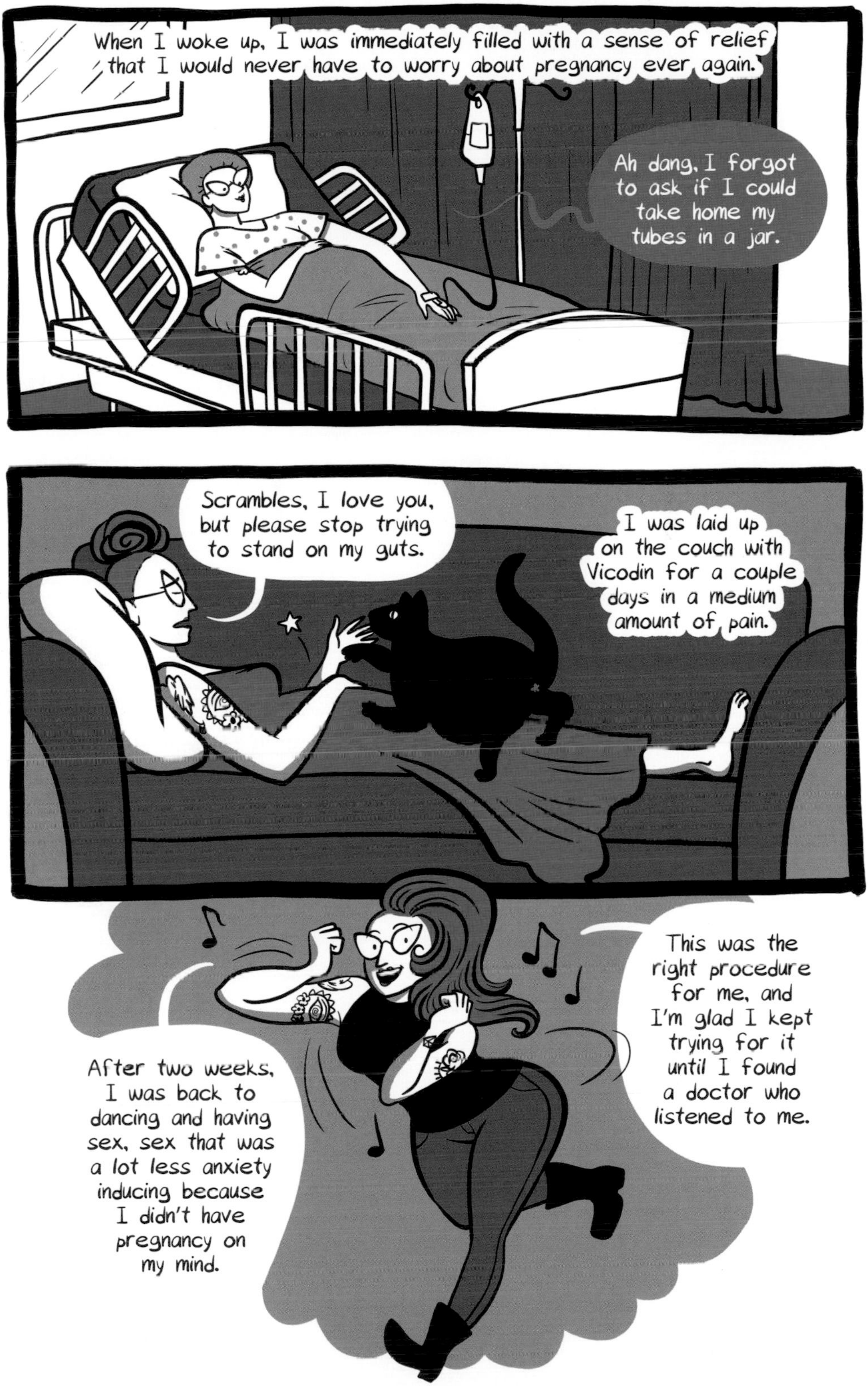
When I woke up, I was immediately filled with a sense of relief that I would never have to worry about pregnancy ever again.
Ah dang, I forgot to ask if I could take home my tubes in a jar.
Scrambles, I love you, but please stop trying to stand on my guts.
I was laid up on the couch with Vicodin for a couple days in a medium amount of pain.
After two weeks, I was back to dancing and having sex, sex that was a lot less anxiety inducing because I didn't have pregnancy on my mind.
This was the right procedure for me, and I'm glad I kept trying for it until I found a doctor who listened to me.

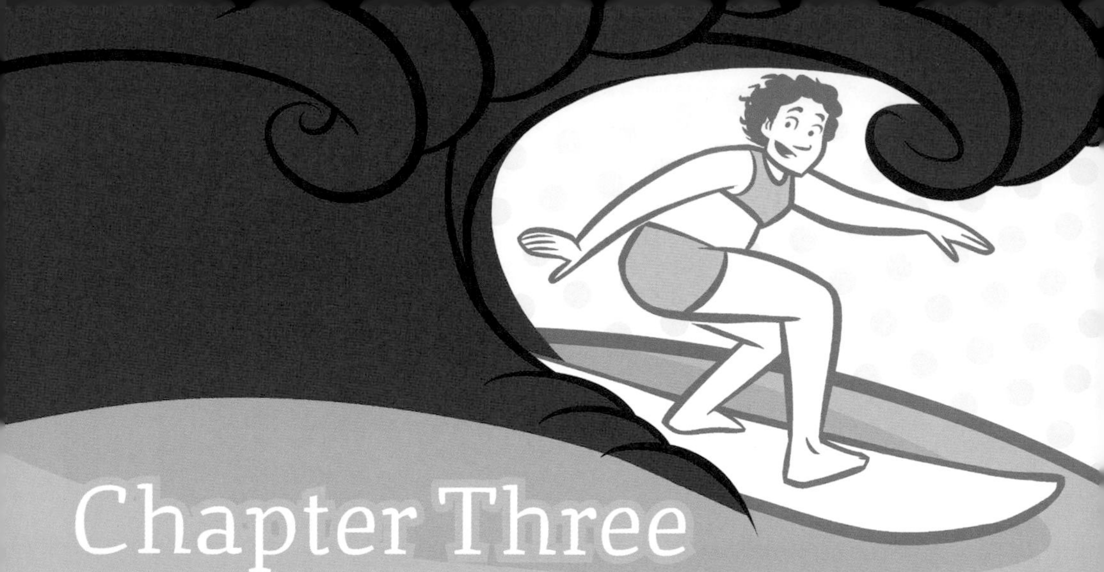

Chapter Three

Menstruation and Menopause

Aunt Flow. Riding the crimson wave. Shark Week. What IS it? Why does it happen? How do you contain it? WHEN WILL IT STOP? ...And what happens after it stops, for good? Half the human population has a uterus, so whether you've got one or not, it's definitely worth reading through this chapter to find out just what exactly is going on in there.

So much attention is paid to the bleeding phase of the menstrual cycle that people forget—or never knew to begin with!— that it's actually a much more involved process that takes up an entire month with very specific stages. About five days to shed the uterus lining, another six-ish for a fresh egg to mature while the uterus lining rebuilds itself, a couple days to pop that matured egg out of the ovary and into the fallopian tube, and then just a bit less than two weeks to work its way down into the uterus, to either implant or not.

If not? Then the body'll go through the same thing again!
On and on, until...

Menopause.

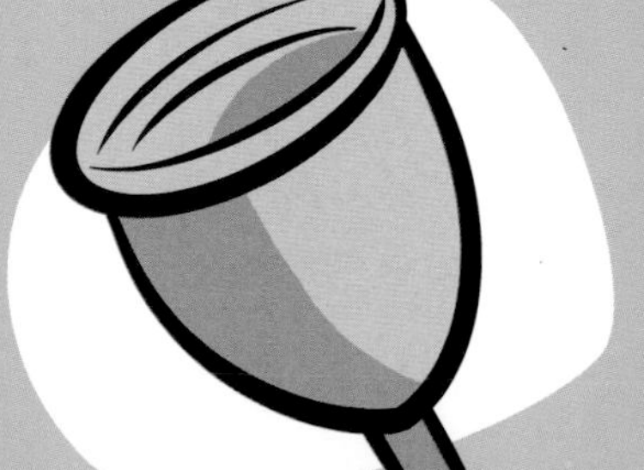

You'd think that turning the works off would be like time-traveling to before your period ever started, but it turns out menopause, whether it's natural or artificially induced, has a whole lot more side effects than you'd guess! Read on to learn what's waiting for future and current menstruators...

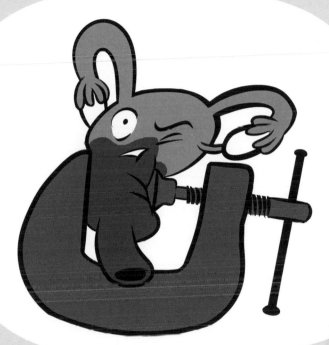

Menstruation

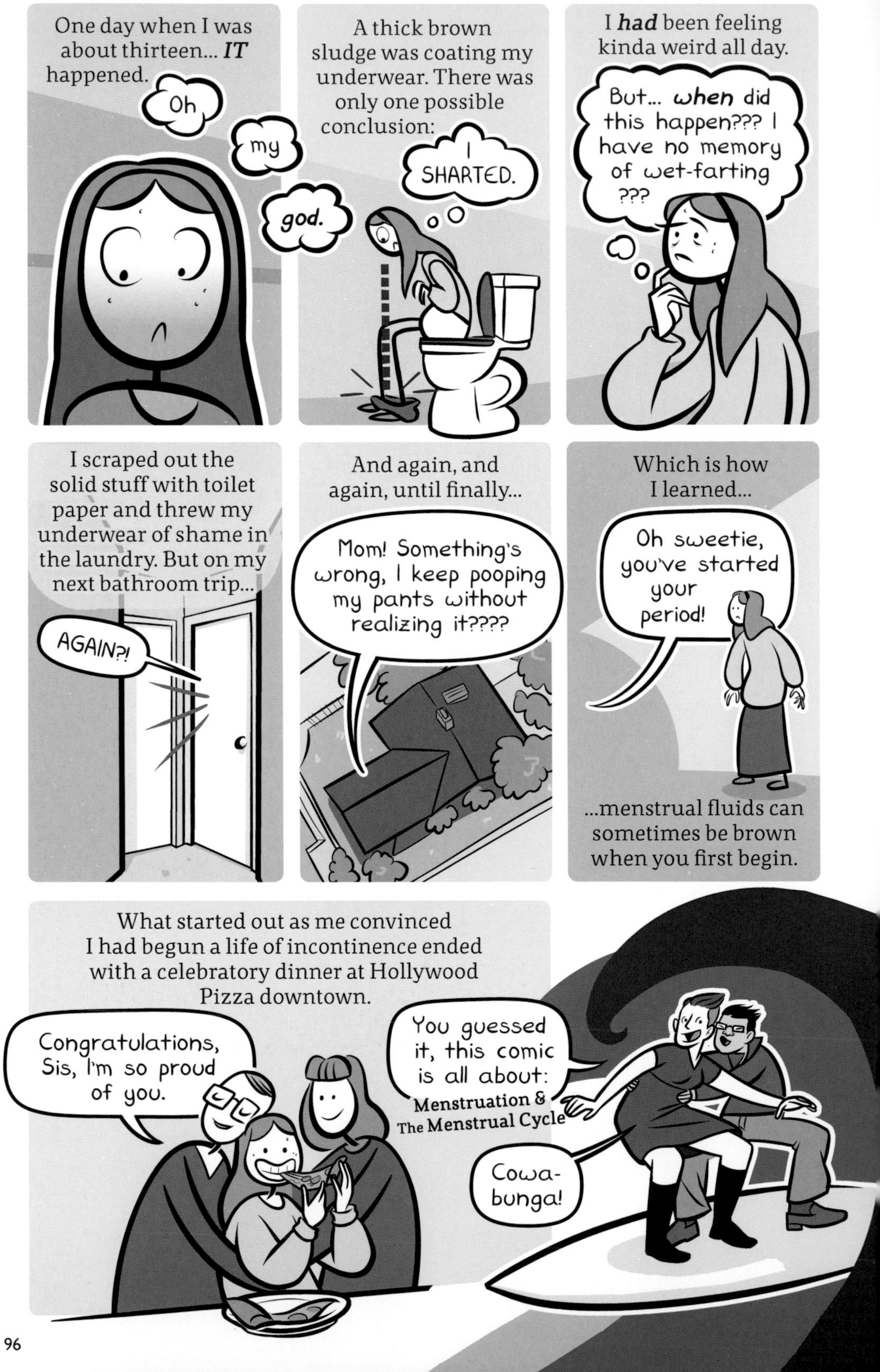
One day when I was about thirteen... ***IT*** happened.
Oh
my
god.
A thick brown sludge was coating my underwear. There was only one possible conclusion:
I SHARTED.
I ***had*** been feeling kinda weird all day.
But... **when** did this happen??? I have no memory of wet-farting ???
I scraped out the solid stuff with toilet paper and threw my underwear of shame in the laundry. But on my next bathroom trip...
AGAIN?!
And again, and again, until finally...
Mom! Something's wrong, I keep pooping my pants without realizing it????
Which is how I learned...
Oh sweetie, you've started your period!
...menstrual fluids can sometimes be brown when you first begin.
What started out as me convinced I had begun a life of incontinence ended with a celebratory dinner at Hollywood Pizza downtown.
Congratulations, Sis, I'm so proud of you.
You guessed it, this comic is all about:
Menstruation & The Menstrual Cycle
Cowa-bunga!

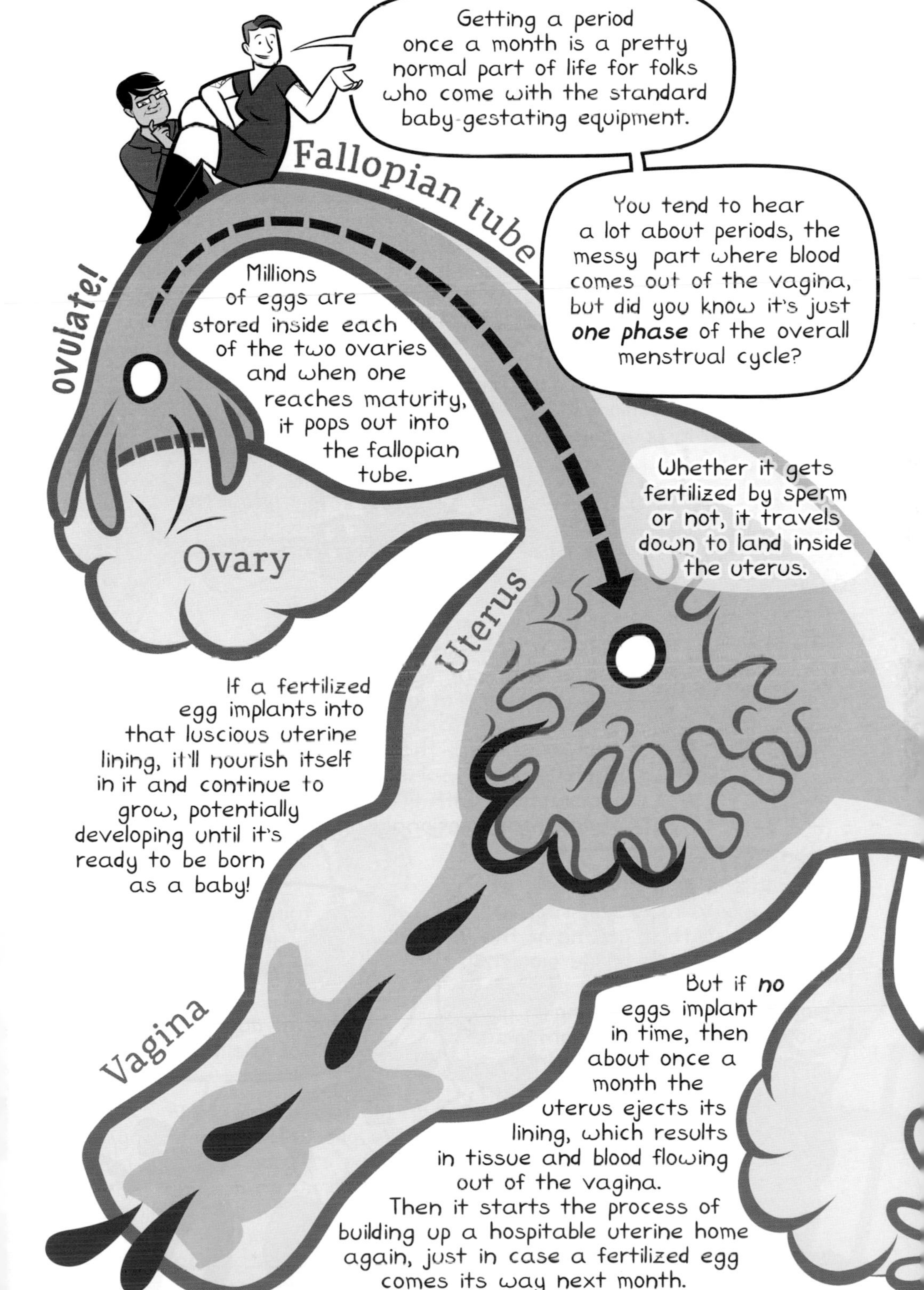
Getting a period once a month is a pretty normal part of life for folks who come with the standard baby-gestating equipment.
You tend to hear a lot about periods, the messy part where blood comes out of the vagina, but did you know it's just ***one phase*** of the overall menstrual cycle?
Fallopian tube
ovulate!
Millions of eggs are stored inside each of the two ovaries and when one reaches maturity, it pops out into the fallopian tube.
Ovary
Whether it gets fertilized by sperm or not, it travels down to land inside the uterus.
Uterus
If a fertilized egg implants into that luscious uterine lining, it'll nourish itself in it and continue to grow, potentially developing until it's ready to be born as a baby!
Vagina
But if ***no*** eggs implant in time, then about once a month the uterus ejects its lining, which results in tissue and blood flowing out of the vagina.
Then it starts the process of building up a hospitable uterine home again, just in case a fertilized egg comes its way next month.

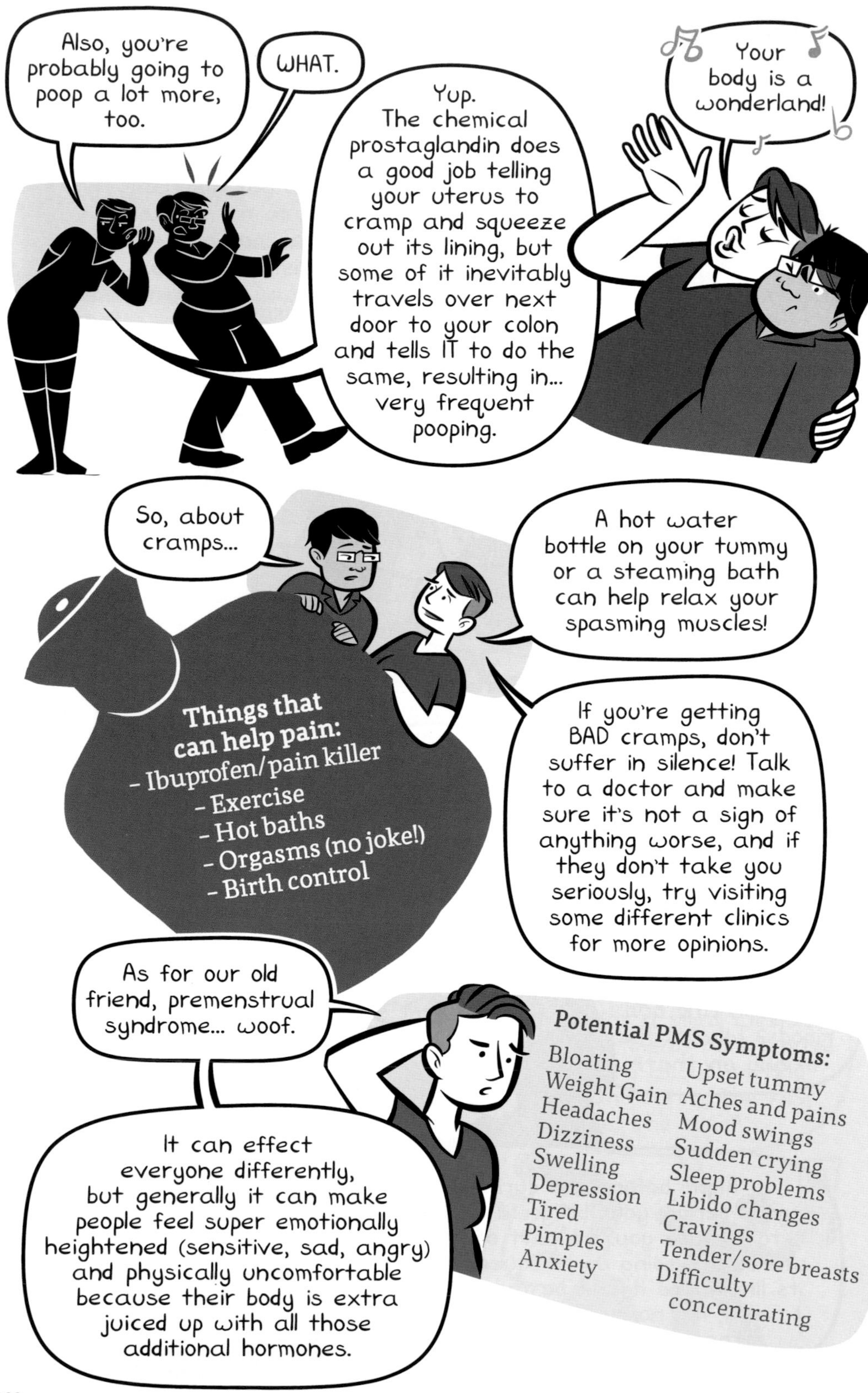
Also, you're probably going to poop a lot more, too.
WHAT.
Yup. The chemical prostaglandin does a good job telling your uterus to cramp and squeeze out its lining, but some of it inevitably travels over next door to your colon and tells IT to do the same, resulting in... very frequent pooping.
Your body is a wonderland!
So, about cramps...
A hot water bottle on your tummy or a steaming bath can help relax your spasming muscles!
Things that can help pain:
- Ibuprofen/pain killer
- Exercise
- Hot baths
- Orgasms (no joke!)
- Birth control
If you're getting BAD cramps, don't suffer in silence! Talk to a doctor and make sure it's not a sign of anything worse, and if they don't take you seriously, try visiting some different clinics for more opinions.
As for our old friend, premenstrual syndrome... woof.
Potential PMS Symptoms:
Bloating
Weight Gain
Headaches
Dizziness
Swelling
Depression
Tired
Pimples
Anxiety
Upset tummy
Aches and pains
Mood swings
Sudden crying
Sleep problems
Libido changes
Cravings
Tender/sore breasts
Difficulty concentrating
It can effect everyone differently, but generally it can make people feel super emotionally heightened (sensitive, sad, angry) and physically uncomfortable because their body is extra juiced up with all those additional hormones.

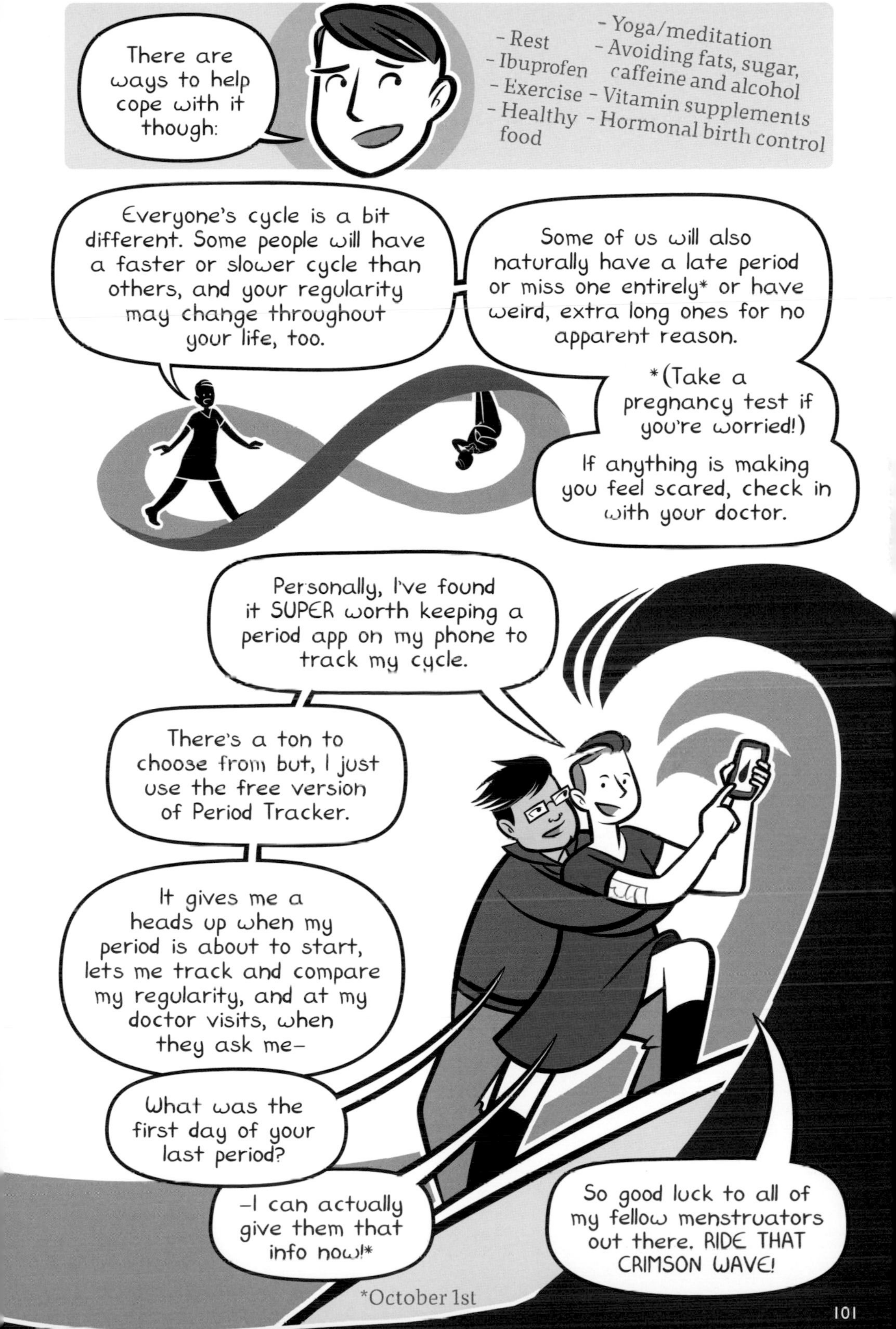
There are ways to help cope with it though:
- Rest
- Ibuprofen
- Exercise
- Healthy food
- Yoga/meditation
- Avoiding fats, sugar, caffeine and alcohol
- Vitamin supplements
- Hormonal birth control
Everyone's cycle is a bit different. Some people will have a faster or slower cycle than others, and your regularity may change throughout your life, too.
Some of us will also naturally have a late period or miss one entirely* or have weird, extra long ones for no apparent reason.
*(Take a pregnancy test if you're worried!)
If anything is making you feel scared, check in with your doctor.
Personally, I've found it SUPER worth keeping a period app on my phone to track my cycle.
There's a ton to choose from but, I just use the free version of Period Tracker.
It gives me a heads up when my period is about to start, lets me track and compare my regularity, and at my doctor visits, when they ask me–
What was the first day of your last period?
–I can actually give them that info now!*
So good luck to all of my fellow menstruators out there. RIDE THAT CRIMSON WAVE!
*October 1st

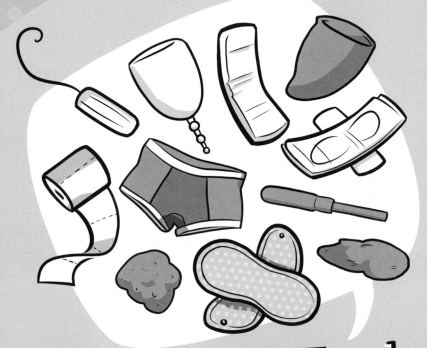

Menstrual Tools

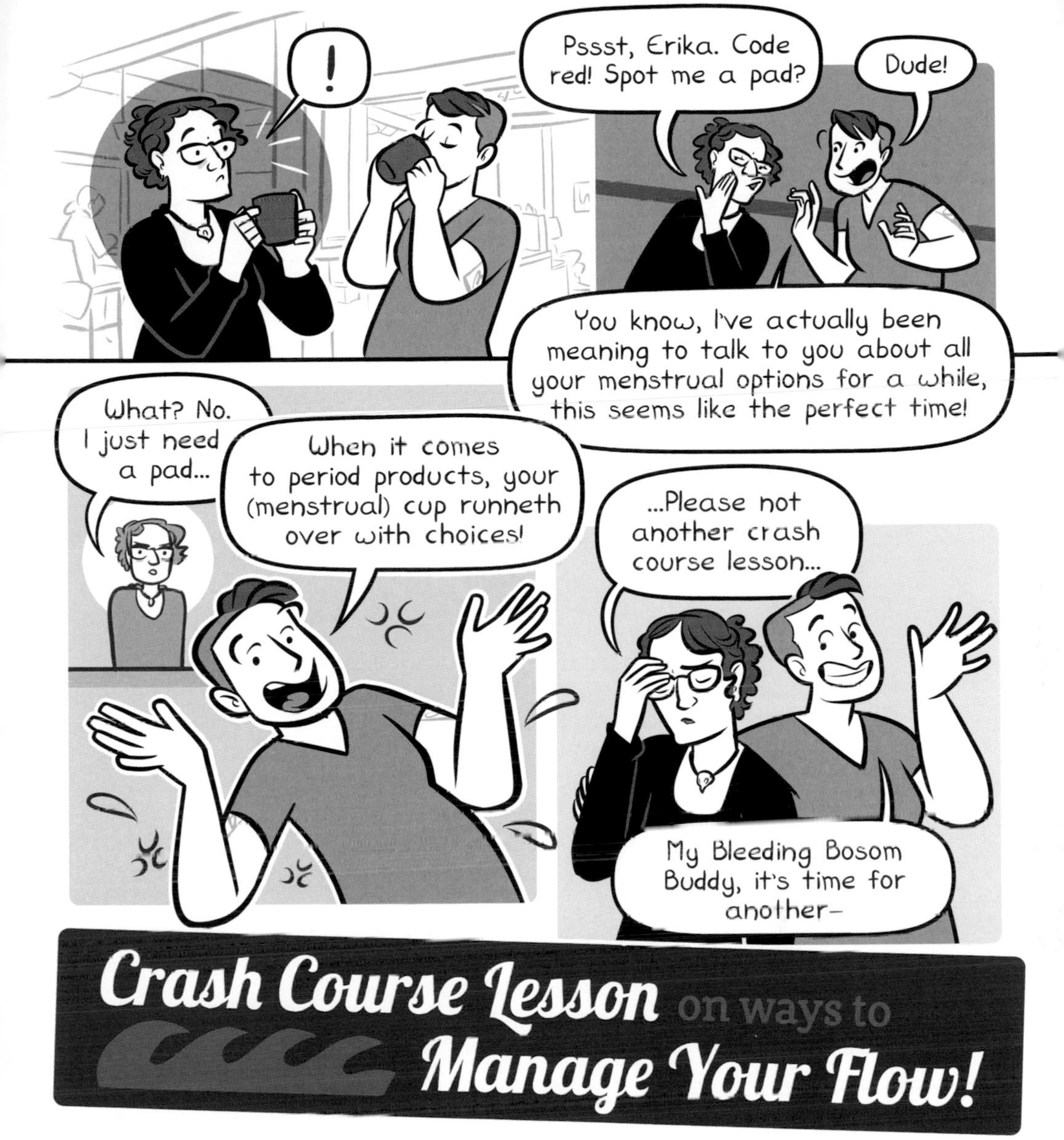
!
Pssst, Erika. Code red! Spot me a pad?
Dude!
You know, I've actually been meaning to talk to you about all your menstrual options for a while, this seems like the perfect time!
What? No. I just need a pad...
When it comes to period products, your (menstrual) cup runneth over with choices!
...Please not another crash course lesson...
My Bleeding Bosom Buddy, it's time for another–

Crash Course Lesson on ways to Manage Your Flow!

Disposable Pads

External Wear
~$7 per box of 36
Plastic and bleached cotton
Single Use
Environment UNfriendly
All-day wear, change every 3-4 hours

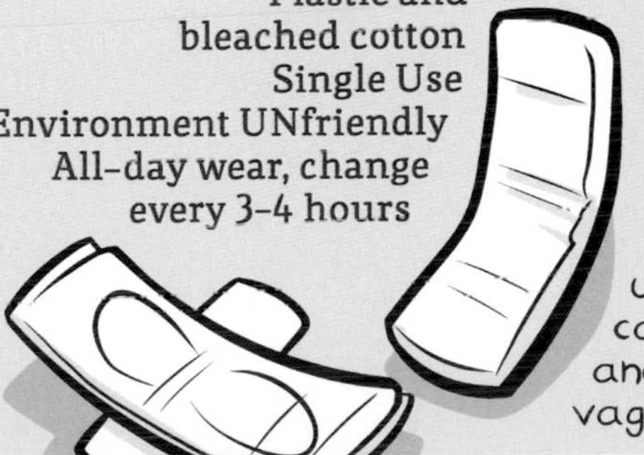

These easy to find single-use pads have an adhesive backing (and sometimes side wings) that stick down into the crotch of your underwear. They only last once and then are tossed into the garbage (boo!). Try and get unscented ones, as fragrances can irritate your delicate zone and mess with your healthy vaginal bacteria.

Washable Reusable Pads

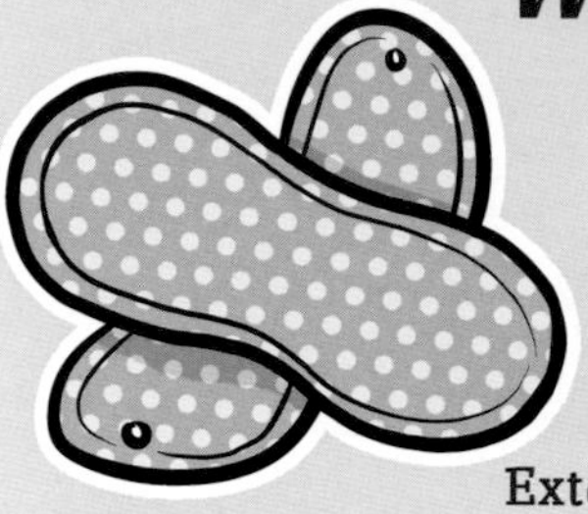

These cotton pads snap around the crotch of your undies and then you just wash them with the rest of your laundry. Some come with padding pockets so you can fill them up with bonus absorbing material on heavier flow days. I love these cuties, as I don't end up contributing as much to the landfill!

External Wear
~$10 per pad
Usually Cotton (Sometimes made out of recycled materials!)
Reusable for years
2-6 hours of wear
Environment friendly

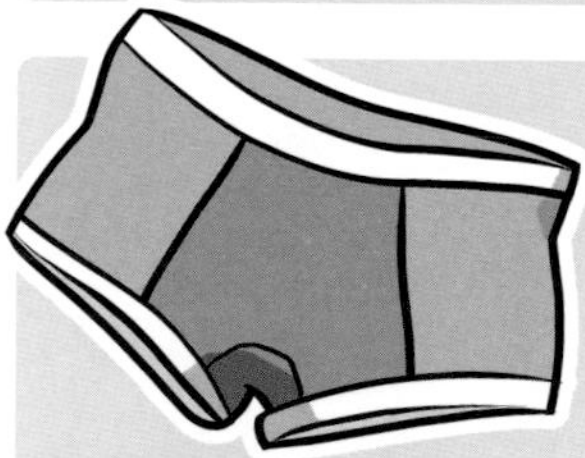

Period Underwear

External Wear
~$30 per undies
Usually cotton
Reusable for years
2-6 hours of wear
Environment friendly

Just like the washable pads, but these are fully formed underwears. A great option if you're always springing leaks from pads or plan on moving around a bunch. Just throw 'em in the regular wash after you've worn 'em!

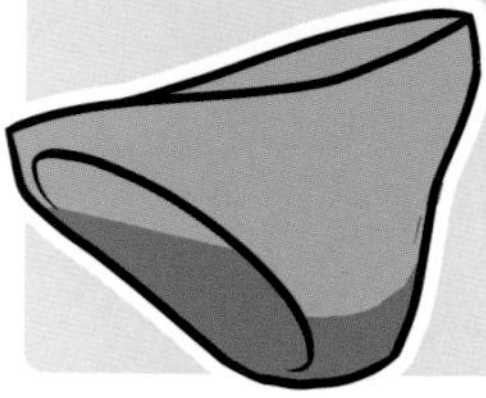

Tampons

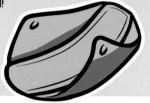

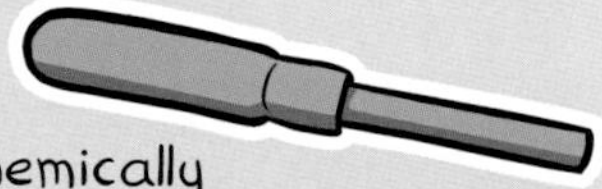

Internal Wear
~$7 per box of 36
Plastic, bleached cotton, rayon fibers
Single use
4-6 hours of wear
Environment UNfriendly

This is a tube of chemically treated cotton that is worn inside the vagina and absorbs your menstrual fluids before they can exit your body. After a few hours, you pull it out by the dangling string and throw it away. You have a choice between just a tampon by itself that you push in with your finger or a tampon that comes with an applicator that can help insert it.

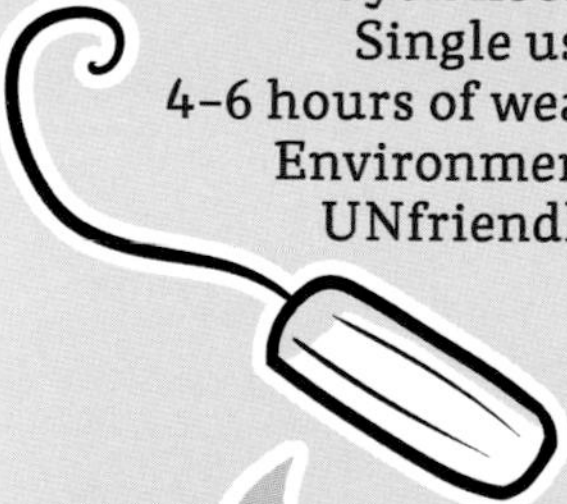

You'll want to stick to unscented ones as fragrances will mess with your healthy vaginal bacteria. If left in too long can irritate your insides or worse, lead to Toxic Shock Syndrome (TSS) which is a whole other kind of might-kill-you-shitshow you'll want to avoid, so pull it out after a few hours. When done, wrap it up and toss it away—don't flush it!

Cups

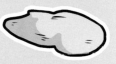

Worn inside the vagina, these flexible, non-porous, silicone or latex cups collect your flow until you remove them and empty their contents down the sink or toilet. Give it a rinse, slip it back in, and you're good to go again. The down side is that it's a bit more trouble to insert than a tampon, especially the first few times, but DOES get easier with practice. Just pinch, fold it in half vertically, and push it in!

Internal Wear
~$30 per cup
Silicon: Reusable for years
Latex: Single Use
12 hours of wear
Active lifestyle friendly
Silicon: Environment friendly
Latex: Environment UNfriendly

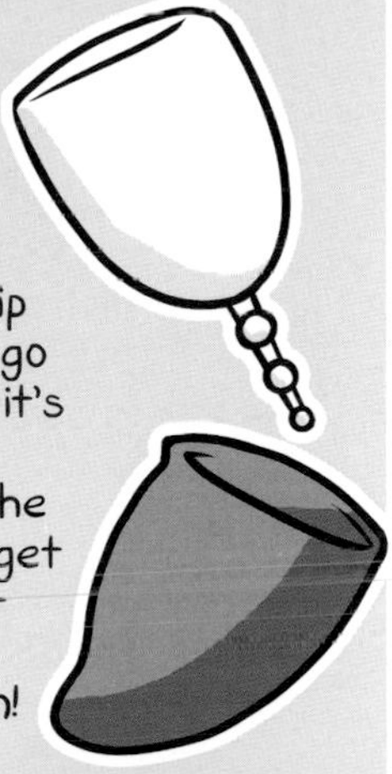

Sponges

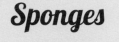

Internal Wear
~$10 per sponge
Natural or synthetic
3 hours of wear
Natural: 6-12 months
Synthetic: Single use
Natural: Environment friendly
Synthetic: Environment UNfriendly
Can be used for blood-free intercourse.

Inserted inside the vagina, this product absorbs your menstrual fluids and after a few hours you just grab an edge to pull it out (a piece of string can be attached to help pull it out too). Sponges need to be washed and sterilized before each use; give it a good scrub/boil/soak in vinegar and tend to start breaking down after a handful of uses, but are biodegradable once thrown out. Synthetic ones are single use before they're tossed. Just like most things, if left in your body for too long, it could cause TSS so make sure you change it out every few hours as well!

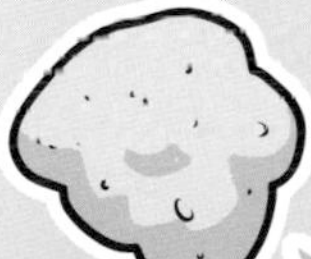

Sponges ARE a hotly debated menstruation tool in some circles, and the FDA restricts how they are to be marketed and sold. But there's a long history of use and anecdotal evidence out there to say they work great as long as you follow instructions. So do your own research if you're considering them!

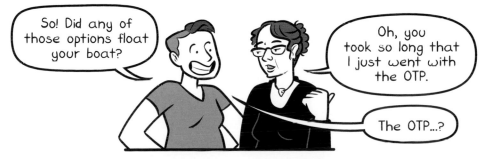

So! Did any of those options float your boat?

Oh, you took so long that I just went with the OTP.

The OTP...?

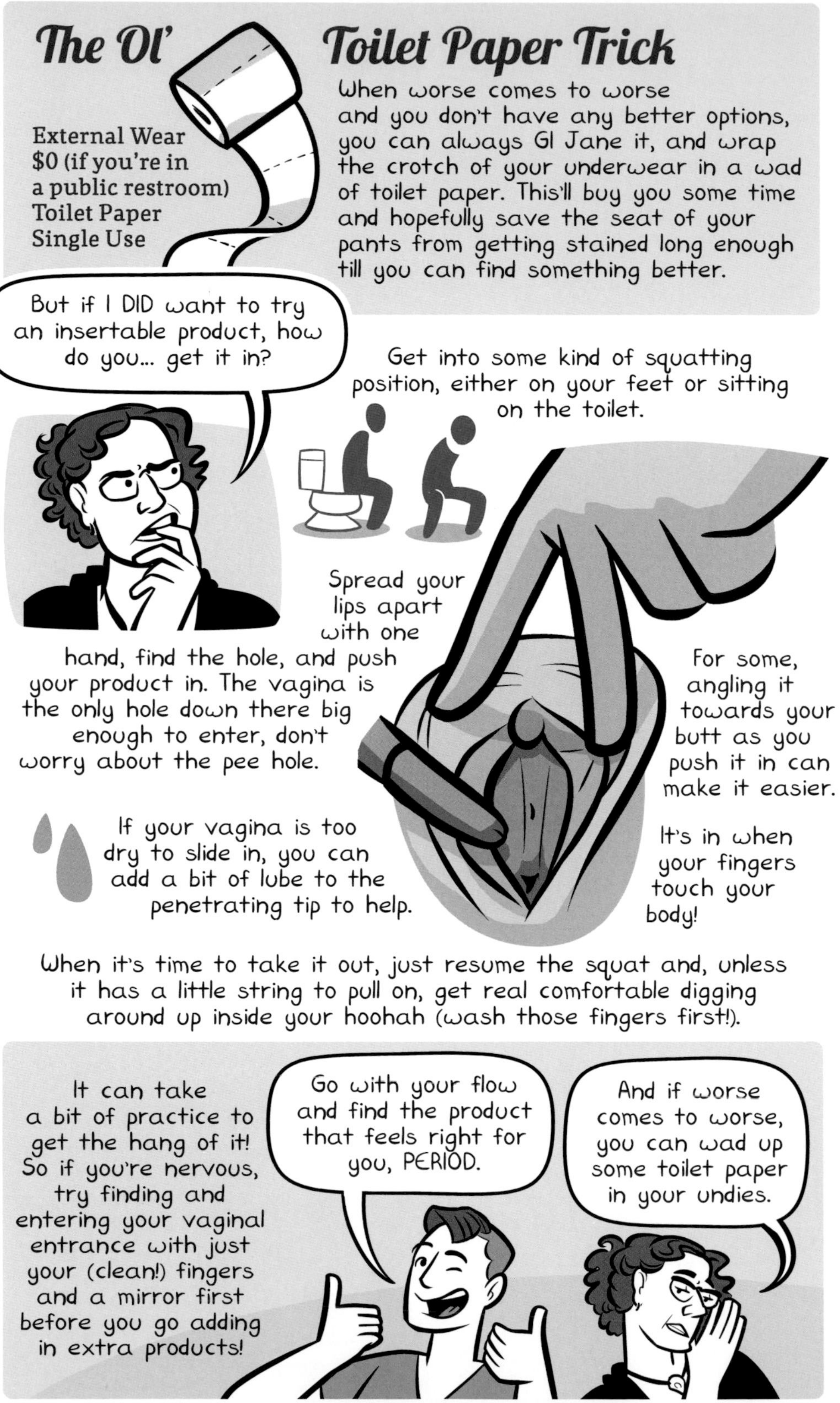
The Ol' Toilet Paper Trick
External Wear
$0 (if you're in a public restroom)
Toilet Paper
Single Use
When worse comes to worse and you don't have any better options, you can always GI Jane it, and wrap the crotch of your underwear in a wad of toilet paper. This'll buy you some time and hopefully save the seat of your pants from getting stained long enough till you can find something better.
But if I DID want to try an insertable product, how do you... get it in?
Get into some kind of squatting position, either on your feet or sitting on the toilet.
Spread your lips apart with one hand, find the hole, and push your product in. The vagina is the only hole down there big enough to enter, don't worry about the pee hole.
For some, angling it towards your butt as you push it in can make it easier.
If your vagina is too dry to slide in, you can add a bit of lube to the penetrating tip to help.
It's in when your fingers touch your body!
When it's time to take it out, just resume the squat and, unless it has a little string to pull on, get real comfortable digging around up inside your hoohah (wash those fingers first!).
It can take a bit of practice to get the hang of it! So if you're nervous, try finding and entering your vaginal entrance with just your (clean!) fingers and a mirror first before you go adding in extra products!
Go with your flow and find the product that feels right for you, PERIOD.
And if worse comes to worse, you can wad up some toilet paper in your undies.

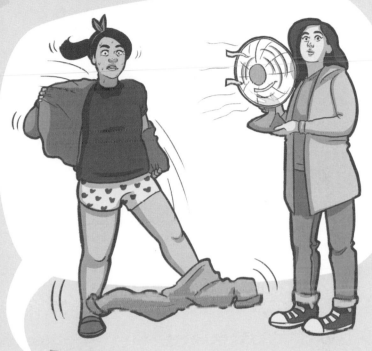

Menopause

By Ashley Guillory
AshleyrGuillory.com

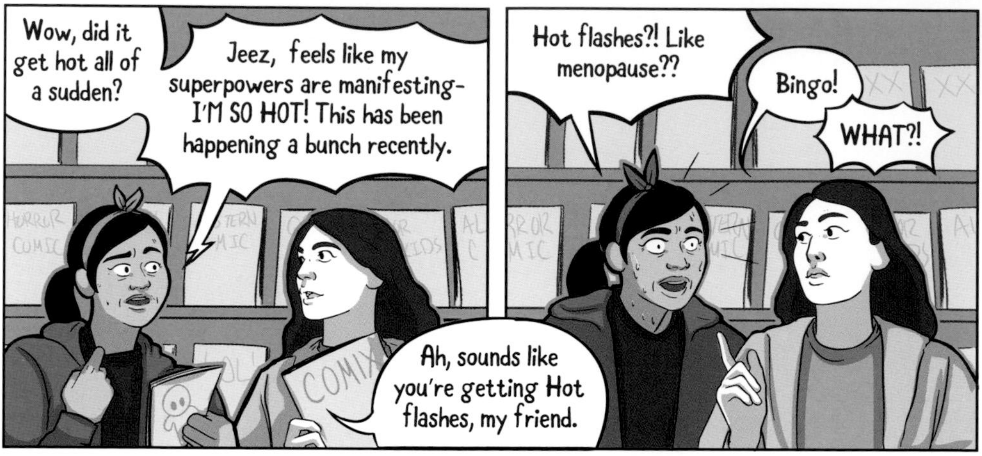
Wow, did it get hot all of a sudden?
Jeez, feels like my superpowers are manifesting-I'M SO HOT! This has been happening a bunch recently.
Ah, sounds like you're getting Hot flashes, my friend.
Hot flashes?! Like menopause??
Bingo!
WHAT?!

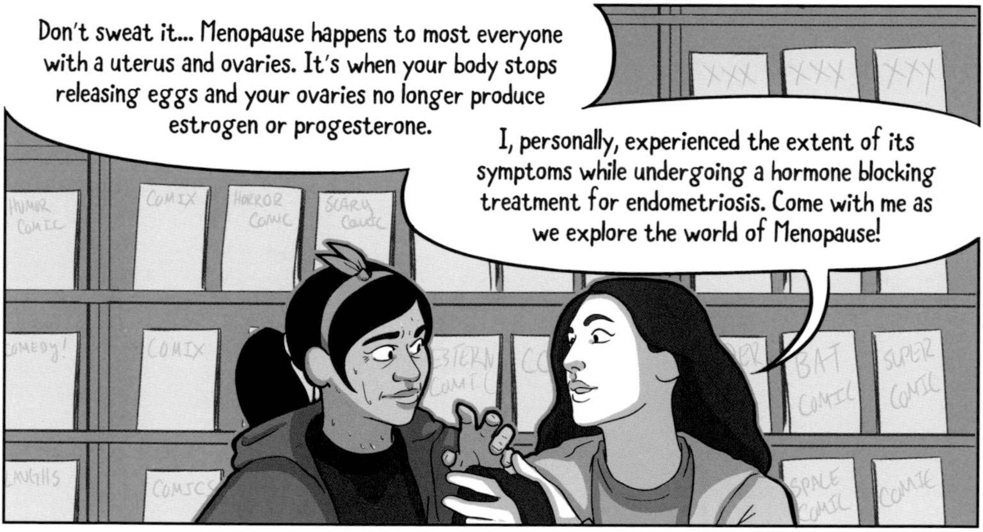
Don't sweat it... Menopause happens to most everyone with a uterus and ovaries. It's when your body stops releasing eggs and your ovaries no longer produce estrogen or progesterone.
I, personally, experienced the extent of its symptoms while undergoing a hormone blocking treatment for endometriosis. Come with me as we explore the world of Menopause!

Menopause generally occurs between the ages of 45-55, but the exact start date can fluctuate depending on the person. Some people have Induced Menopause which is menopause due to a medical procedure like a bilateral oophorectomy.*

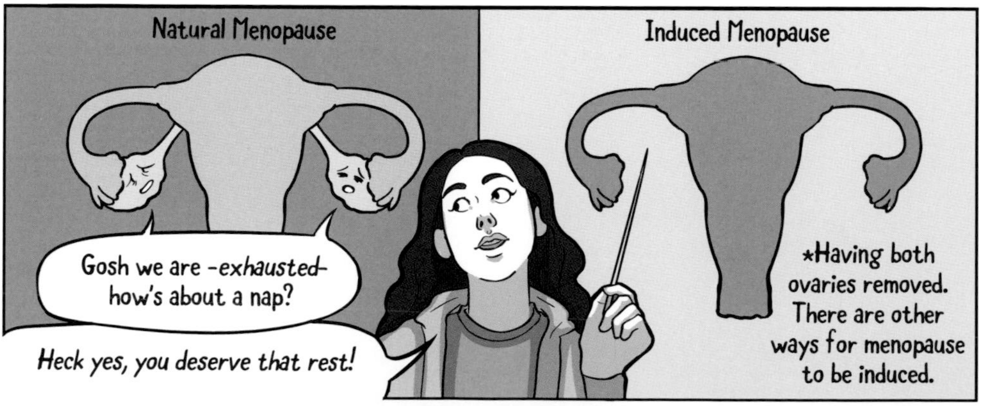
Natural Menopause
Induced Menopause
Gosh we are -*exhausted*- how's about a nap?
Heck yes, you deserve that rest!
*Having both ovaries removed. There are other ways for menopause to be induced.

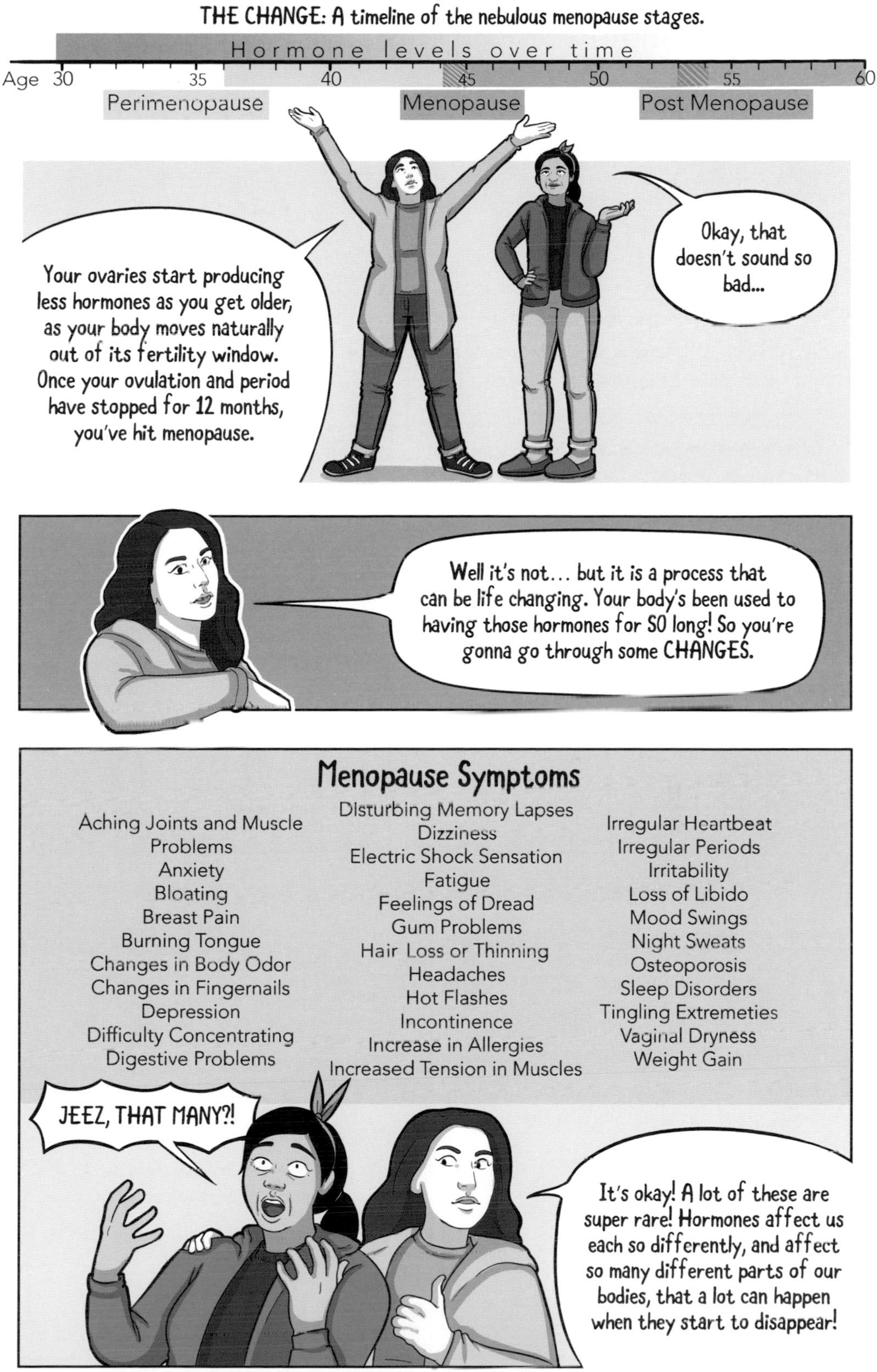
THE CHANGE: A timeline of the nebulous menopause stages.
Hormone levels over time
Age 30 35 40 45 50 55 60
Perimenopause
Menopause
Post Menopause
Your ovaries start producing less hormones as you get older, as your body moves naturally out of its fertility window. Once your ovulation and period have stopped for 12 months, you've hit menopause.
Okay, that doesn't sound so bad...
Well it's not... but it is a process that can be life changing. Your body's been used to having those hormones for SO long! So you're gonna go through some CHANGES.
Menopause Symptoms
Aching Joints and Muscle Problems
Anxiety
Bloating
Breast Pain
Burning Tongue
Changes in Body Odor
Changes in Fingernails
Depression
Difficulty Concentrating
Digestive Problems
Disturbing Memory Lapses
Dizziness
Electric Shock Sensation
Fatigue
Feelings of Dread
Gum Problems
Hair Loss or Thinning
Headaches
Hot Flashes
Incontinence
Increase in Allergies
Increased Tension in Muscles
Irregular Heartbeat
Irregular Periods
Irritability
Loss of Libido
Mood Swings
Night Sweats
Osteoporosis
Sleep Disorders
Tingling Extremeties
Vaginal Dryness
Weight Gain
JEEZ, THAT MANY?!
It's okay! A lot of these are super rare! Hormones affect us each so differently, and affect so many different parts of our bodies, that a lot can happen when they start to disappear!

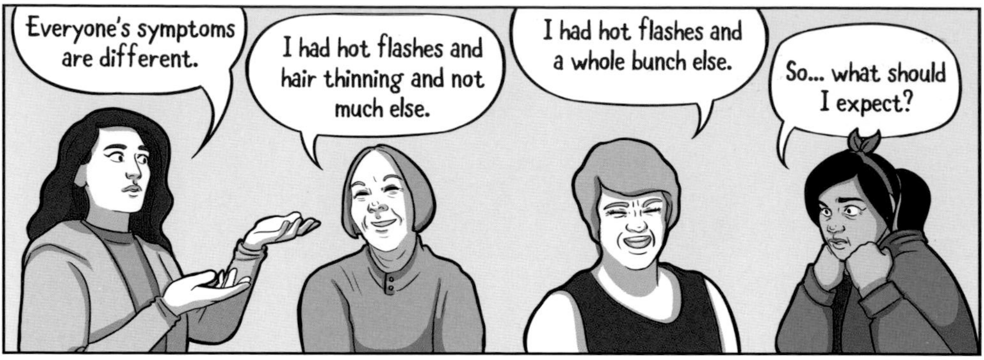
Everyone's symptoms are different.
I had hot flashes and hair thinning and not much else.
I had hot flashes and a whole bunch else.
So... what should I expect?

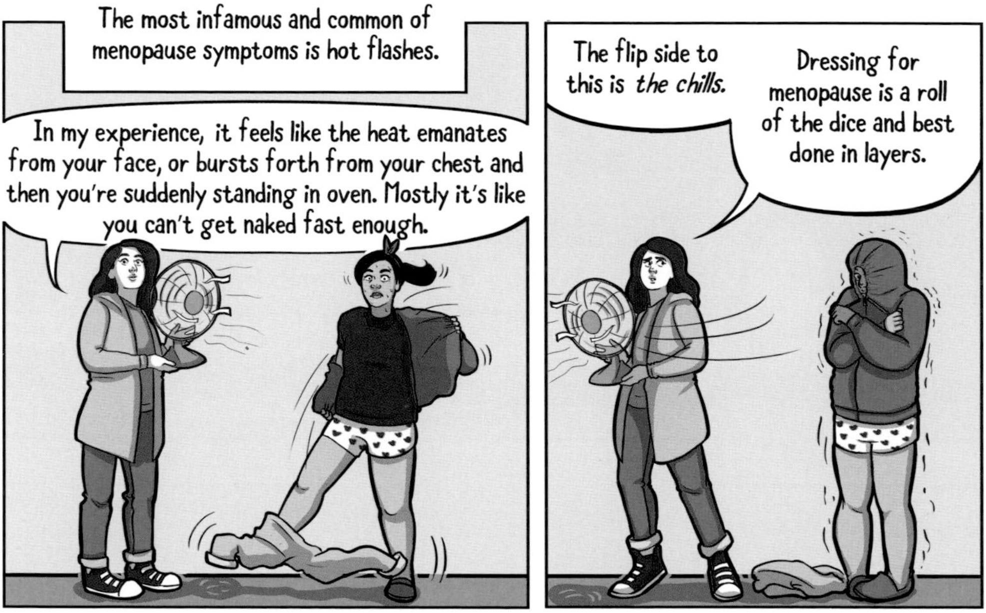
The most infamous and common of menopause symptoms is hot flashes.
In my experience, it feels like the heat emanates from your face, or bursts forth from your chest and then you're suddenly standing in oven. Mostly it's like you can't get naked fast enough.
The flip side to this is *the chills.*
Dressing for menopause is a roll of the dice and best done in layers.

Insomnia or sleep disruption go directly hand in hand with hot flashes.

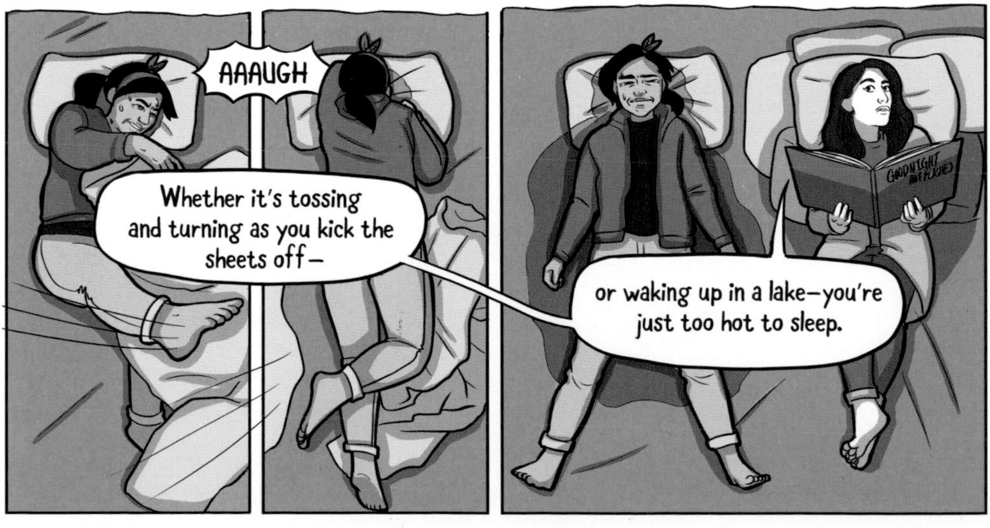
AAAUGH
Whether it's tossing and turning as you kick the sheets off—
or waking up in a lake—you're just too hot to sleep.

Some of the other common symptoms take a bit longer to set in.

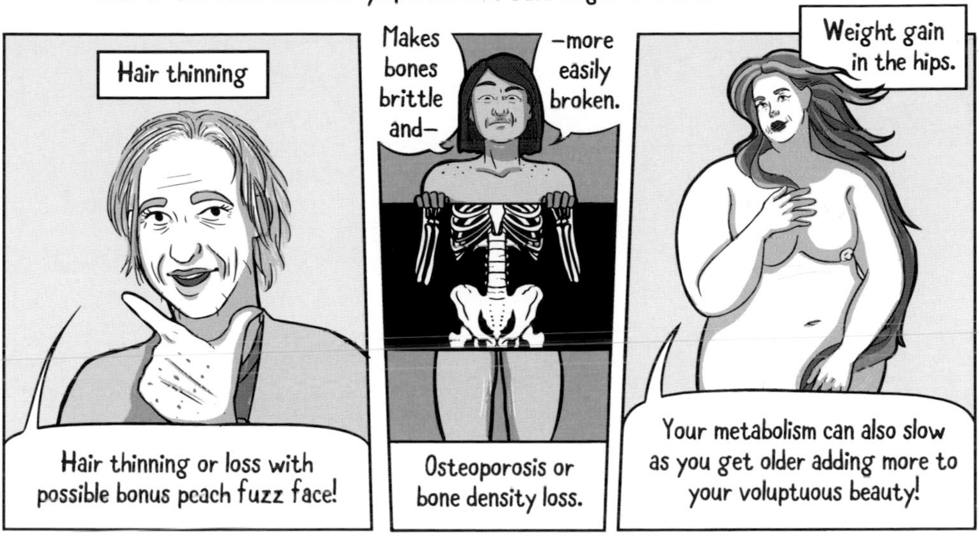
Hair thinning
Hair thinning or loss with possible bonus peach fuzz face!
Makes bones brittle and–
–more easily broken.
Osteoporosis or bone density loss.
Weight gain in the hips.
Your metabolism can also slow as you get older adding more to your voluptuous beauty!

Along with physical changes there are also mental ones. Menopause can cause forgetfulness.

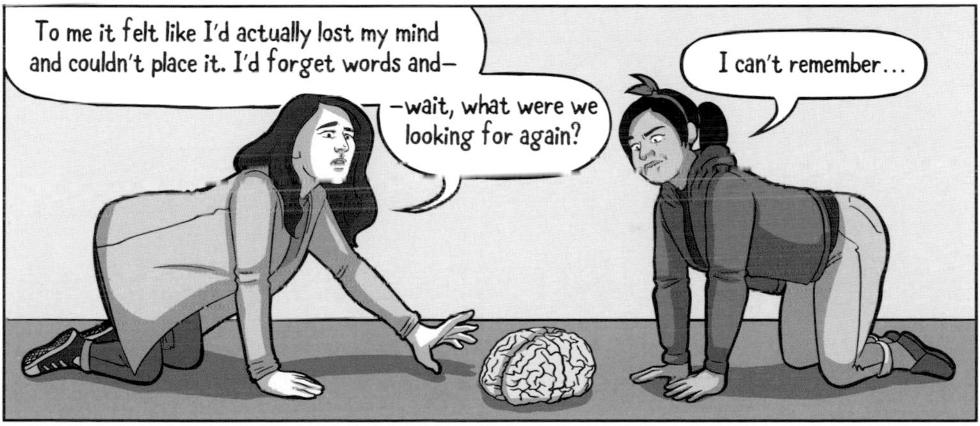
To me it felt like I'd actually lost my mind and couldn't place it. I'd forget words and–
–wait, what were we looking for again?
I can't remember...

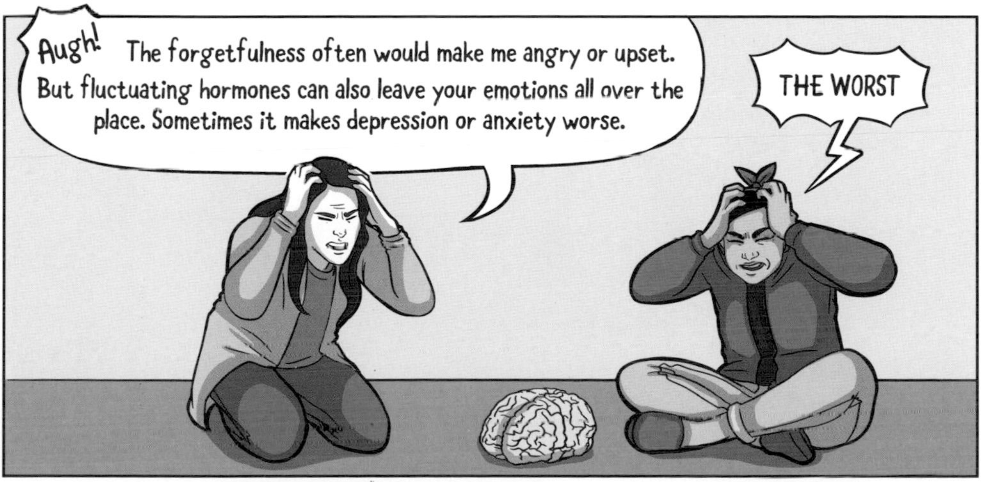
Augh! The forgetfulness often would make me angry or upset. But fluctuating hormones can also leave your emotions all over the place. Sometimes it makes depression or anxiety worse.
THE WORST

For me, the most impactful side effect after hot flashes was Vaginal Dryness and Atrophy.

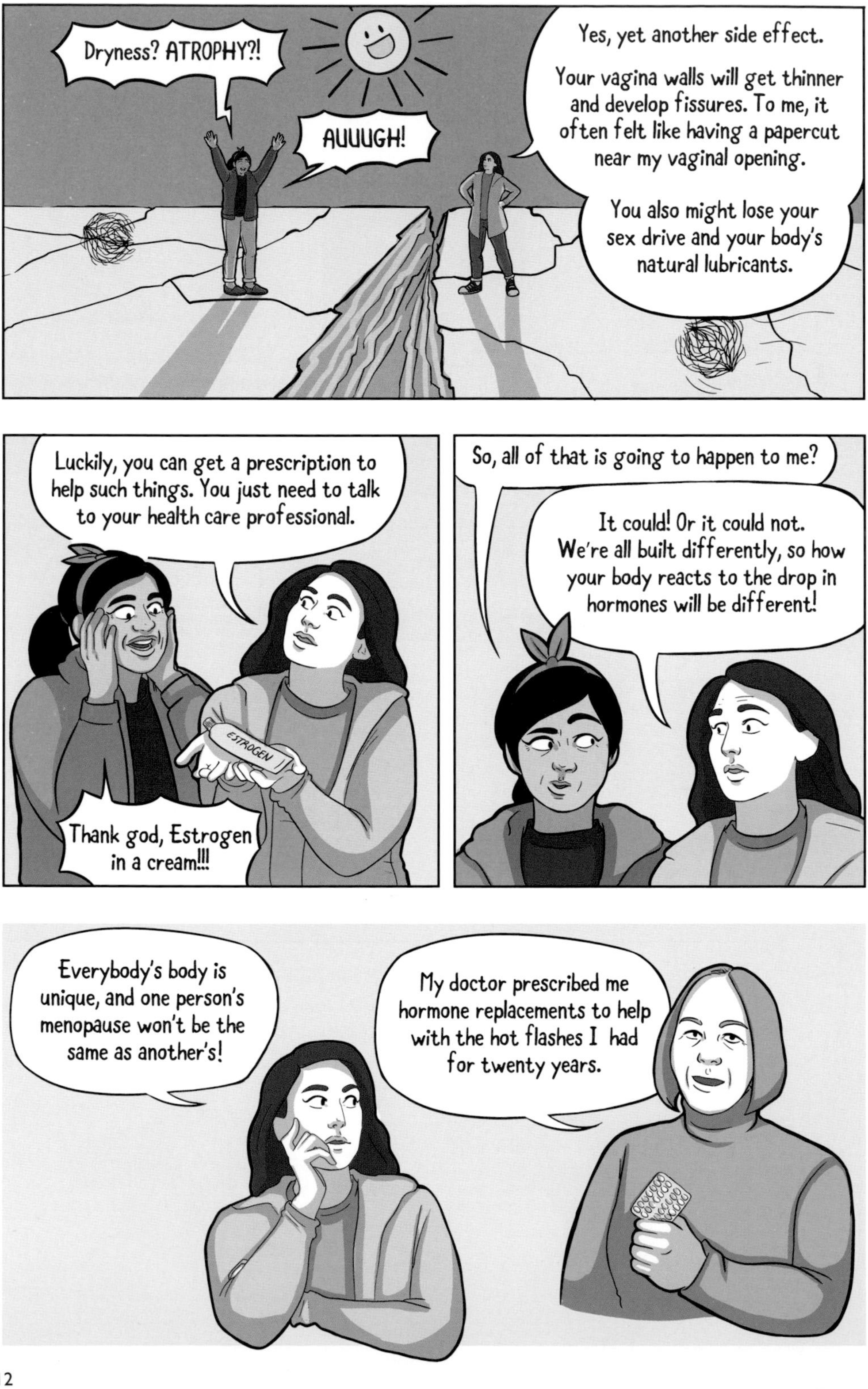
Dryness? ATROPHY?!
AUUUGH!
Yes, yet another side effect.
Your vagina walls will get thinner and develop fissures. To me, it often felt like having a papercut near my vaginal opening.
You also might lose your sex drive and your body's natural lubricants.
Luckily, you can get a prescription to help such things. You just need to talk to your health care professional.
ESTROGEN
Thank god, Estrogen in a cream!!!
So, all of that is going to happen to me?
It could! Or it could not. We're all built differently, so how your body reacts to the drop in hormones will be different!
Everybody's body is unique, and one person's menopause won't be the same as another's!
My doctor prescribed me hormone replacements to help with the hot flashes I had for twenty years.

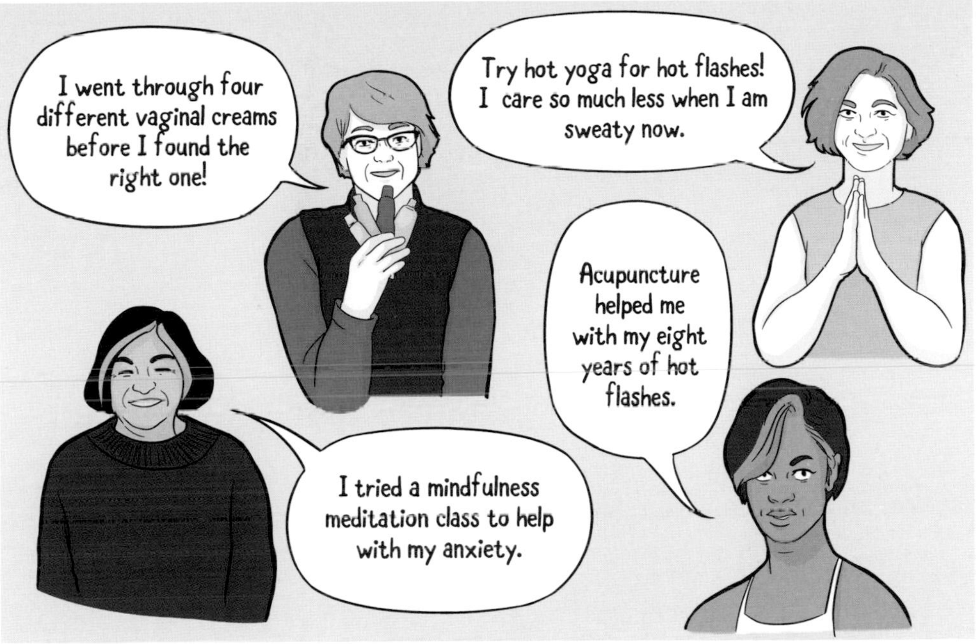

I went through four different vaginal creams before I found the right one!
Try hot yoga for hot flashes! I care so much less when I am sweaty now.
Acupuncture helped me with my eight years of hot flashes.
I tried a mindfulness meditation class to help with my anxiety.

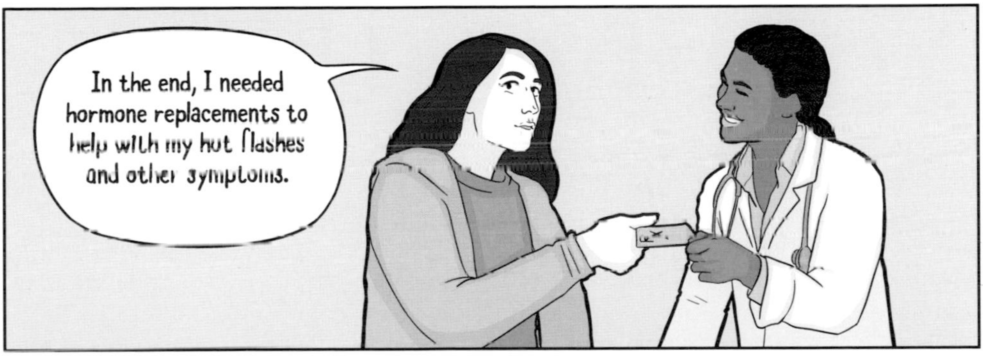

In the end, I needed hormone replacements to help with my hot flashes and other symptoms.

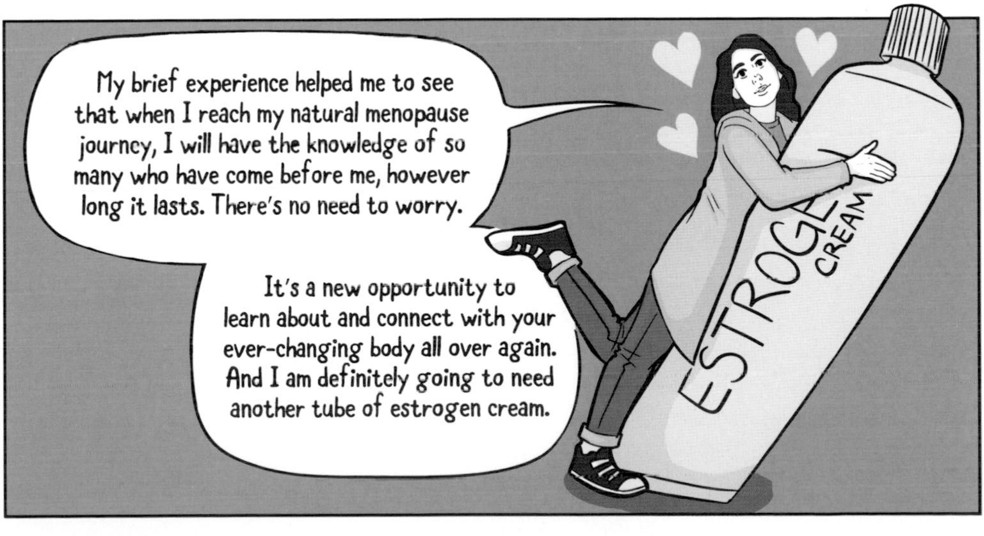

My brief experience helped me to see that when I reach my natural menopause journey, I will have the knowledge of so many who have come before me, however long it lasts. There's no need to worry.
It's a new opportunity to learn about and connect with your ever-changing body all over again. And I am definitely going to need another tube of estrogen cream.
ESTROGE
CREAM

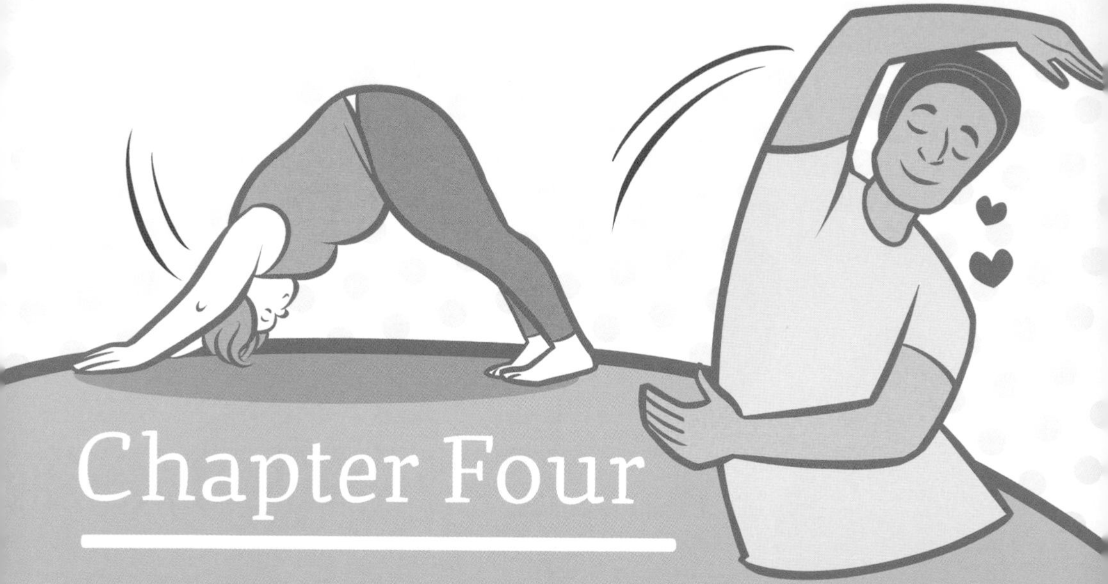

Chapter Four

Taking Care of Your health

You are an amazing but, ah, complicated machine! A machine that's gonna go haywire, occasionally break, and probably need tune-ups. But that's OK, because we *all* catch something or break-down over time – it's a normal part of life!

In this chapter, we talk about some of the more common ways our sexy bodies can go wrong, annnnd some of the examinations and treatments that can help. We also look at some of the more common things you'll need to see a doctor for, from temporary itchy and smelly infections to conditions that need ongoing care.

Breasts, balls, penises, bladders, vulvas... if it's a soft and sensitive place, chances are that it's going to need some extra TLC to keep it running smoothly. If you take away nothing else from this chapter, let it be to PEE AFTER SEX. Just. For real. Flush that ol' tube out. Trust me, you'll thank me later.

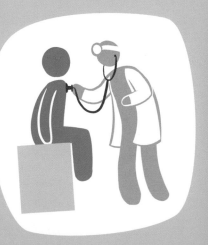

And if you take a second thing away from this chapter, let it also be that YOU ARE NOT ALONE. So many others are dealing with the exact same physical difficulties as you, and there is no reason to feel shame. If something doesn't feel right or is causing you pain, drop everything and check in with a doctor.

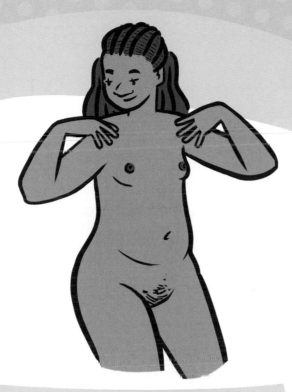

Checking Your Breasts

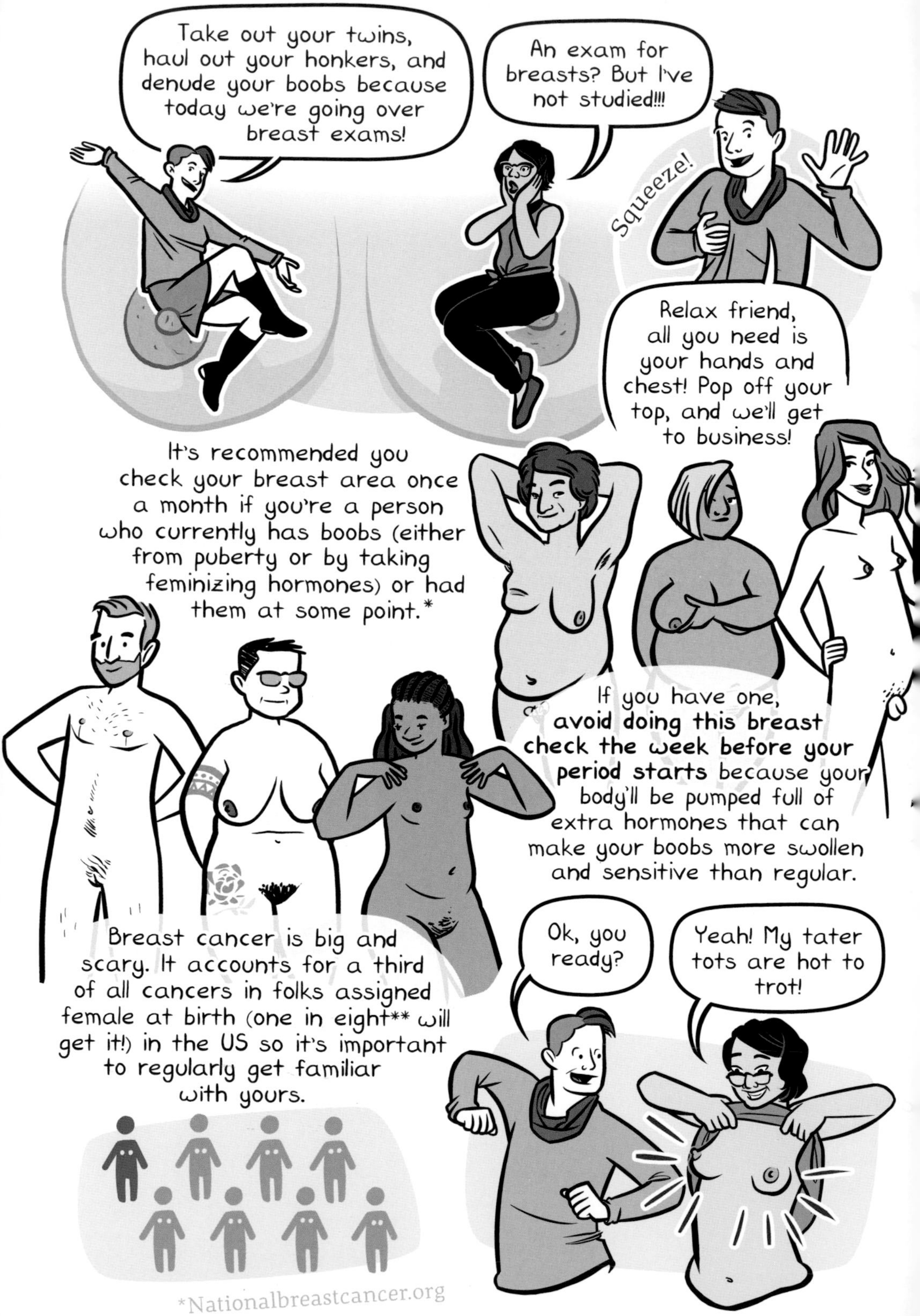

Take out your twins, haul out your honkers, and denude your boobs because today we're going over breast exams!
An exam for breasts? But I've not studied!!!
Squeeze!
Relax friend, all you need is your hands and chest! Pop off your top, and we'll get to business!
It's recommended you check your breast area once a month if you're a person who currently has boobs (either from puberty or by taking feminizing hormones) or had them at some point.*
If you have one, **avoid doing this breast check the week before your period starts** because your body'll be pumped full of extra hormones that can make your boobs more swollen and sensitive than regular.
Breast cancer is big and scary. It accounts for a third of all cancers in folks assigned female at birth (one in eight** will get it!) in the US so it's important to regularly get familiar with yours.
Ok, you ready?
Yeah! My tater tots are hot to trot!

*Nationalbreastcancer.org

**Cancer.gov

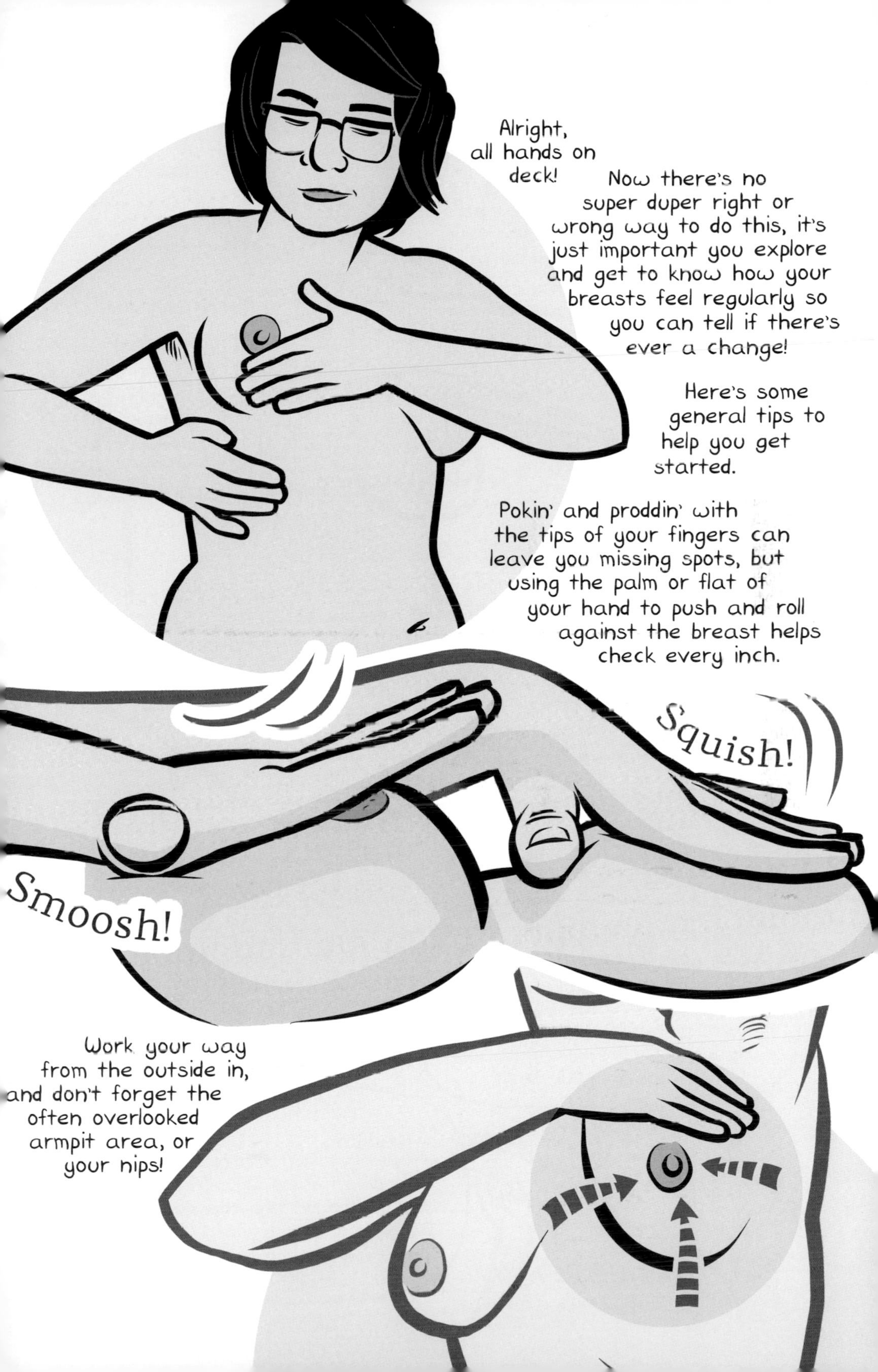

Alright, all hands on deck!
Now there's no super duper right or wrong way to do this, it's just important you explore and get to know how your breasts feel regularly so you can tell if there's ever a change!
Here's some general tips to help you get started.
Pokin' and proddin' with the tips of your fingers can leave you missing spots, but using the palm or flat of your hand to push and roll against the breast helps check every inch.
Squish!
Smoosh!
Work your way from the outside in, and don't forget the often overlooked armpit area, or your nips!

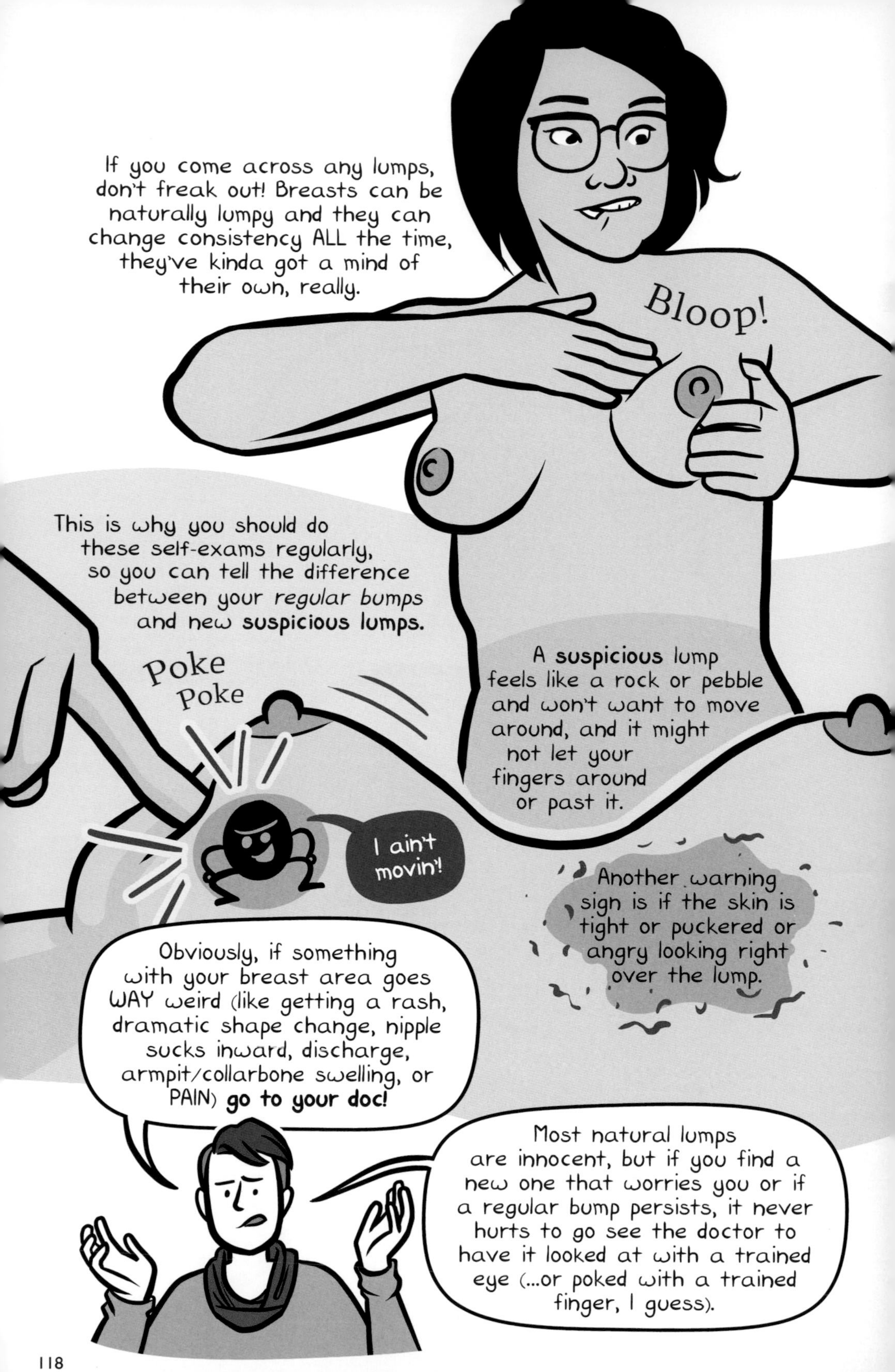
If you come across any lumps, don't freak out! Breasts can be naturally lumpy and they can change consistency ALL the time, they've kinda got a mind of their own, really.
Bloop!
This is why you should do these self-exams regularly, so you can tell the difference between your *regular bumps* and new **suspicious lumps.**
Poke Poke
A **suspicious** lump feels like a rock or pebble and won't want to move around, and it might not let your fingers around or past it.
I ain't movin'!
Another warning sign is if the skin is tight or puckered or angry looking right over the lump.
Obviously, if something with your breast area goes WAY weird (like getting a rash, dramatic shape change, nipple sucks inward, discharge, armpit/collarbone swelling, or PAIN) **go to your doc!**
Most natural lumps are innocent, but if you find a new one that worries you or if a regular bump persists, it never hurts to go see the doctor to have it looked at with a trained eye (...or poked with a trained finger, I guess).

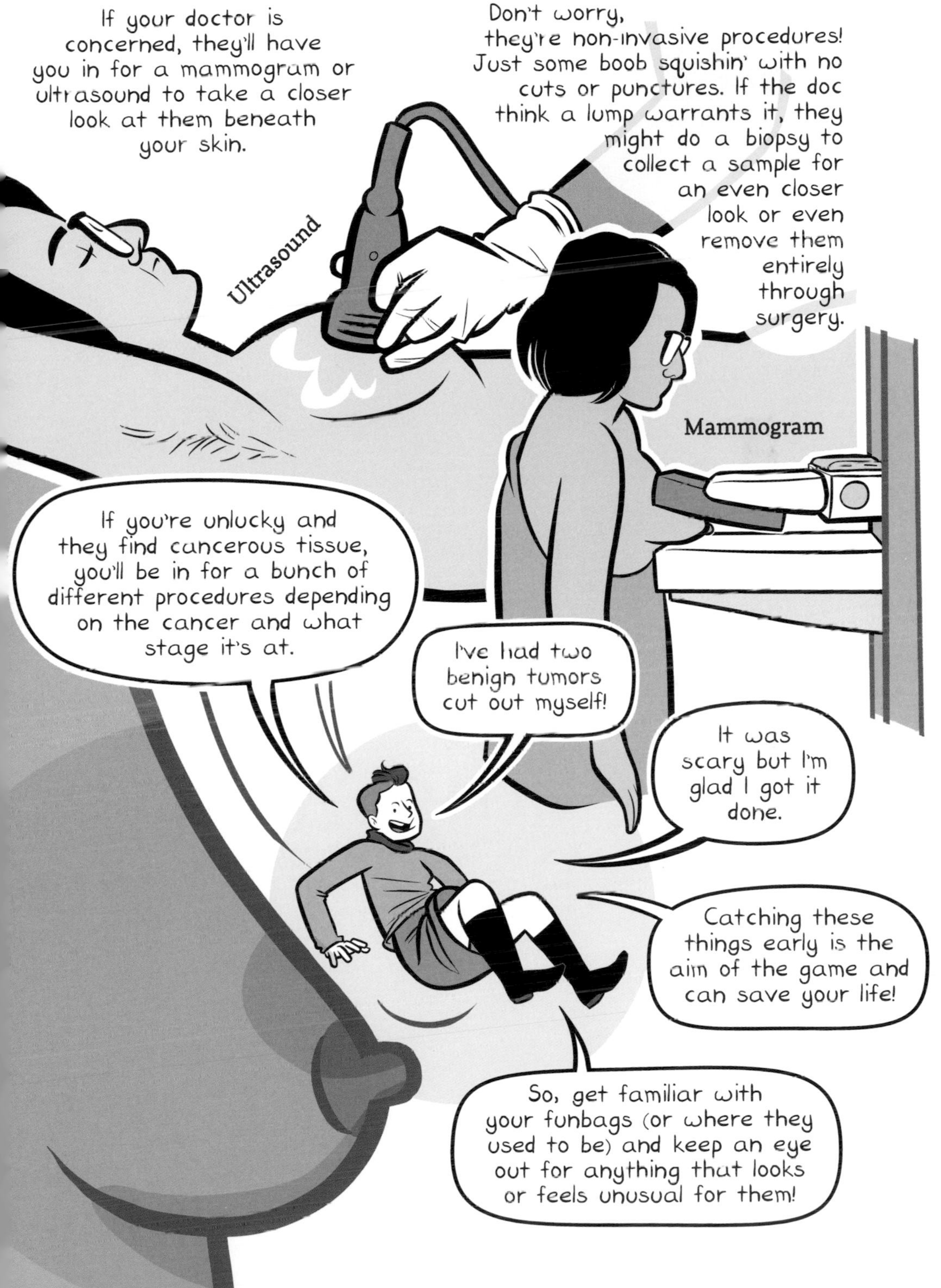

If your doctor is concerned, they'll have you in for a mammogram or ultrasound to take a closer look at them beneath your skin.
Don't worry, they're non-invasive procedures! Just some boob squishin' with no cuts or punctures. If the doc think a lump warrants it, they might do a biopsy to collect a sample for an even closer look or even remove them entirely through surgery.
Ultrasound
Mammogram
If you're unlucky and they find cancerous tissue, you'll be in for a bunch of different procedures depending on the cancer and what stage it's at.
I've had two benign tumors cut out myself!
It was scary but I'm glad I got it done.
Catching these things early is the aim of the game and can save your life!
So, get familiar with your funbags (or where they used to be) and keep an eye out for anything that looks or feels unusual for them!

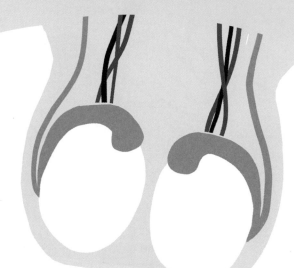

Checking Your Balls

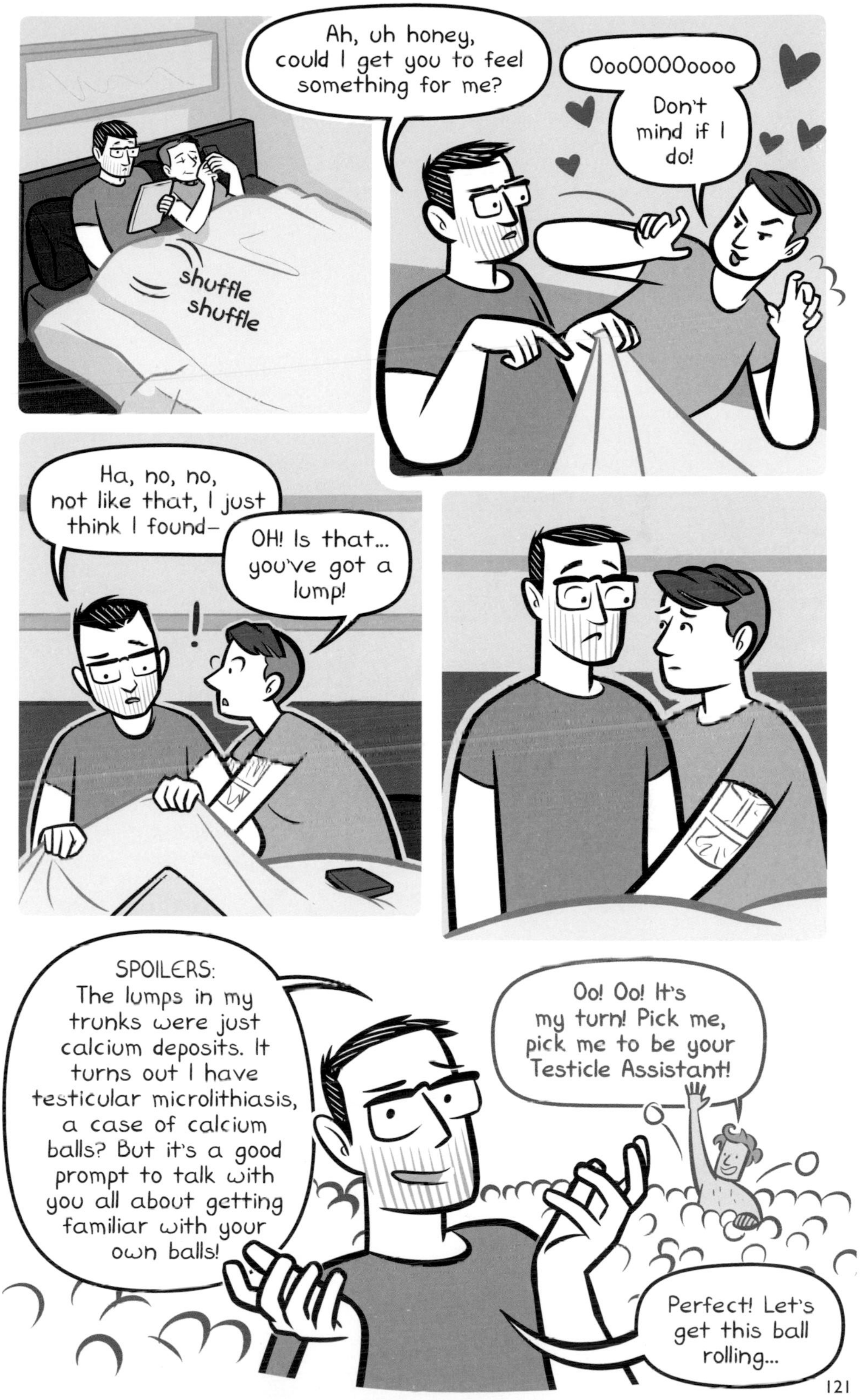
shuffle shuffle
Ah, uh honey, could I get you to feel something for me?
OooOOOOoooo
Don't mind if I do!
Ha, no, no, not like that, I just think I found–
OH! Is that... you've got a lump!
!
SPOILERS: The lumps in my trunks were just calcium deposits. It turns out I have testicular microlithiasis, a case of calcium balls? But it's a good prompt to talk with you all about getting familiar with your own balls!
Oo! Oo! It's my turn! Pick me, pick me to be your Testicle Assistant!
Perfect! Let's get this ball rolling...

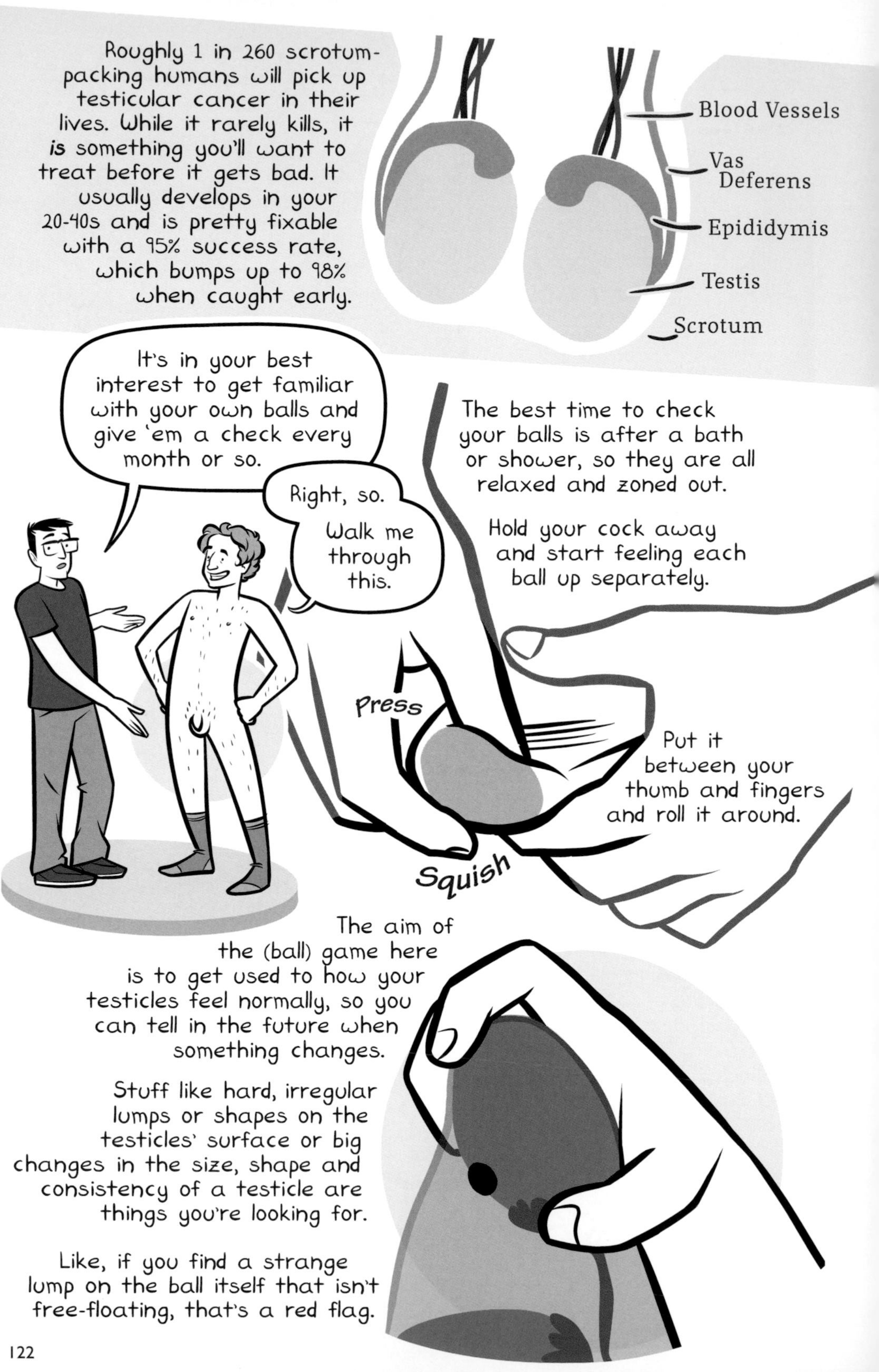
Roughly 1 in 260 scrotum-packing humans will pick up testicular cancer in their lives. While it rarely kills, it *is* something you'll want to treat before it gets bad. It usually develops in your 20-40s and is pretty fixable with a 95% success rate, which bumps up to 98% when caught early.
Blood Vessels
Vas Deferens
Epididymis
Testis
Scrotum
It's in your best interest to get familiar with your own balls and give 'em a check every month or so.
Right, so.
Walk me through this.
The best time to check your balls is after a bath or shower, so they are all relaxed and zoned out.
Hold your cock away and start feeling each ball up separately.
Press
Put it between your thumb and fingers and roll it around.
Squish
The aim of the (ball) game here is to get used to how your testicles feel normally, so you can tell in the future when something changes.
Stuff like hard, irregular lumps or shapes on the testicles' surface or big changes in the size, shape and consistency of a testicle are things you're looking for.
Like, if you find a strange lump on the ball itself that isn't free-floating, that's a red flag.

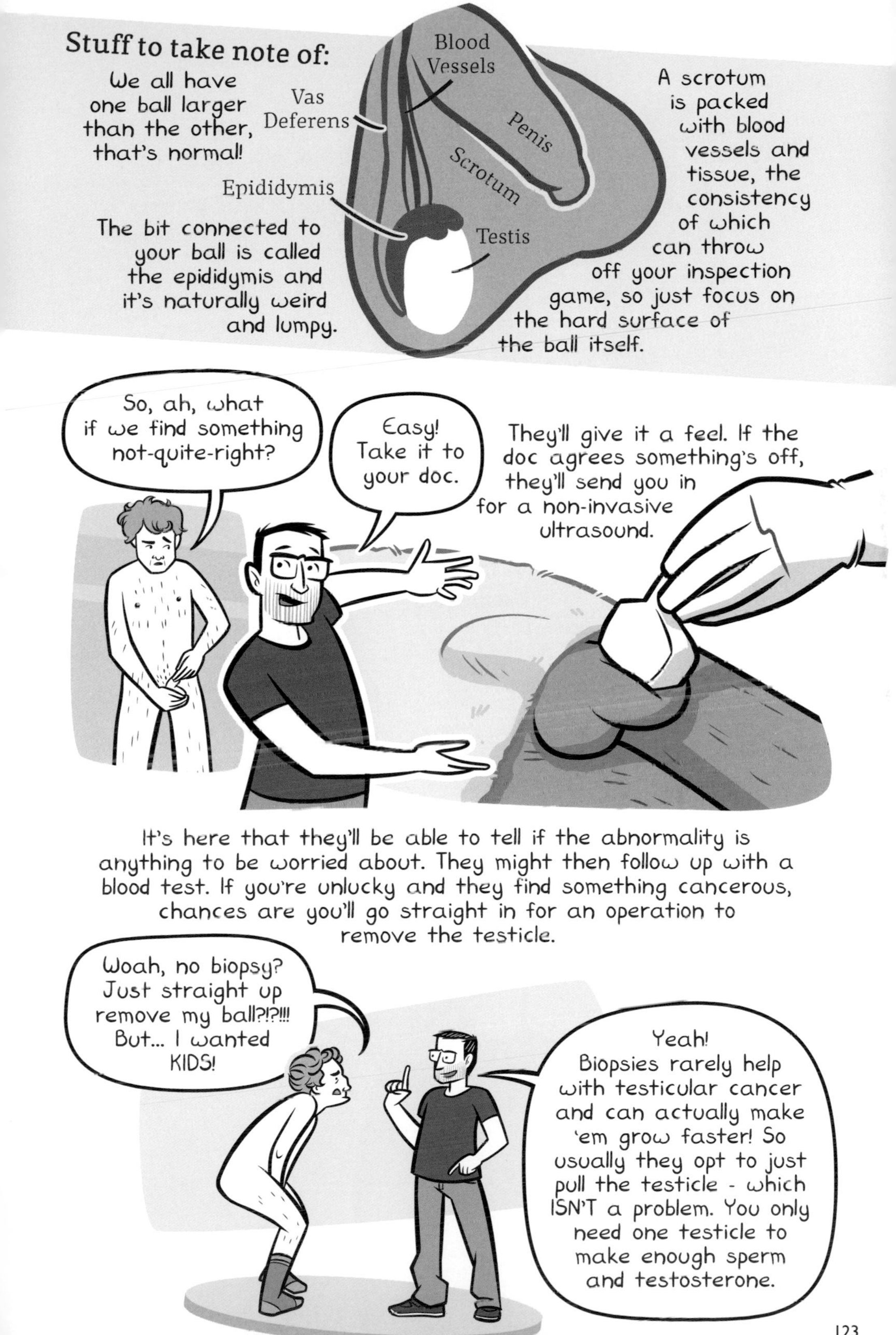
Stuff to take note of:
We all have one ball larger than the other, that's normal!
Blood Vessels
Vas Deferens
Penis
Scrotum
Epididymis
Testis
The bit connected to your ball is called the epididymis and it's naturally weird and lumpy.
A scrotum is packed with blood vessels and tissue, the consistency of which can throw off your inspection game, so just focus on the hard surface of the ball itself.
So, ah, what if we find something not-quite-right?
Easy! Take it to your doc.
They'll give it a feel. If the doc agrees something's off, they'll send you in for a non-invasive ultrasound.
It's here that they'll be able to tell if the abnormality is anything to be worried about. They might then follow up with a blood test. If you're unlucky and they find something cancerous, chances are you'll go straight in for an operation to remove the testicle.
Woah, no biopsy? Just straight up remove my ball?!?!!! But... I wanted KIDS!
Yeah! Biopsies rarely help with testicular cancer and can actually make 'em grow faster! So usually they opt to just pull the testicle - which ISN'T a problem. You only need one testicle to make enough sperm and testosterone.

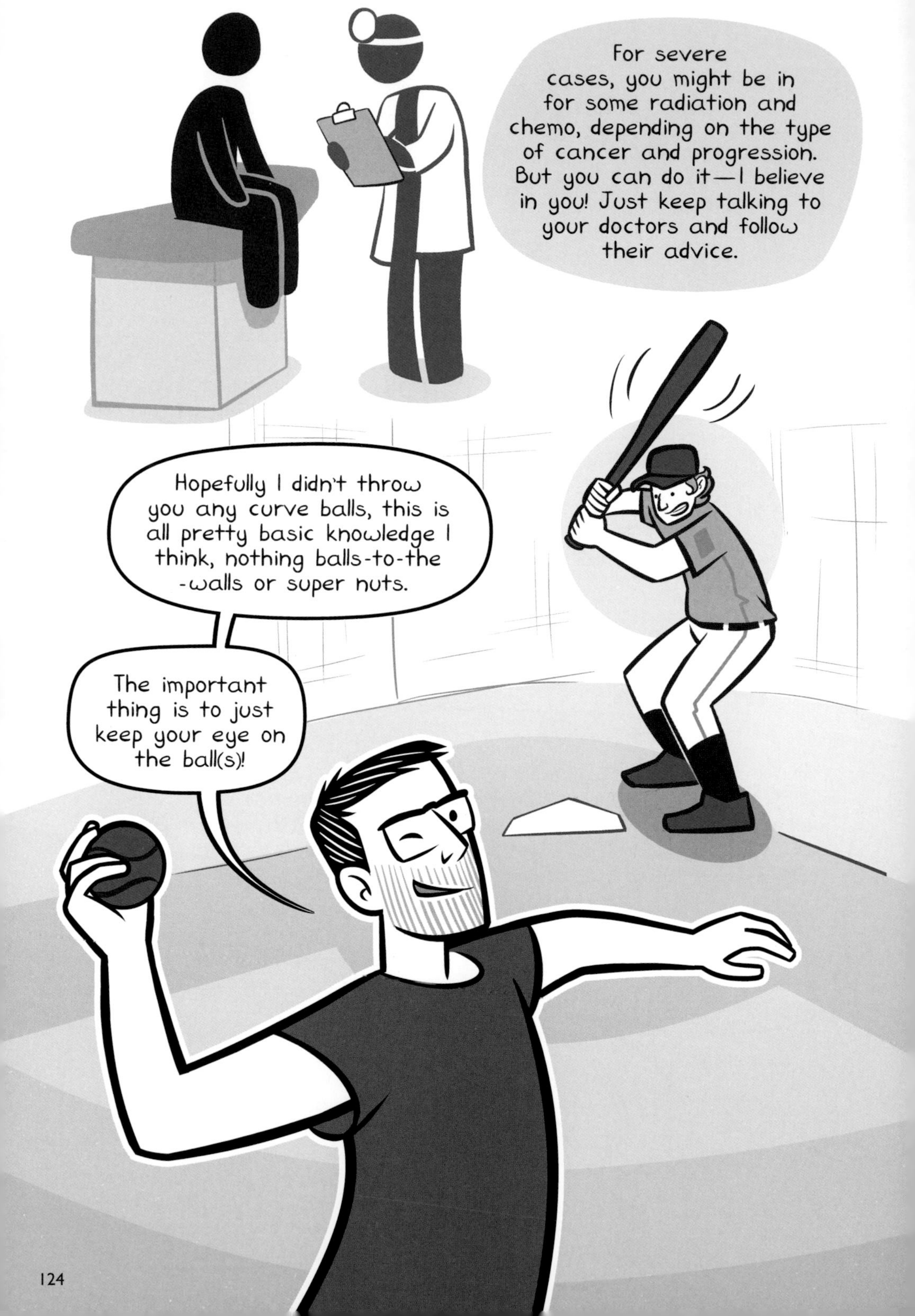
For severe cases, you might be in for some radiation and chemo, depending on the type of cancer and progression. But you can do it—I believe in you! Just keep talking to your doctors and follow their advice.
Hopefully I didn't throw you any curve balls, this is all pretty basic knowledge I think, nothing balls-to-the-walls or super nuts.
The important thing is to just keep your eye on the ball(s)!

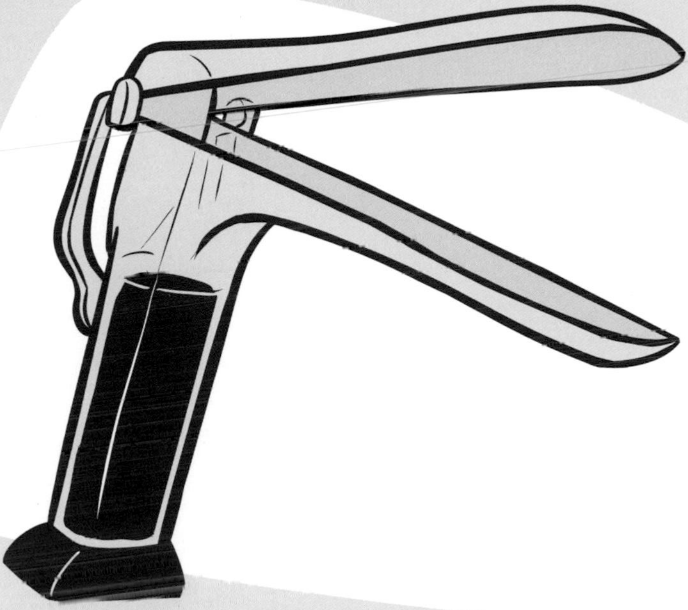

Gyno Exam

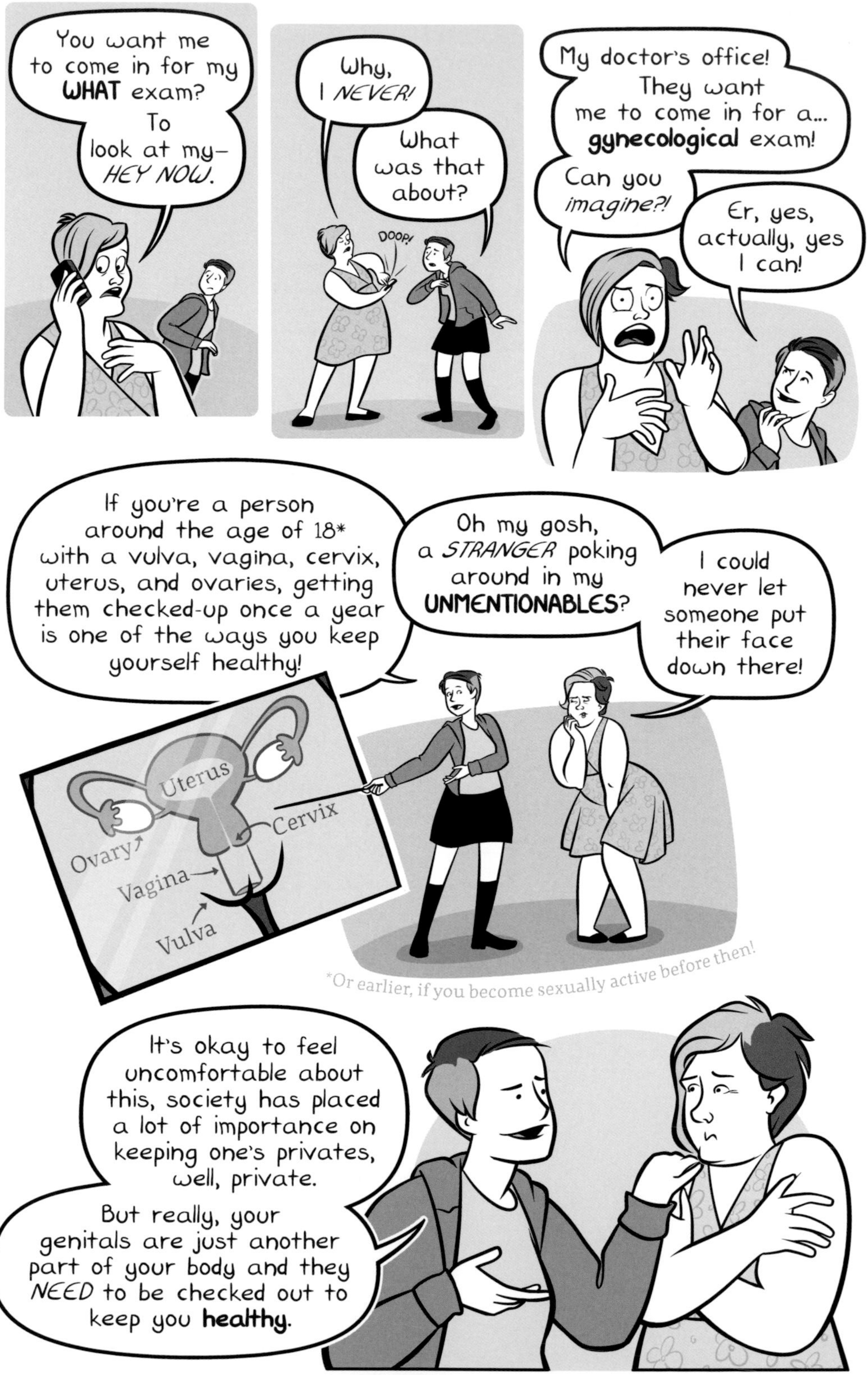
You want me to come in for my **WHAT** exam? To look at my— *HEY NOW*.
Why, I *NEVER!*
DOOP!
What was that about?
My doctor's office! They want me to come in for a... **gynecological** exam!
Can you *imagine?!*
Er, yes, actually, yes I can!
If you're a person around the age of 18* with a vulva, vagina, cervix, uterus, and ovaries, getting them checked-up once a year is one of the ways you keep yourself healthy!
Oh my gosh, a *STRANGER* poking around in my **UNMENTIONABLES**?
I could never let someone put their face down there!
Uterus
Cervix
Ovary
Vagina
Vulva
*Or earlier, if you become sexually active before then!
It's okay to feel uncomfortable about this, society has placed a lot of importance on keeping one's privates, well, private.
But really, your genitals are just another part of your body and they *NEED* to be checked out to keep you **healthy**.

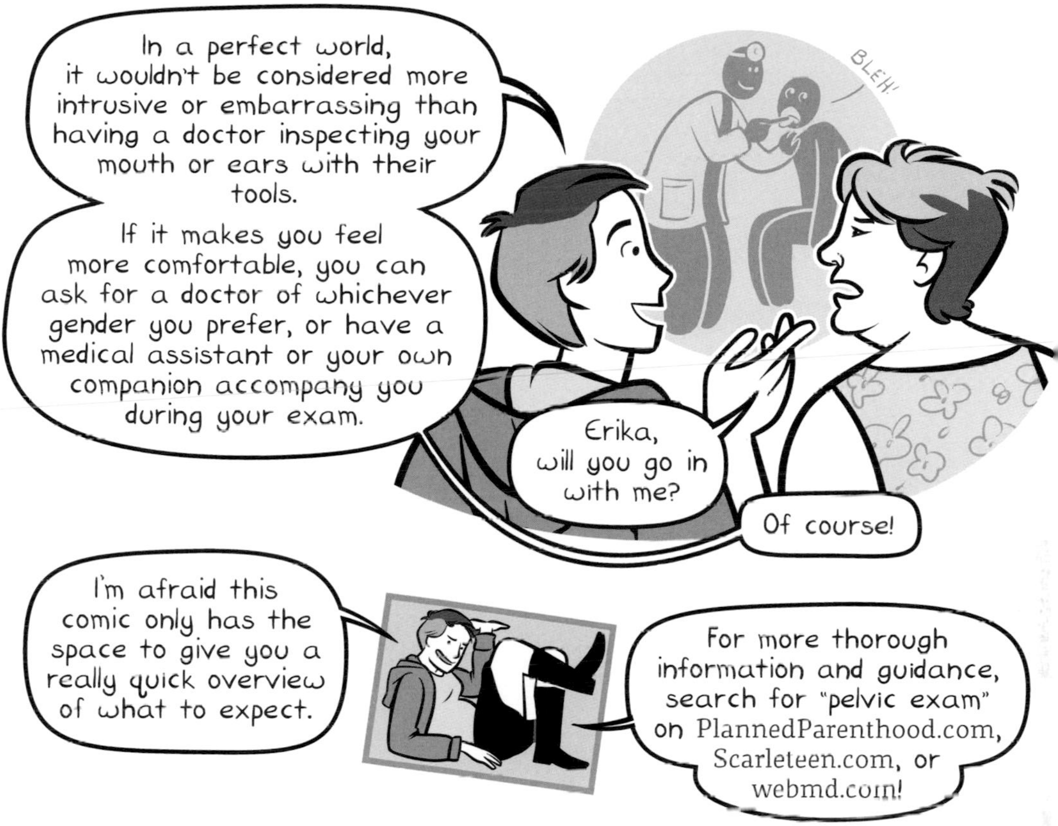
In a perfect world, it wouldn't be considered more intrusive or embarrassing than having a doctor inspecting your mouth or ears with their tools.
If it makes you feel more comfortable, you can ask for a doctor of whichever gender you prefer, or have a medical assistant or your own companion accompany you during your exam.
BLEH!
Erika, will you go in with me?
Of course!
I'm afraid this comic only has the space to give you a really quick overview of what to expect.
For more thorough information and guidance, search for "pelvic exam" on PlannedParenthood.com, Scarleteen.com, or webmd.com!

General Checkup

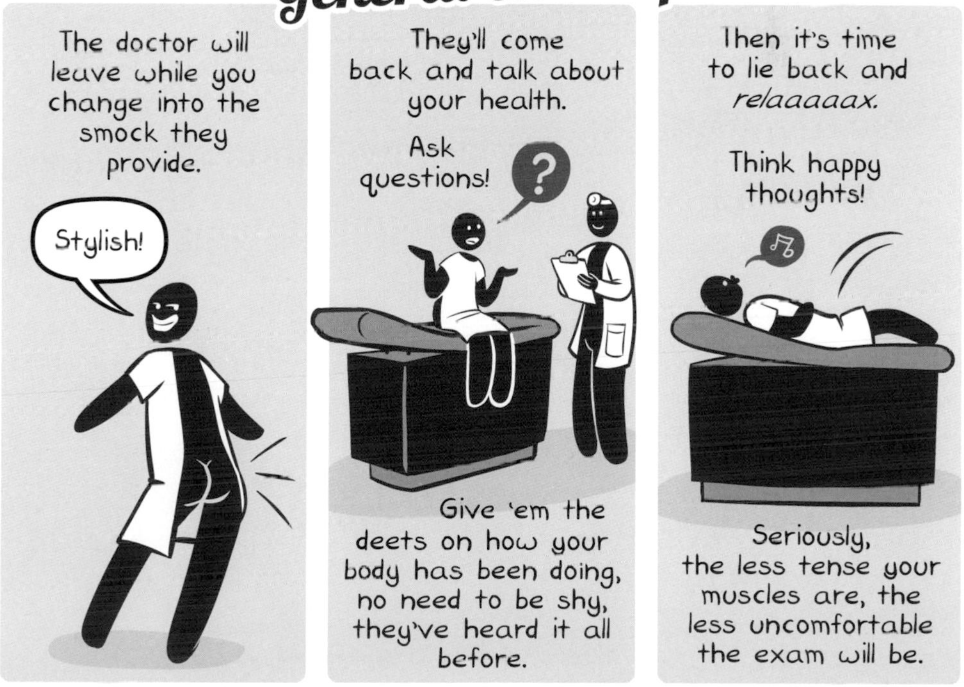
The doctor will leave while you change into the smock they provide.
Stylish!
They'll come back and talk about your health.
Ask questions!
?
Give 'em the deets on how your body has been doing, no need to be shy, they've heard it all before.
Then it's time to lie back and *relaaaaax.*
Think happy thoughts!
Seriously, the less tense your muscles are, the less uncomfortable the exam will be.

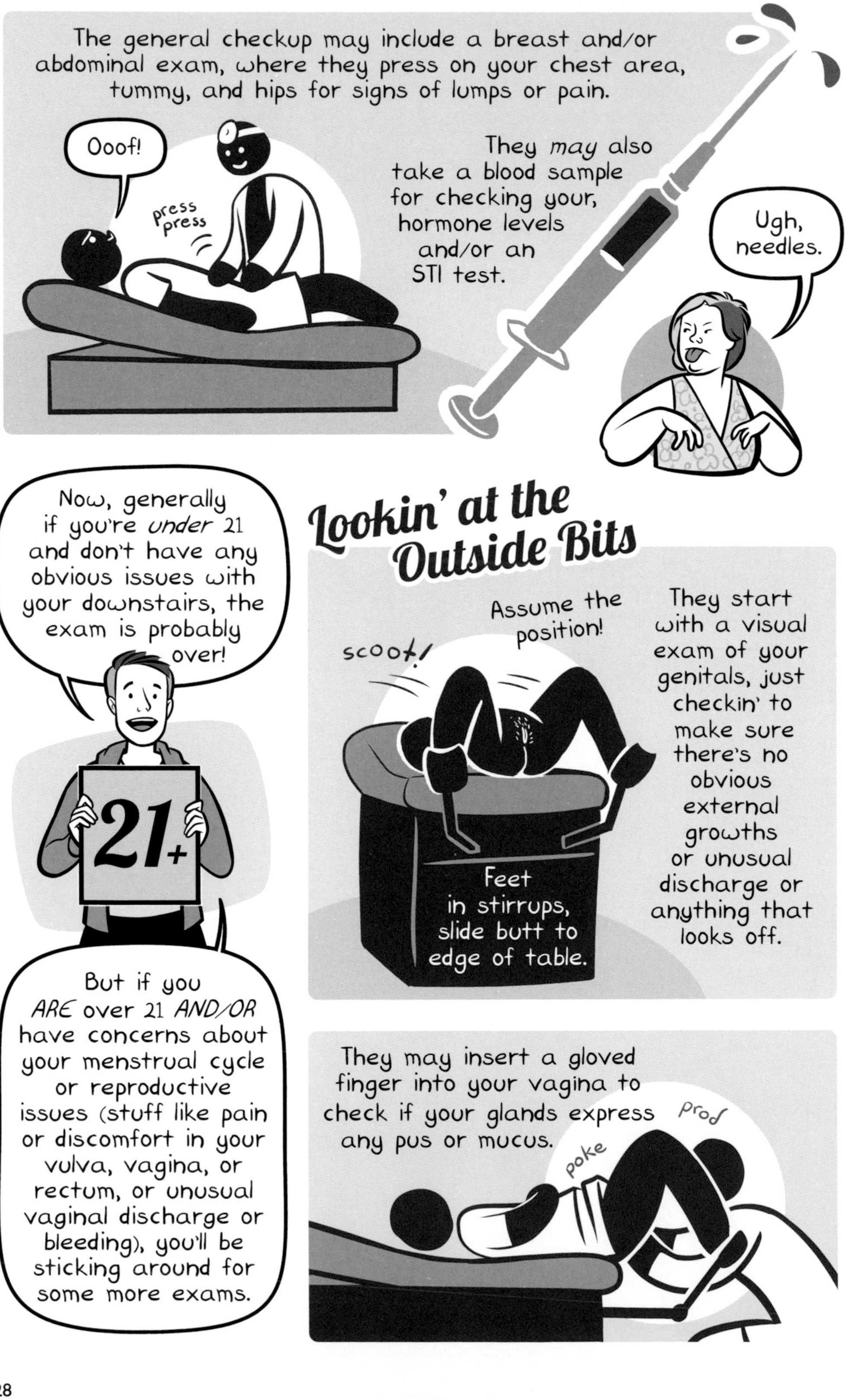

The general checkup may include a breast and/or abdominal exam, where they press on your chest area, tummy, and hips for signs of lumps or pain.
Ooof!
press press
They *may* also take a blood sample for checking your, hormone levels and/or an STI test.
Ugh, needles.
Now, generally if you're *under* 21 and don't have any obvious issues with your downstairs, the exam is probably over!
21+
Lookin' at the Outside Bits
Assume the position!
scoot!
Feet in stirrups, slide butt to edge of table.
They start with a visual exam of your genitals, just checkin' to make sure there's no obvious external growths or unusual discharge or anything that looks off.
But if you *ARE* over 21 *AND/OR* have concerns about your menstrual cycle or reproductive issues (stuff like pain or discomfort in your vulva, vagina, or rectum, or unusual vaginal discharge or bleeding), you'll be sticking around for some more exams.
They may insert a gloved finger into your vagina to check if your glands express any pus or mucus.
prod
poke

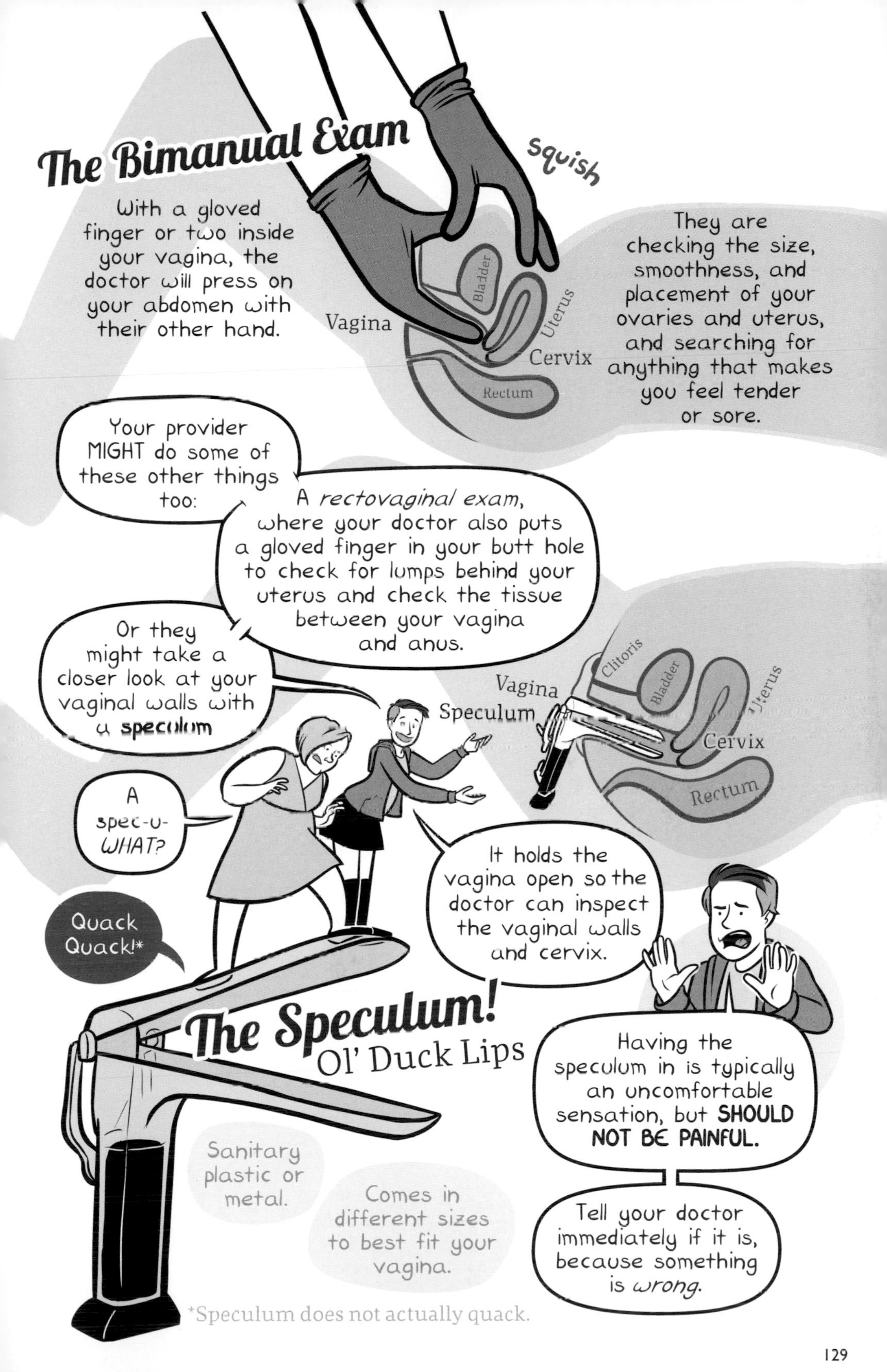
The Bimanual Exam
squish
With a gloved finger or two inside your vagina, the doctor will press on your abdomen with their other hand.
Bladder
Uterus
Vagina
Cervix
Rectum
They are checking the size, smoothness, and placement of your ovaries and uterus, and searching for anything that makes you feel tender or sore.
Your provider MIGHT do some of these other things too:
A *rectovaginal exam*, where your doctor also puts a gloved finger in your butt hole to check for lumps behind your uterus and check the tissue between your vagina and anus.
Or they might take a closer look at your vaginal walls with a **speculum**
Clitoris
Bladder
Uterus
Vagina
Speculum
Cervix
Rectum
A spec-u-*WHAT?*
It holds the vagina open so the doctor can inspect the vaginal walls and cervix.
Quack Quack!*
The Speculum!
Ol' Duck Lips
Having the speculum in is typically an uncomfortable sensation, but **SHOULD NOT BE PAINFUL.**
Sanitary plastic or metal.
Comes in different sizes to best fit your vagina.
Tell your doctor immediately if it is, because something is *wrong*.
*Speculum does not actually quack.

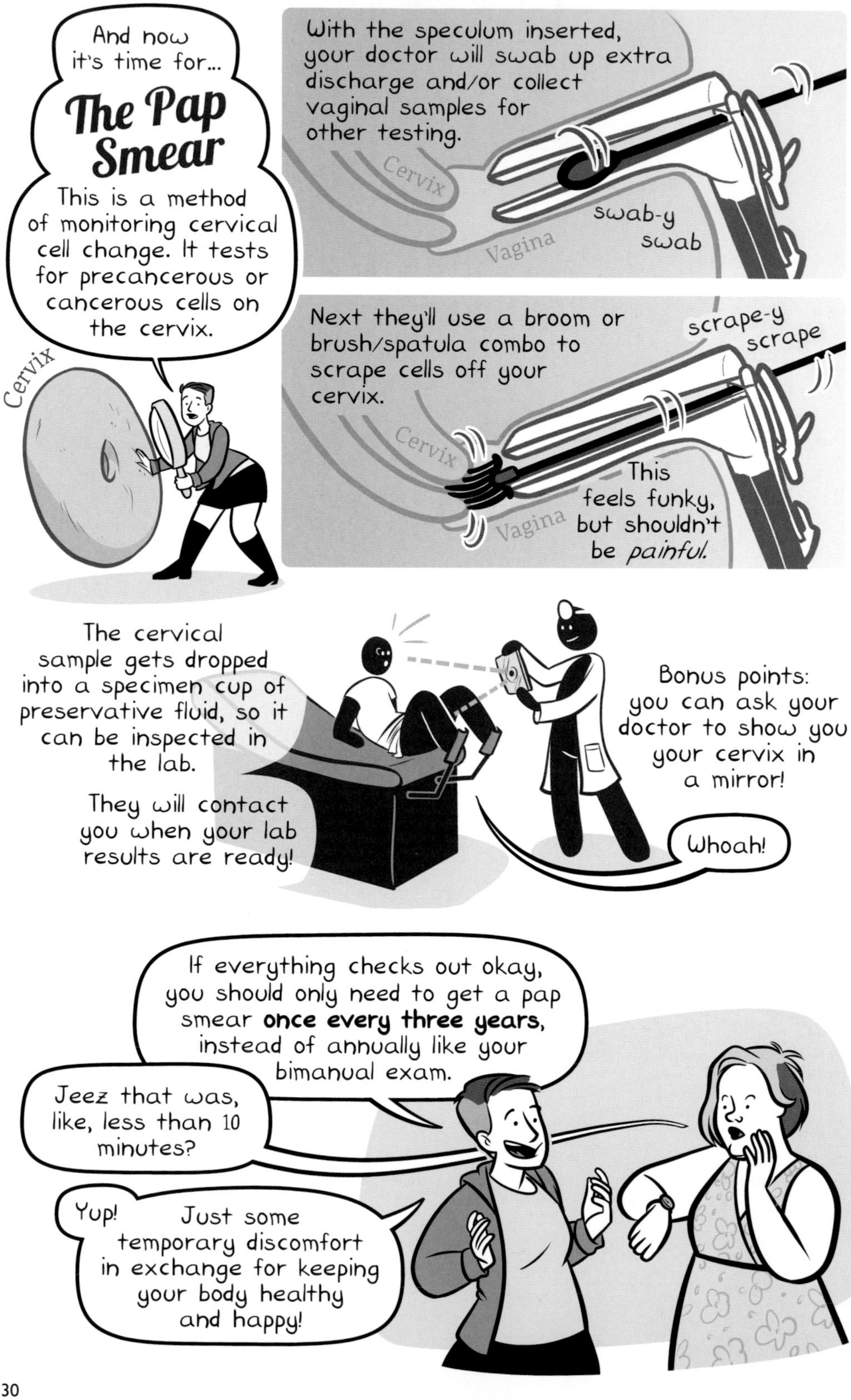
And now it's time for...
The Pap Smear
This is a method of monitoring cervical cell change. It tests for precancerous or cancerous cells on the cervix.
Cervix
With the speculum inserted, your doctor will swab up extra discharge and/or collect vaginal samples for other testing.
Cervix
Vagina
swab-y swab
Next they'll use a broom or brush/spatula combo to scrape cells off your cervix.
scrape-y scrape
Cervix
Vagina
This feels funky, but shouldn't be *painful.*
The cervical sample gets dropped into a specimen cup of preservative fluid, so it can be inspected in the lab.
They will contact you when your lab results are ready!
Bonus points: you can ask your doctor to show you your cervix in a mirror!
Whoah!
If everything checks out okay, you should only need to get a pap smear **once every three years**, instead of annually like your bimanual exam.
Jeez that was, like, less than 10 minutes?
Yup!
Just some temporary discomfort in exchange for keeping your body healthy and happy!

I can't
BREATHE!

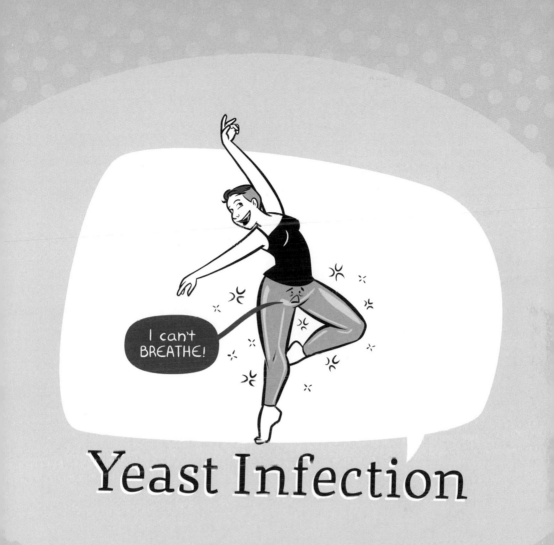

Yeast Infection

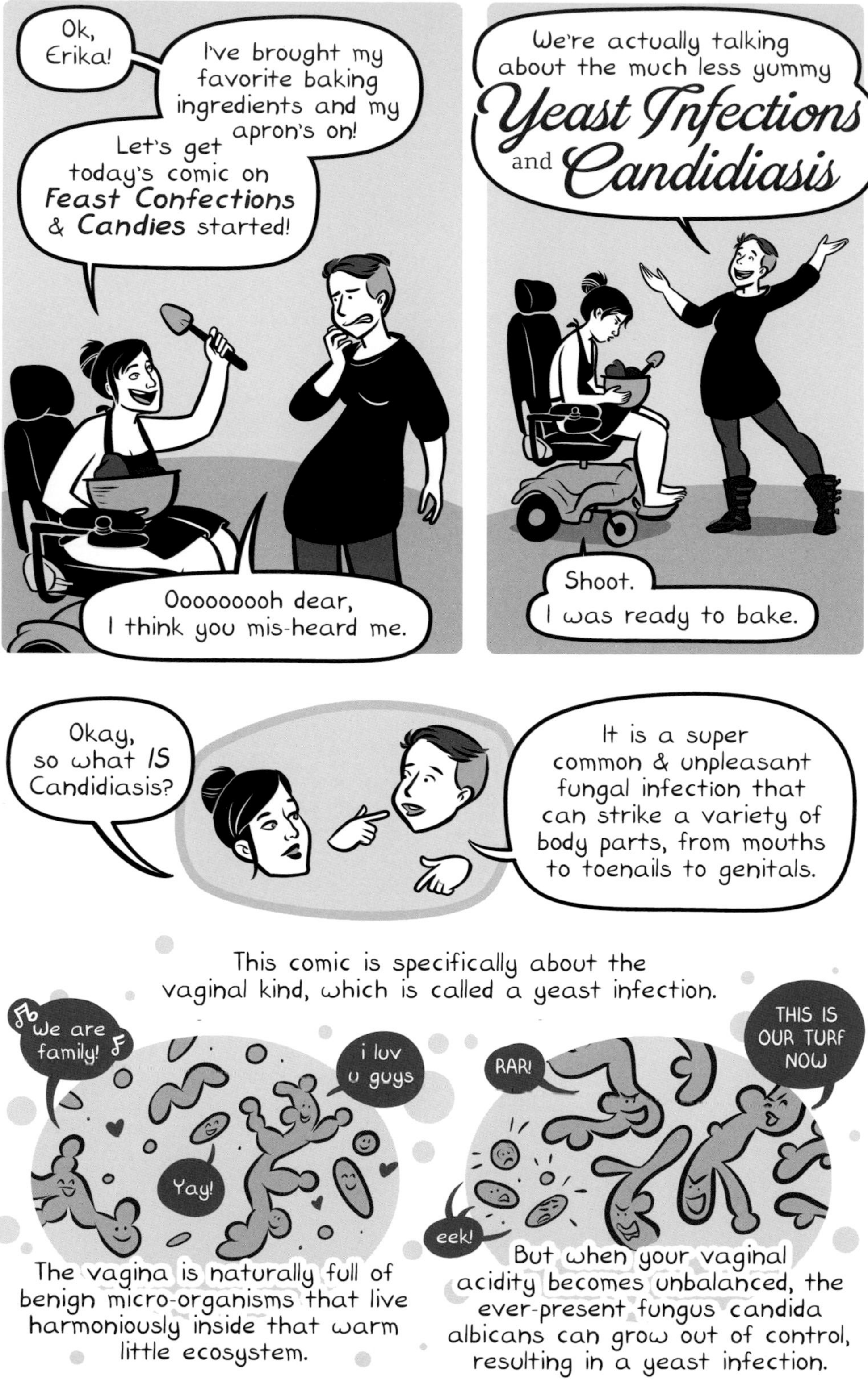

Ok, Erika!
I've brought my favorite baking ingredients and my apron's on!
Let's get today's comic on Feast Confections & Candies started!
Oooooooh dear, I think you mis-heard me.
We're actually talking about the much less yummy Yeast Infections and Candidiasis
Shoot. I was ready to bake.
Okay, so what IS Candidiasis?
It is a super common & unpleasant fungal infection that can strike a variety of body parts, from mouths to toenails to genitals.
This comic is specifically about the vaginal kind, which is called a yeast infection.
We are family!
i luv u guys
Yay!
The vagina is naturally full of benign micro-organisms that live harmoniously inside that warm little ecosystem.
RAR!
THIS IS OUR TURF NOW
eek!
But when your vaginal acidity becomes unbalanced, the ever-present fungus candida albicans can grow out of control, resulting in a yeast infection.

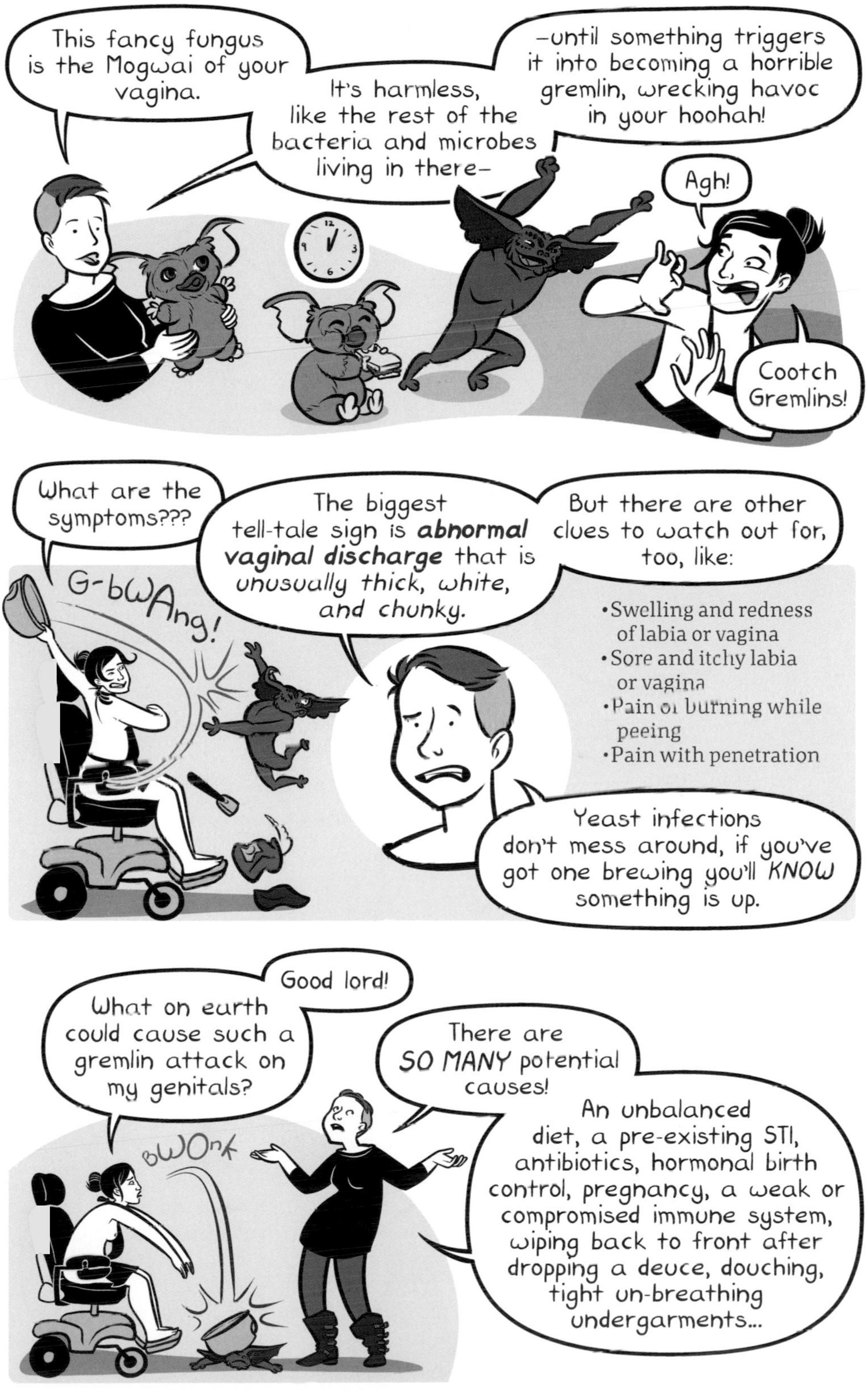

This fancy fungus is the Mogwai of your vagina.
It's harmless, like the rest of the bacteria and microbes living in there–
–until something triggers it into becoming a horrible gremlin, wrecking havoc in your hoohah!
Agh!
Cootch Gremlins!
What are the symptoms???
The biggest tell-tale sign is **abnormal vaginal discharge** that is *unusually thick, white, and chunky.*
G-bWAng!
But there are other clues to watch out for, too, like:
•Swelling and redness of labia or vagina
•Sore and itchy labia or vagina
•Pain or burning while peeing
•Pain with penetration
Yeast infections don't mess around, if you've got one brewing you'll *KNOW* something is up.
Good lord!
What on earth could cause such a gremlin attack on my genitals?
BWOnk
There are *SO MANY* potential causes!
An unbalanced diet, a pre-existing STI, antibiotics, hormonal birth control, pregnancy, a weak or compromised immune system, wiping back to front after dropping a deuce, douching, tight un-breathing undergarments...

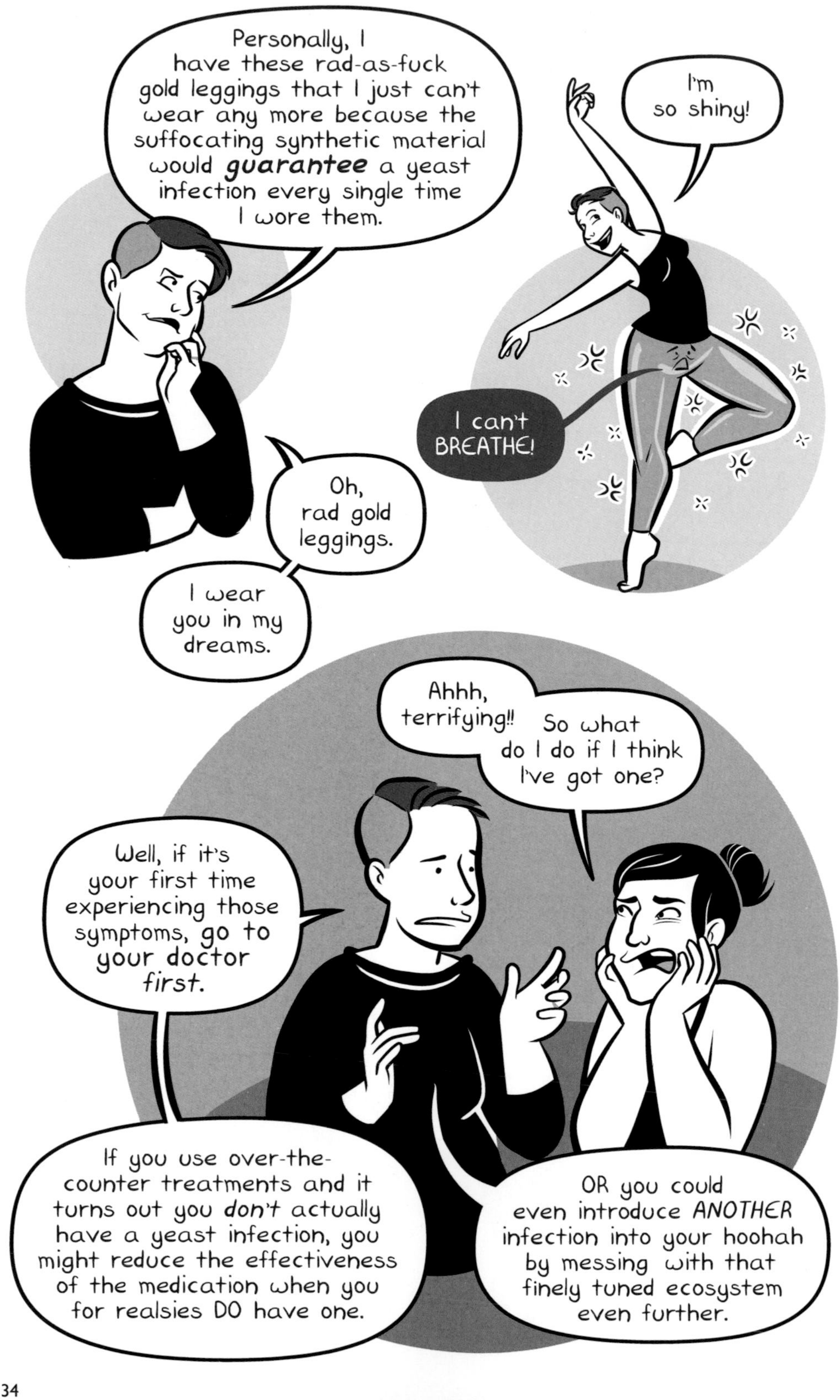
Personally, I have these rad-as-fuck gold leggings that I just can't wear any more because the suffocating synthetic material would **guarantee** a yeast infection every single time I wore them.
I'm so shiny!
I can't BREATHE!
Oh, rad gold leggings.
I wear you in my dreams.
Ahhh, terrifying!!
So what do I do if I think I've got one?
Well, if it's your first time experiencing those symptoms, go to your doctor first.
If you use over-the-counter treatments and it turns out you *don't* actually have a yeast infection, you might reduce the effectiveness of the medication when you for realsies DO have one.
OR you could even introduce *ANOTHER* infection into your hoohah by messing with that finely tuned ecosystem even further.

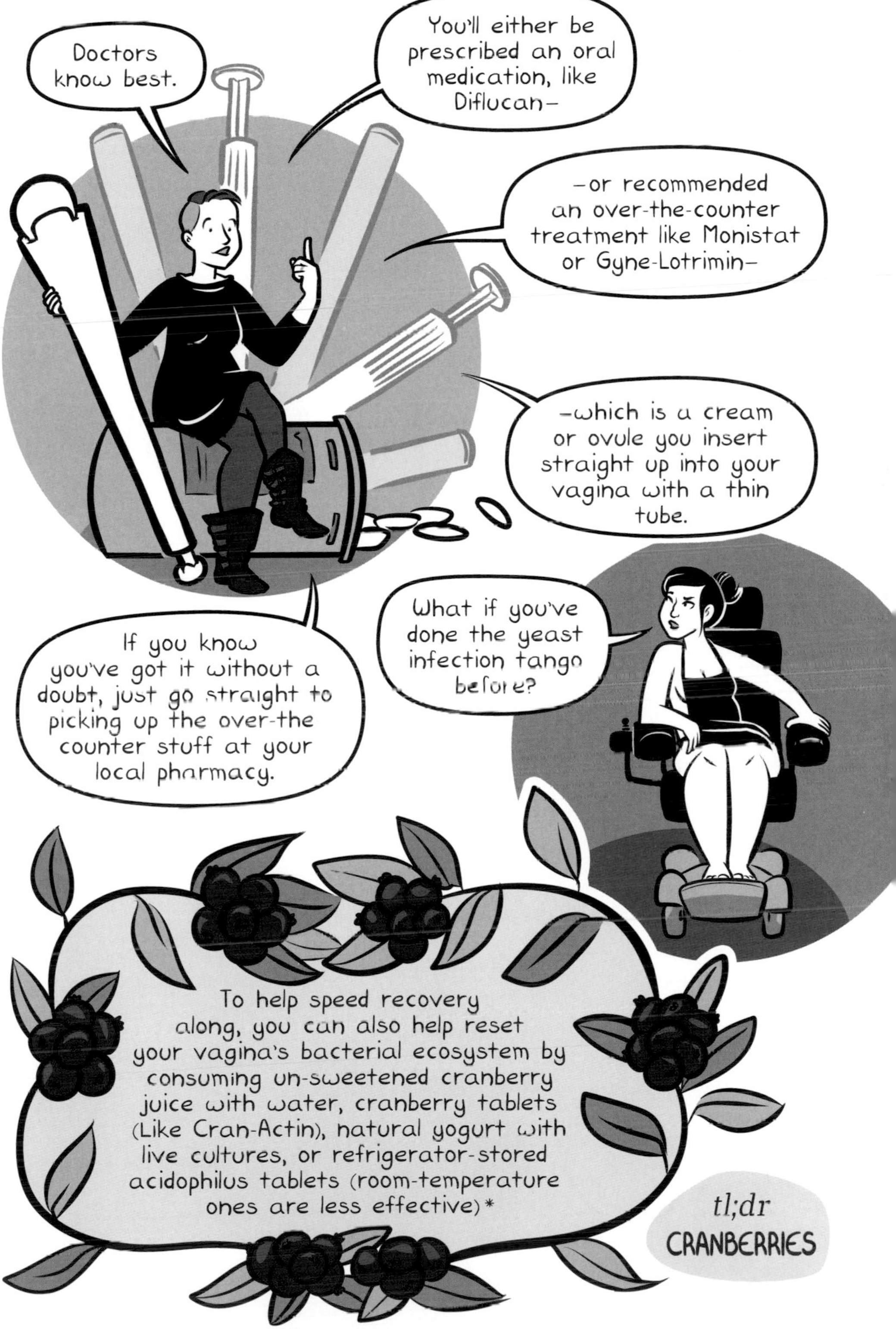

Doctors know best.
You'll either be prescribed an oral medication, like Diflucan–
–or recommended an over-the-counter treatment like Monistat or Gyne-Lotrimin–
–which is a cream or ovule you insert straight up into your vagina with a thin tube.
If you know you've got it without a doubt, just go straight to picking up the over-the counter stuff at your local pharmacy.
What if you've done the yeast infection tango before?
To help speed recovery along, you can also help reset your vagina's bacterial ecosystem by consuming un-sweetened cranberry juice with water, cranberry tablets (Like Cran-Actin), natural yogurt with live cultures, or refrigerator-stored acidophilus tablets (room-temperature ones are less effective)*
tl;dr
CRANBERRIES

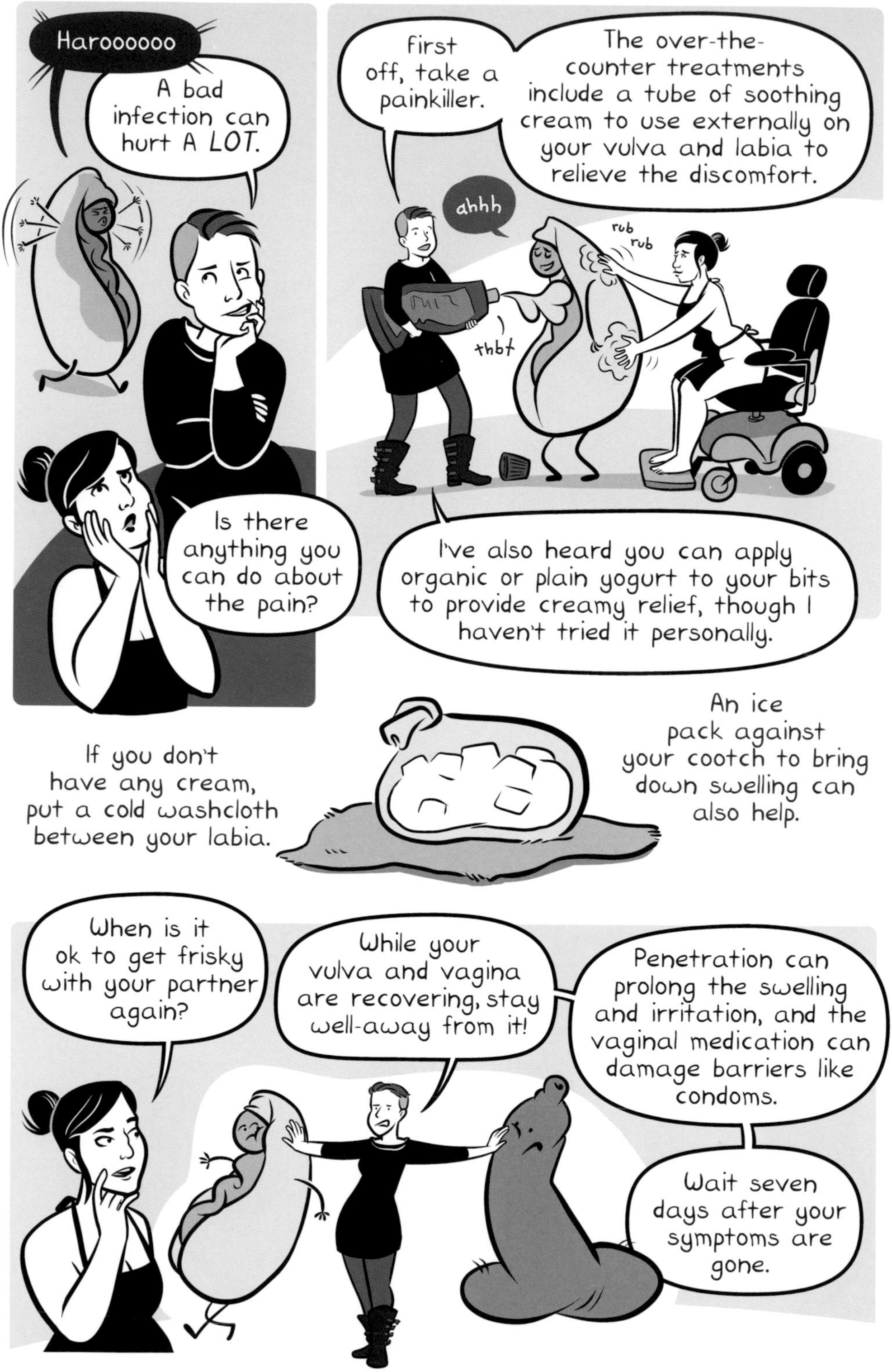
Harooooo
A bad infection can hurt A LOT.
Is there anything you can do about the pain?
First off, take a painkiller.
The over-the-counter treatments include a tube of soothing cream to use externally on your vulva and labia to relieve the discomfort.
ahhh
rub rub
thbt
I've also heard you can apply organic or plain yogurt to your bits to provide creamy relief, though I haven't tried it personally.
If you don't have any cream, put a cold washcloth between your labia.
An ice pack against your cootch to bring down swelling can also help.
When is it ok to get frisky with your partner again?
While your vulva and vagina are recovering, stay well-away from it!
Penetration can prolong the swelling and irritation, and the vaginal medication can damage barriers like condoms.
Wait seven days after your symptoms are gone.

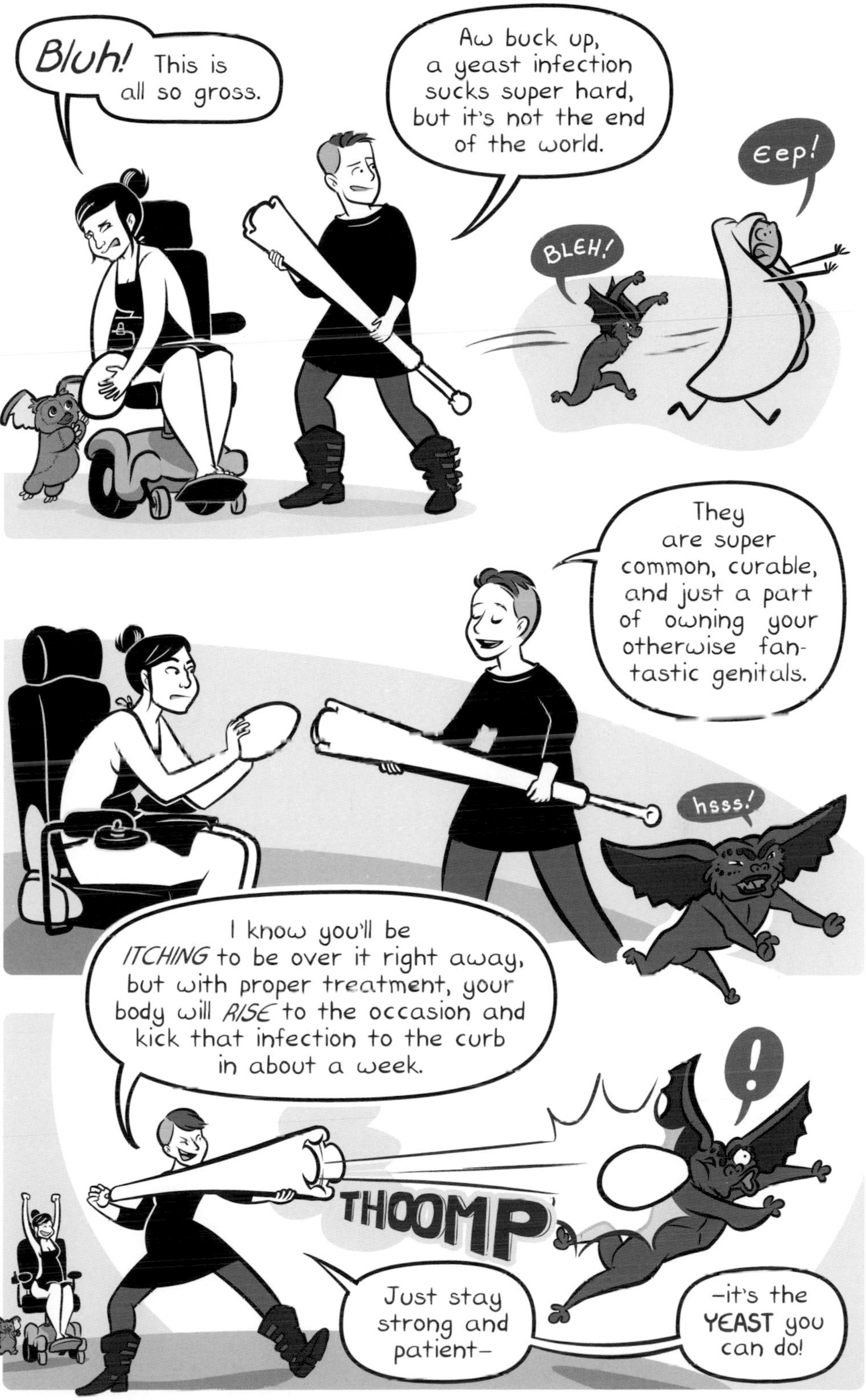
Bluh! This is all so gross.
Aw buck up, a yeast infection sucks super hard, but it's not the end of the world.
Eep!
BLEH!
They are super common, curable, and just a part of owning your otherwise fan-tastic genitals.
hsss!
I know you'll be ITCHING to be over it right away, but with proper treatment, your body will RISE to the occasion and kick that infection to the curb in about a week.
!
THOOMP
Just stay strong and patient–
–it's the YEAST you can do!

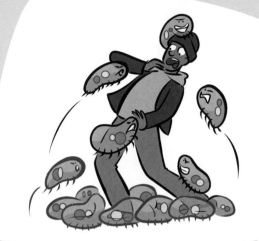

Urinary Tract Infection (UTI)

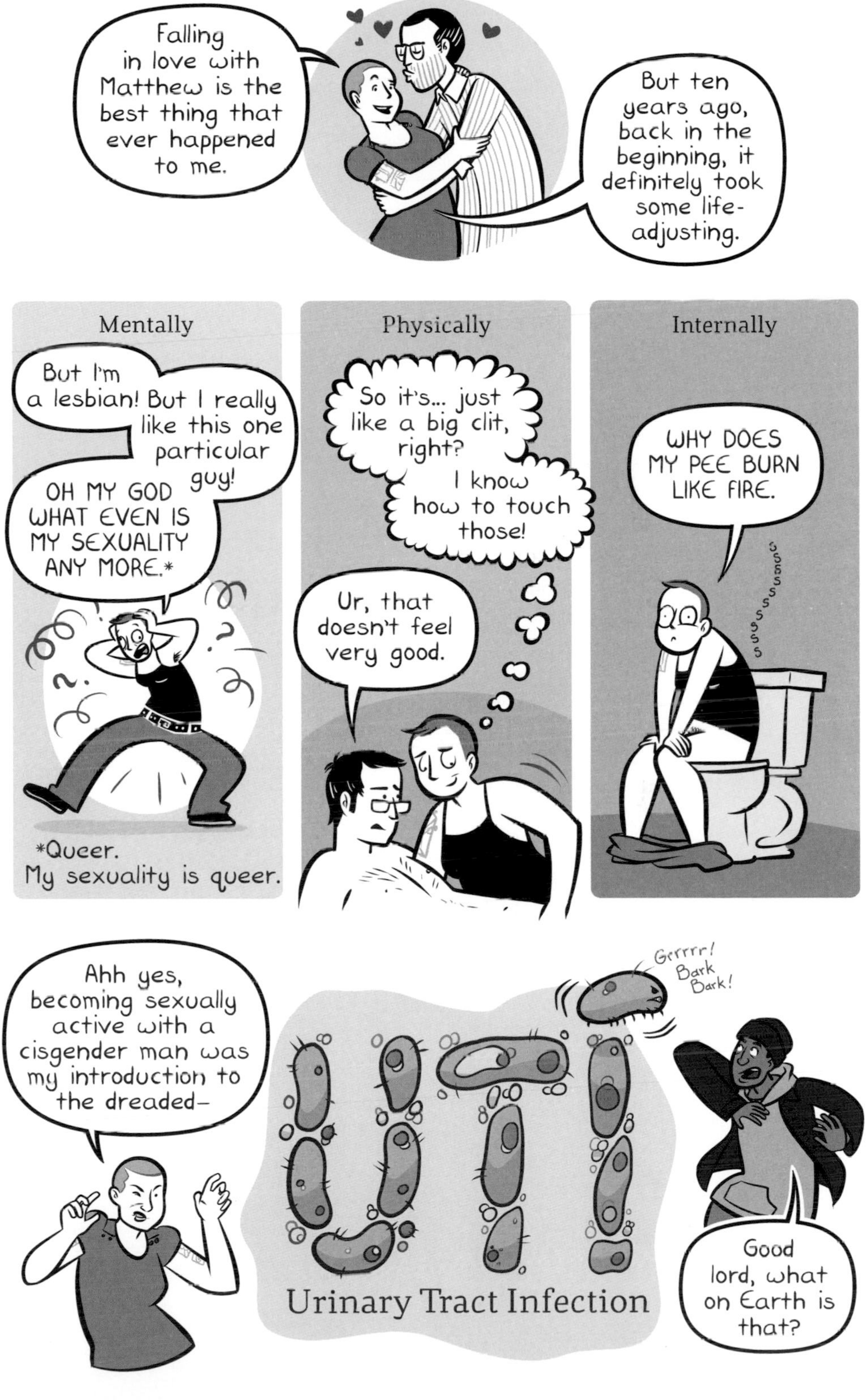
Falling in love with Matthew is the best thing that ever happened to me.
But ten years ago, back in the beginning, it definitely took some life-adjusting.
Mentally
But I'm a lesbian! But I really like this one particular guy!
OH MY GOD WHAT EVEN IS MY SEXUALITY ANY MORE.*
*Queer. My sexuality is queer.
Physically
So it's... just like a big clit, right?
I know how to touch those!
Ur, that doesn't feel very good.
Internally
WHY DOES MY PEE BURN LIKE FIRE.
Ahh yes, becoming sexually active with a cisgender man was my introduction to the dreaded–
UTI
Urinary Tract Infection
Grrrrr! Bark Bark!
Good lord, what on Earth is that?

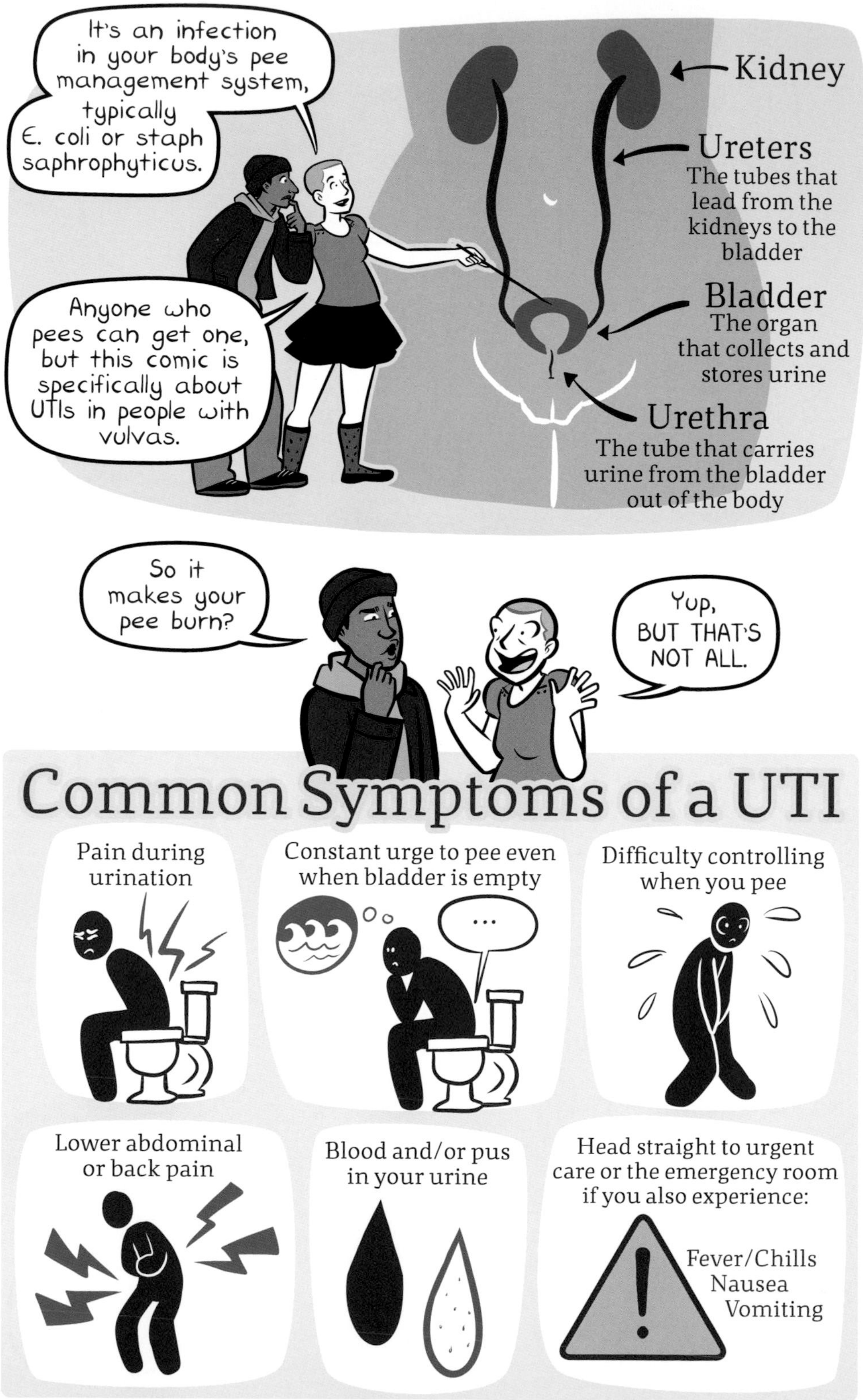
It's an infection in your body's pee management system, typically E. coli or staph saphrophyticus.
Kidney
Ureters
The tubes that lead from the kidneys to the bladder
Bladder
The organ that collects and stores urine
Urethra
The tube that carries urine from the bladder out of the body
Anyone who pees can get one, but this comic is specifically about UTIs in people with vulvas.
So it makes your pee burn?
Yup, BUT THAT'S NOT ALL.
Common Symptoms of a UTI
Pain during urination
Constant urge to pee even when bladder is empty
...
Difficulty controlling when you pee
Lower abdominal or back pain
Blood and/or pus in your urine
Head straight to urgent care or the emergency room if you also experience:
Fever/Chills
Nausea
Vomiting

I remember one particular flare up when I was on my way to interview for an apartment....

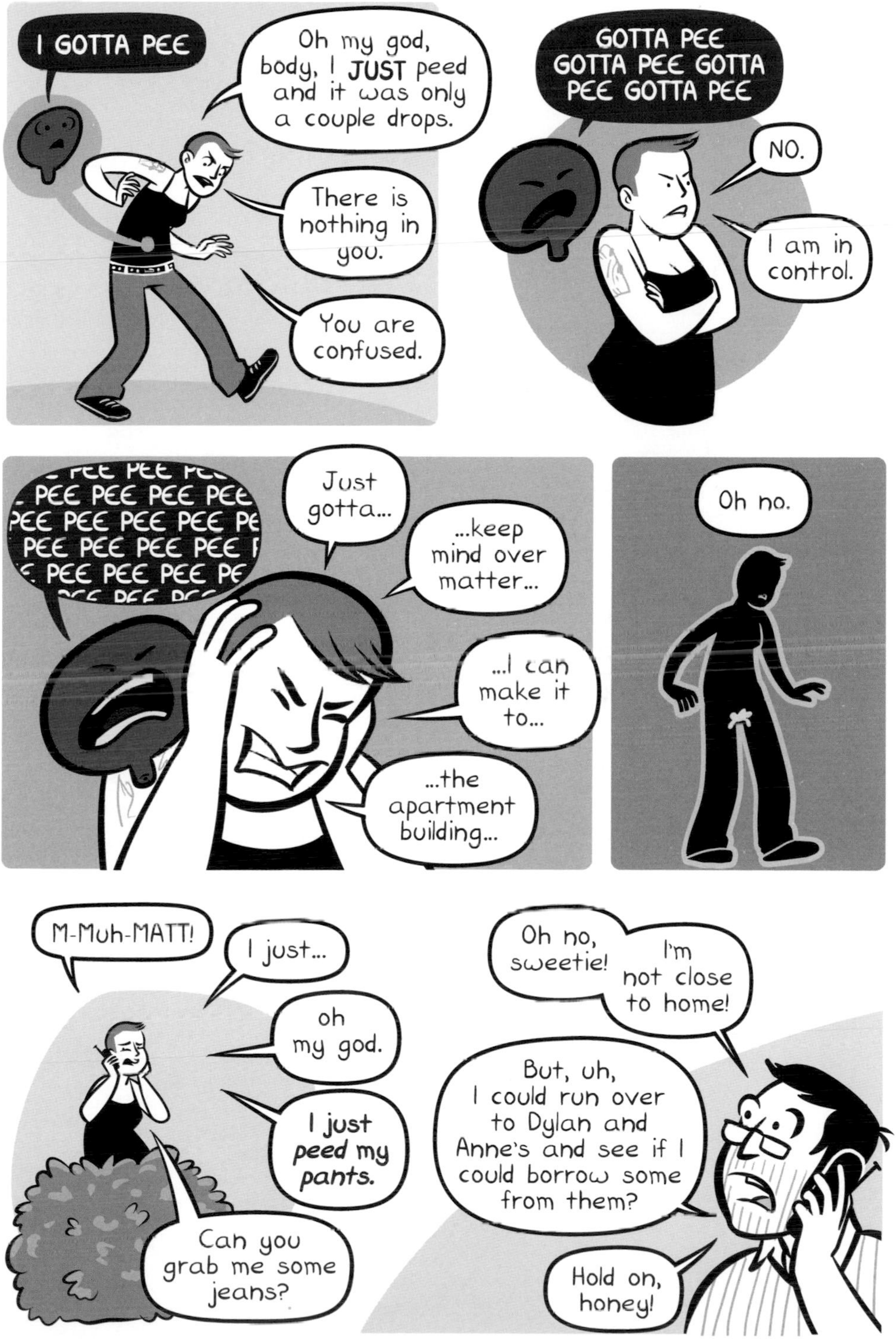
I GOTTA PEE
Oh my god, body, I JUST peed and it was only a couple drops.
There is nothing in you.
You are confused.
GOTTA PEE GOTTA PEE GOTTA PEE GOTTA PEE
NO.
I am in control.
PEE PEE PEE PEE PEE PEE PEE PEE PEE PEE PEE PEE PEE PEE PEE PEE
Just gotta...
...keep mind over matter...
...I can make it to...
...the apartment building...
Oh no.
M-Muh-MATT!
I just...
oh my god.
I just *peed* my *pants.*
Can you grab me some jeans?
Oh no, sweetie!
I'm not close to home!
But, uh, I could run over to Dylan and Anne's and see if I could borrow some from them?
Hold on, honey!

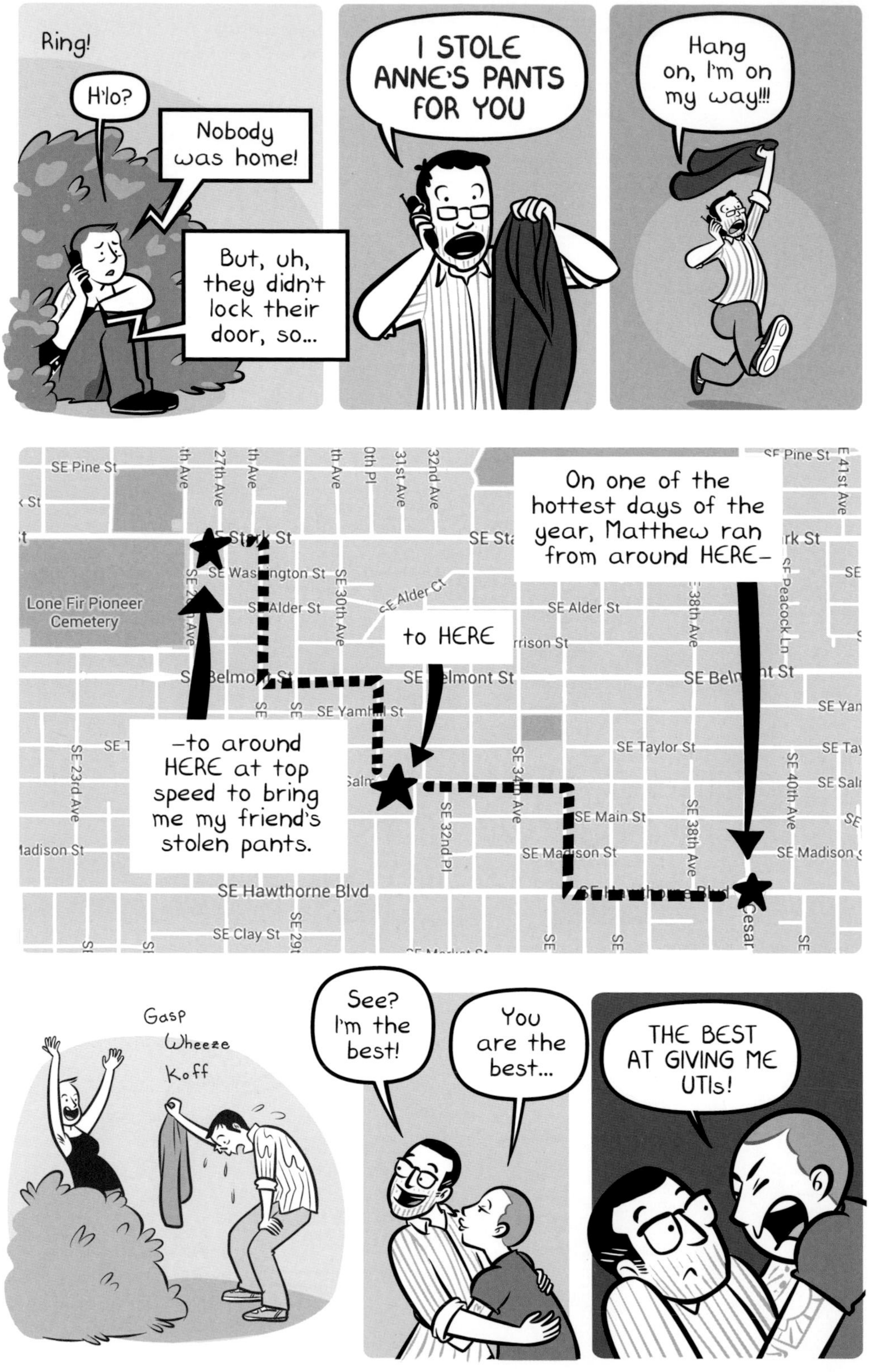
Ring!
H'lo?
Nobody was home!
But, uh, they didn't lock their door, so...
I STOLE ANNE'S PANTS FOR YOU
Hang on, I'm on my way!!!
SE Pine St
27th Ave
31st Ave
32nd Ave
Lone Fir Pioneer Cemetery
SE Alder St
SE 30th Ave
SE Alder Ct
SE Alder St
SE 38th Ave
SE Peacock Ln
On one of the hottest days of the year, Matthew ran from around HERE–
to HERE
–to around HERE at top speed to bring me my friend's stolen pants.
SE Belmont St
SE Taylor St
SE 23rd Ave
SE 32nd Pl
SE Main St
SE 38th Ave
SE 40th Ave
SE Madison St
SE Hawthorne Blvd
SE Clay St
Gasp
Wheeze
Koff
See? I'm the best!
You are the best...
THE BEST AT GIVING ME UTIs!

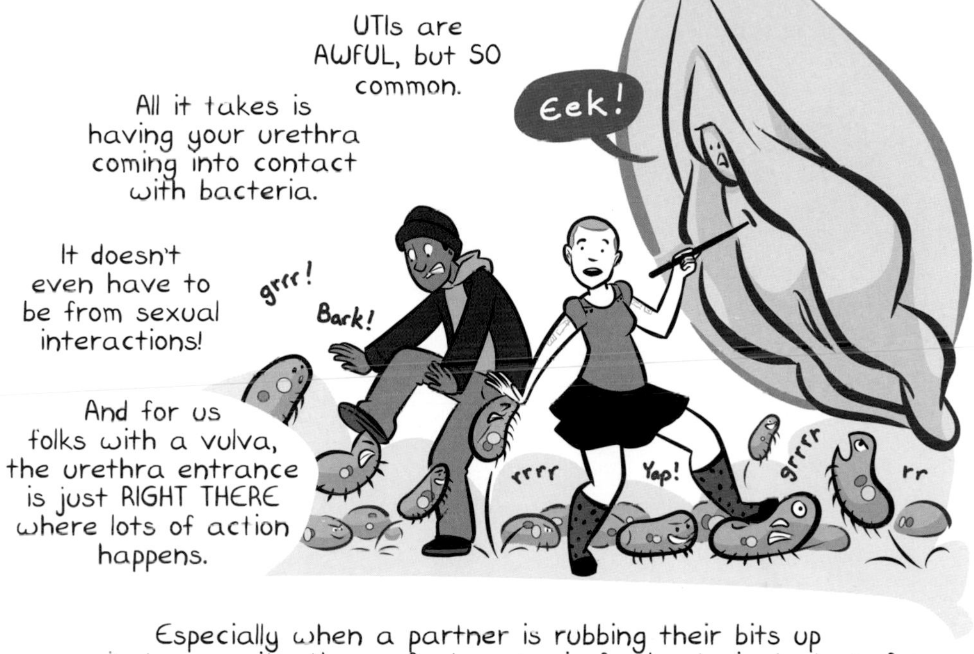
UTIs are AWFUL, but SO common.
All it takes is having your urethra coming into contact with bacteria.
Eek!
It doesn't even have to be from sexual interactions!
grrr!
Bark!
And for us folks with a vulva, the urethra entrance is just RIGHT THERE where lots of action happens.
rrrr
Yap!
grrrr
rr

Especially when a partner is rubbing their bits up against yours, it's the perfect scenario for bacteria to transfer off of them, or for your own bacteria to be pushed directly into your urethral opening, during all that grinding motion.

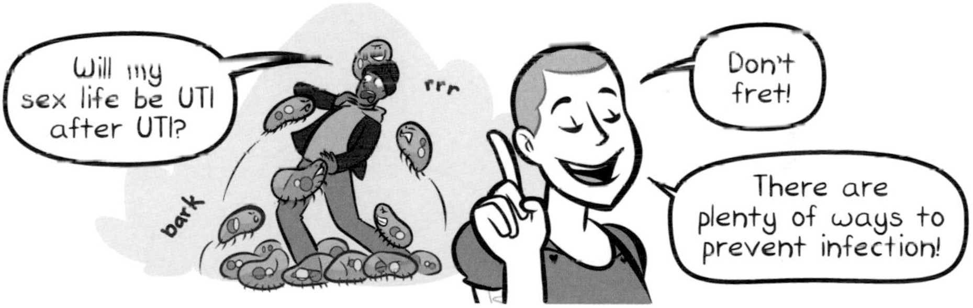
Will my sex life be UTI after UTI?
rrr
bark
Don't fret!
There are plenty of ways to prevent infection!

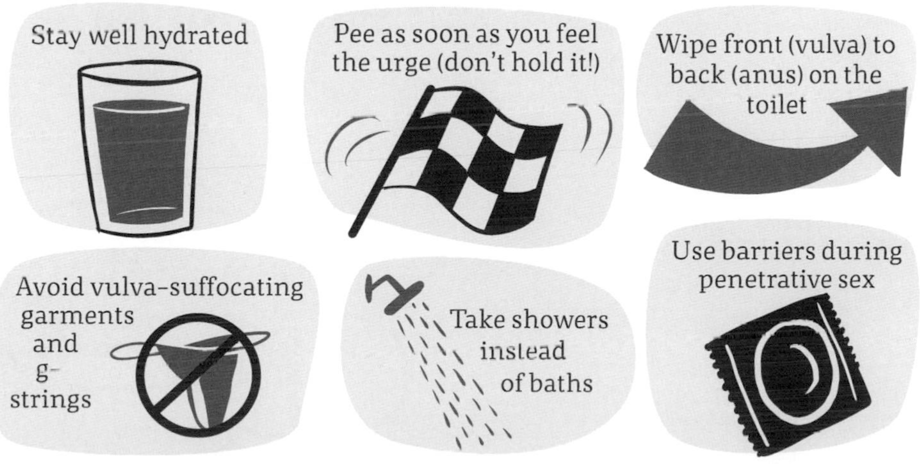
Stay well hydrated
Pee as soon as you feel the urge (don't hold it!)
Wipe front (vulva) to back (anus) on the toilet
Avoid vulva-suffocating garments and g-strings
Take showers instead of baths
Use barriers during penetrative sex

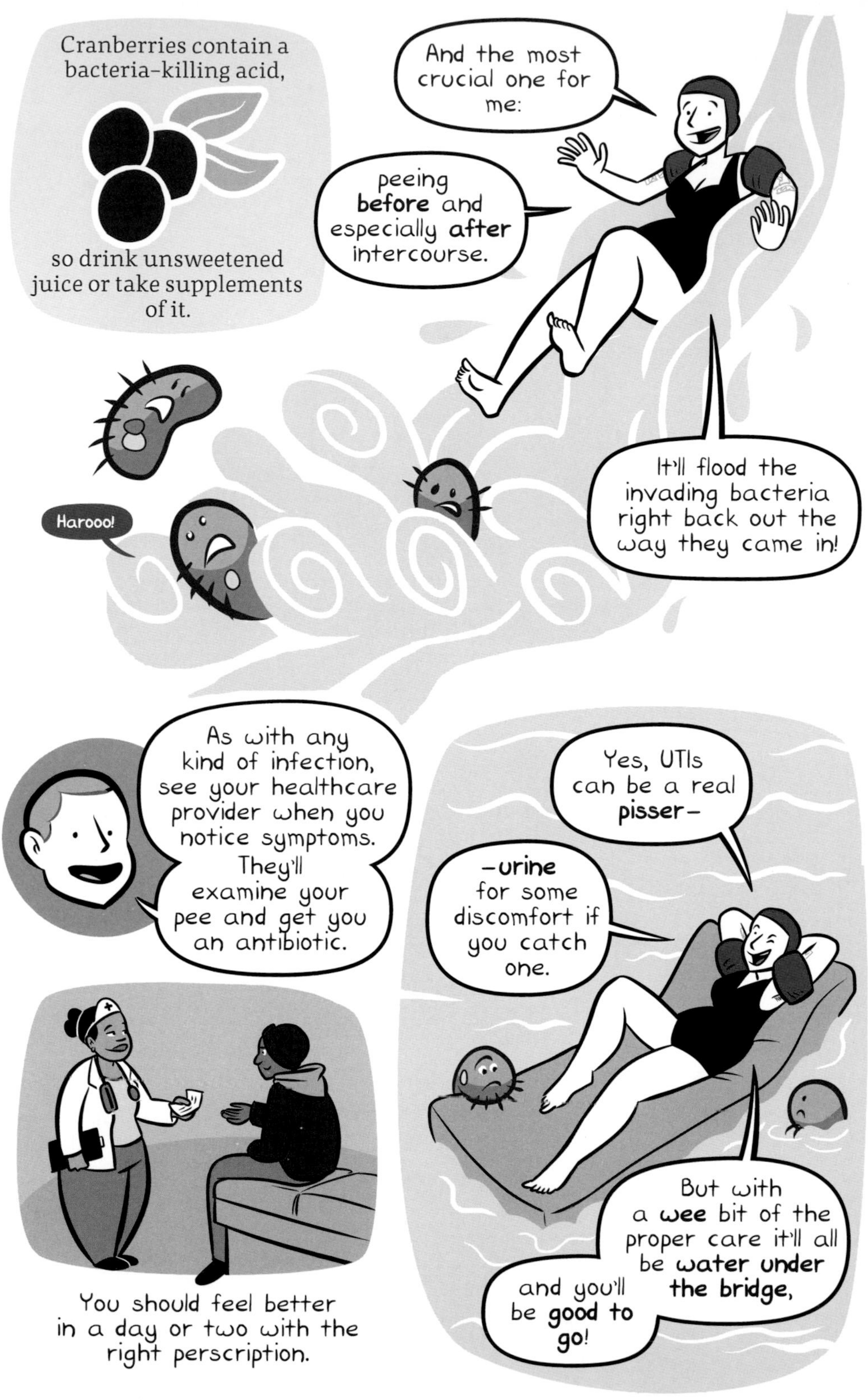
Cranberries contain a bacteria-killing acid,
so drink unsweetened juice or take supplements of it.
And the most crucial one for me:
peeing **before** and especially **after** intercourse.
It'll flood the invading bacteria right back out the way they came in!
Harooo!
As with any kind of infection, see your healthcare provider when you notice symptoms. They'll examine your pee and get you an antibiotic.
You should feel better in a day or two with the right perscription.
Yes, UTIs can be a real **pisser**–
–**urine** for some discomfort if you catch one.
But with a **wee** bit of the proper care it'll all be **water under the bridge**,
and you'll be **good to go**!

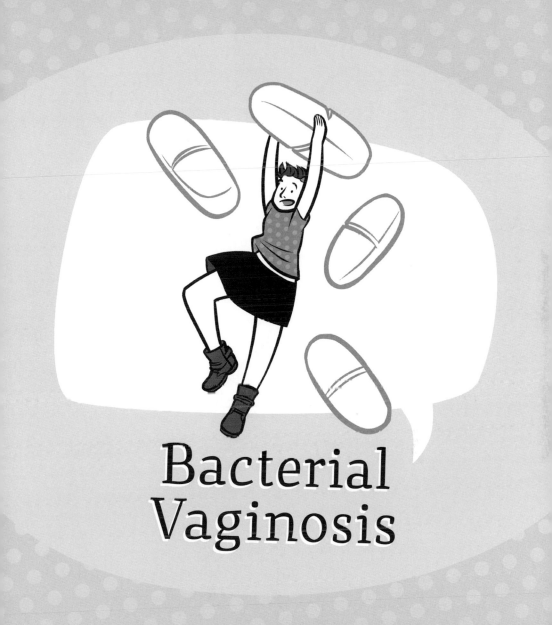

Bacterial
Vaginosis

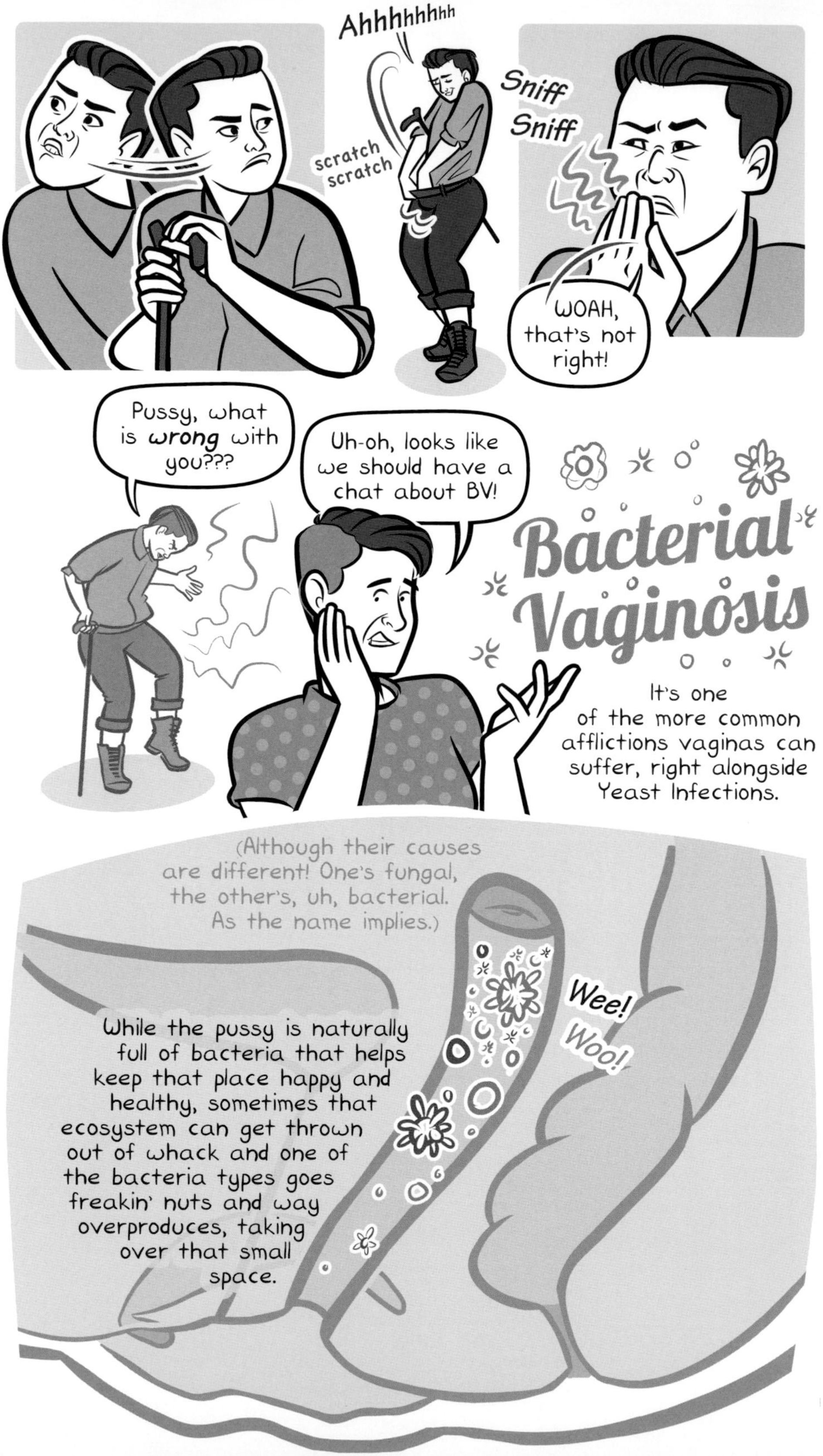

Ahhhhhhhh
scratch scratch
Sniff
Sniff
WOAH, that's not right!
Pussy, what is **wrong** with you???
Uh-oh, looks like we should have a chat about BV!
Bacterial Vaginosis
It's one of the more common afflictions vaginas can suffer, right alongside Yeast Infections.
(Although their causes are different! One's fungal, the other's, uh, bacterial. As the name implies.)
Wee!
Woo!
While the pussy is naturally full of bacteria that helps keep that place happy and healthy, sometimes that ecosystem can get thrown out of whack and one of the bacteria types goes freakin' nuts and way overproduces, taking over that small space.

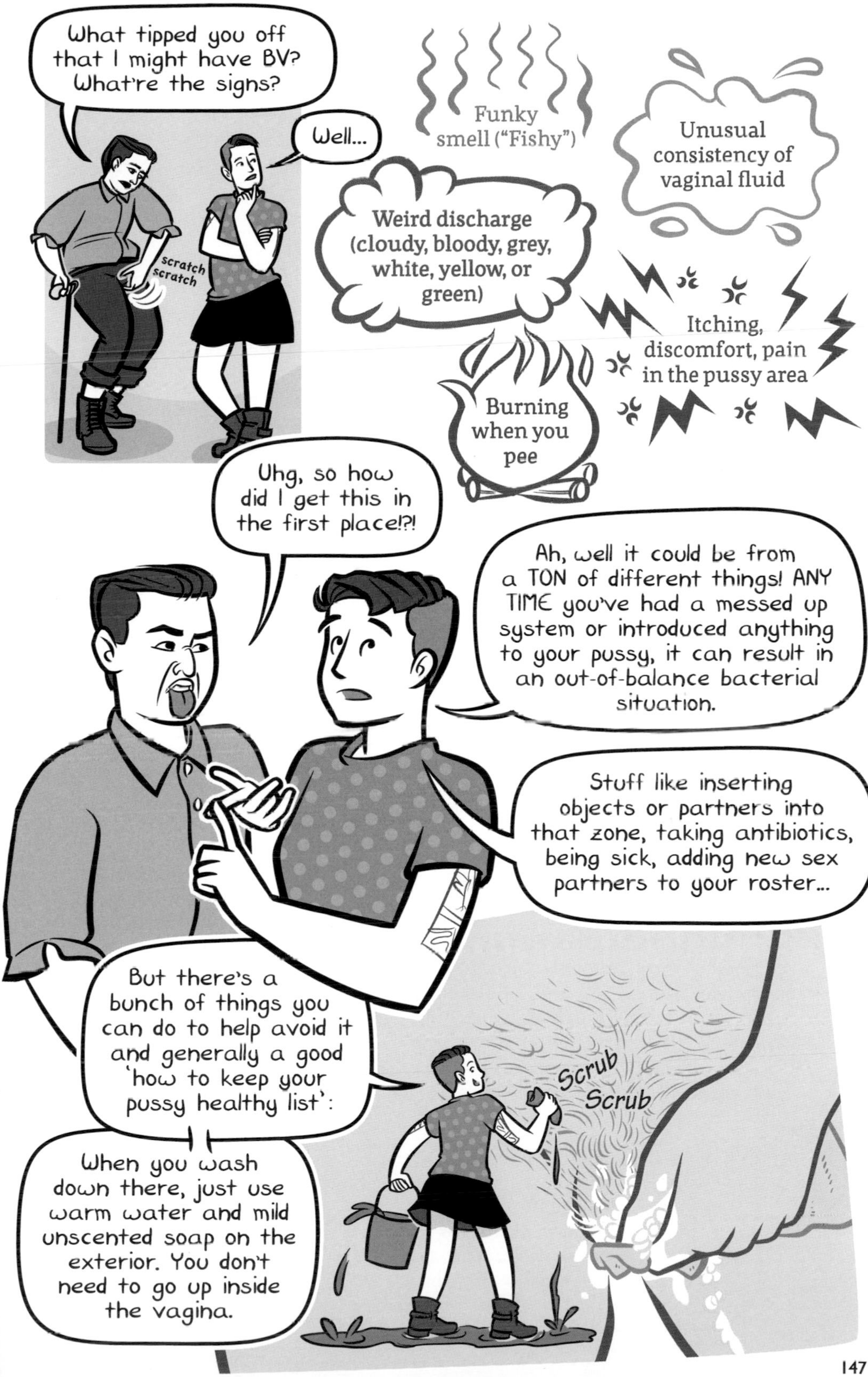

What tipped you off that I might have BV? What're the signs?
Well...
scratch scratch
Funky smell ("Fishy")
Unusual consistency of vaginal fluid
Weird discharge (cloudy, bloody, grey, white, yellow, or green)
Itching, discomfort, pain in the pussy area
Burning when you pee
Uhg, so how did I get this in the first place!?!
Ah, well it could be from a TON of different things! ANY TIME you've had a messed up system or introduced anything to your pussy, it can result in an out-of-balance bacterial situation.
Stuff like inserting objects or partners into that zone, taking antibiotics, being sick, adding new sex partners to your roster...
But there's a bunch of things you can do to help avoid it and generally a good 'how to keep your pussy healthy list':
When you wash down there, just use warm water and mild unscented soap on the exterior. You don't need to go up inside the vagina.
Scrub
Scrub

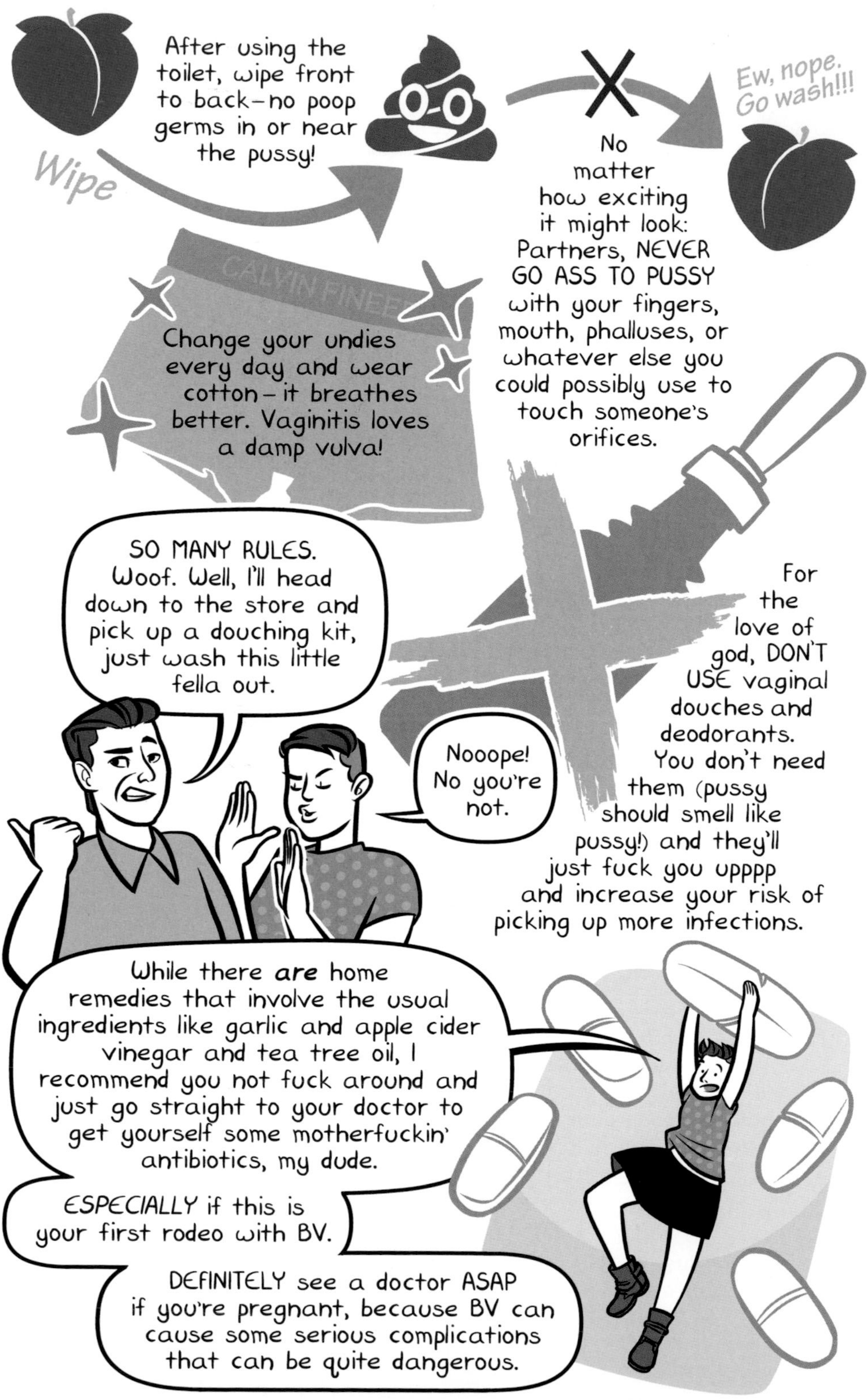
After using the toilet, wipe front to back—no poop germs in or near the pussy!
Wipe
Ew, nope. Go wash!!!
No matter how exciting it might look: Partners, NEVER GO ASS TO PUSSY with your fingers, mouth, phalluses, or whatever else you could possibly use to touch someone's orifices.
CALVIN FINEE
Change your undies every day and wear cotton – it breathes better. Vaginitis loves a damp vulva!
SO MANY RULES. Woof. Well, I'll head down to the store and pick up a douching kit, just wash this little fella out.
Nooope! No you're not.
For the love of god, DON'T USE vaginal douches and deodorants. You don't need them (pussy should smell like pussy!) and they'll just fuck you upppp and increase your risk of picking up more infections.
While there **are** home remedies that involve the usual ingredients like garlic and apple cider vinegar and tea tree oil, I recommend you not fuck around and just go straight to your doctor to get yourself some motherfuckin' antibiotics, my dude.
ESPECIALLY if this is your first rodeo with BV.
DEFINITELY see a doctor ASAP if you're pregnant, because BV can cause some serious complications that can be quite dangerous.

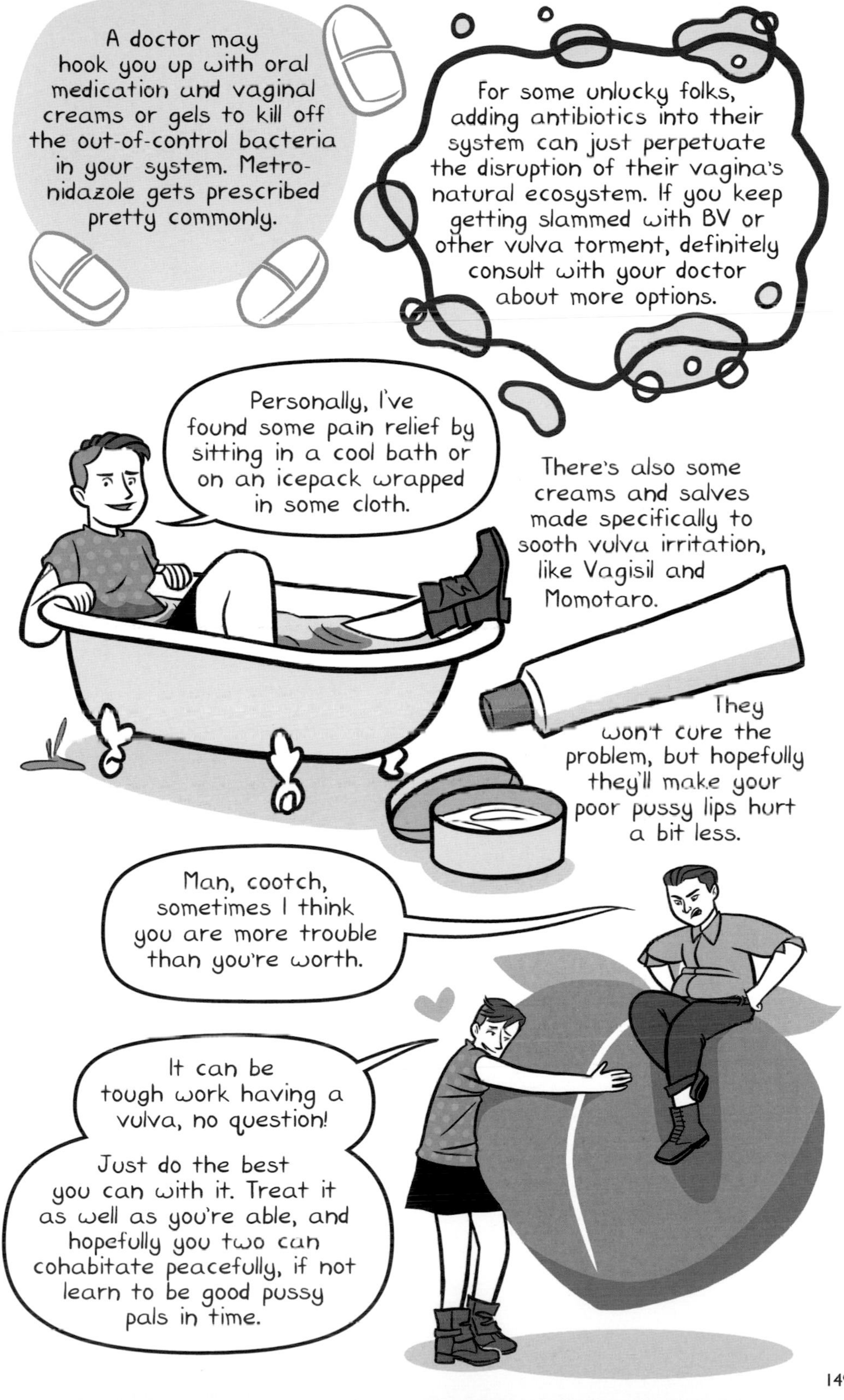
A doctor may hook you up with oral medication and vaginal creams or gels to kill off the out-of-control bacteria in your system. Metronidazole gets prescribed pretty commonly.
For some unlucky folks, adding antibiotics into their system can just perpetuate the disruption of their vagina's natural ecosystem. If you keep getting slammed with BV or other vulva torment, definitely consult with your doctor about more options.
Personally, I've found some pain relief by sitting in a cool bath or on an icepack wrapped in some cloth.
There's also some creams and salves made specifically to sooth vulva irritation, like Vagisil and Momotaro.
They won't cure the problem, but hopefully they'll make your poor pussy lips hurt a bit less.
Man, cootch, sometimes I think you are more trouble than you're worth.
It can be tough work having a vulva, no question!
Just do the best you can with it. Treat it as well as you're able, and hopefully you two can cohabitate peacefully, if not learn to be good pussy pals in time.

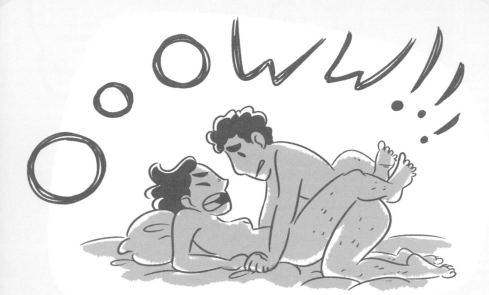

Vestibulodynia

By Alex Assan
AlexAssanart.com

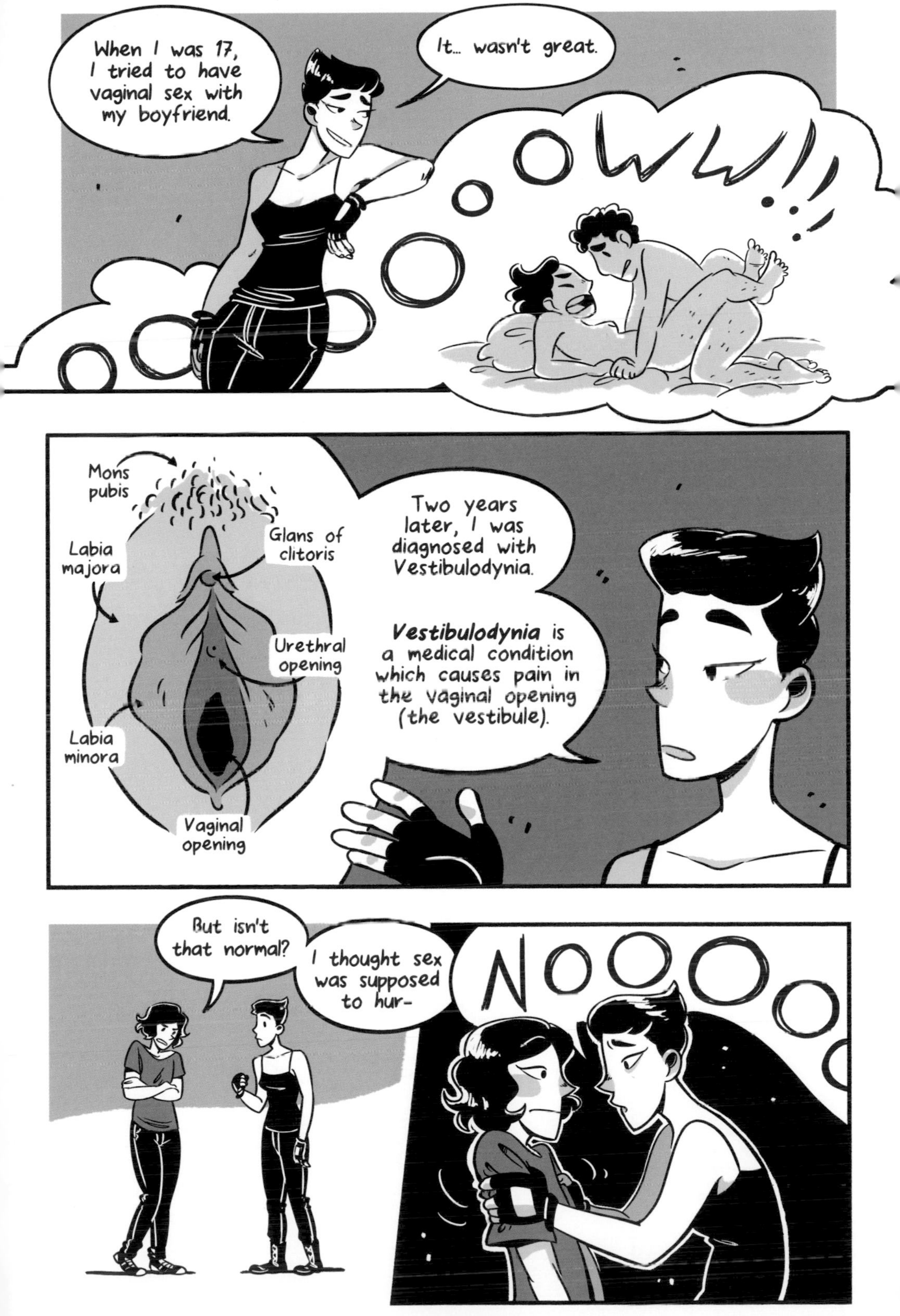

When I was 17, I tried to have vaginal sex with my boyfriend.
It... wasn't great.
OOOOWW!!!
Mons pubis
Glans of clitoris
Labia majora
Urethral opening
Labia minora
Vaginal opening
Two years later, I was diagnosed with Vestibulodynia.
Vestibulodynia is a medical condition which causes pain in the vaginal opening (the vestibule).
But isn't that normal?
I thought sex was supposed to hur-
NOOOOO

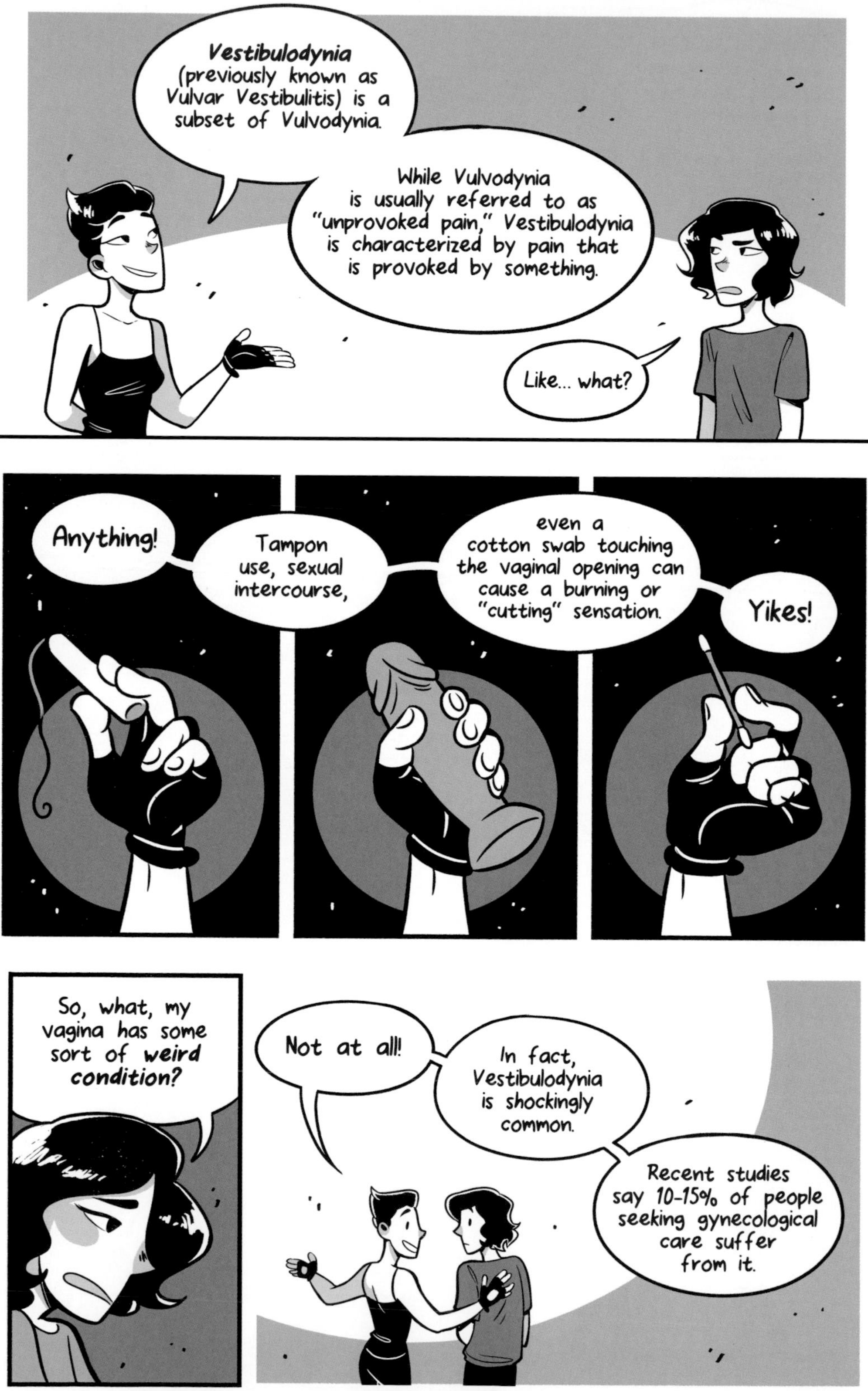

Vestibulodynia (previously known as Vulvar Vestibulitis) is a subset of Vulvodynia.
While Vulvodynia is usually referred to as "unprovoked pain," Vestibulodynia is characterized by pain that is provoked by something.
Like... what?
Anything!
Tampon use, sexual intercourse,
even a cotton swab touching the vaginal opening can cause a burning or "cutting" sensation.
Yikes!
So, what, my vagina has some sort of **weird condition?**
Not at all!
In fact, Vestibulodynia is shockingly common.
Recent studies say 10-15% of people seeking gynecological care suffer from it.

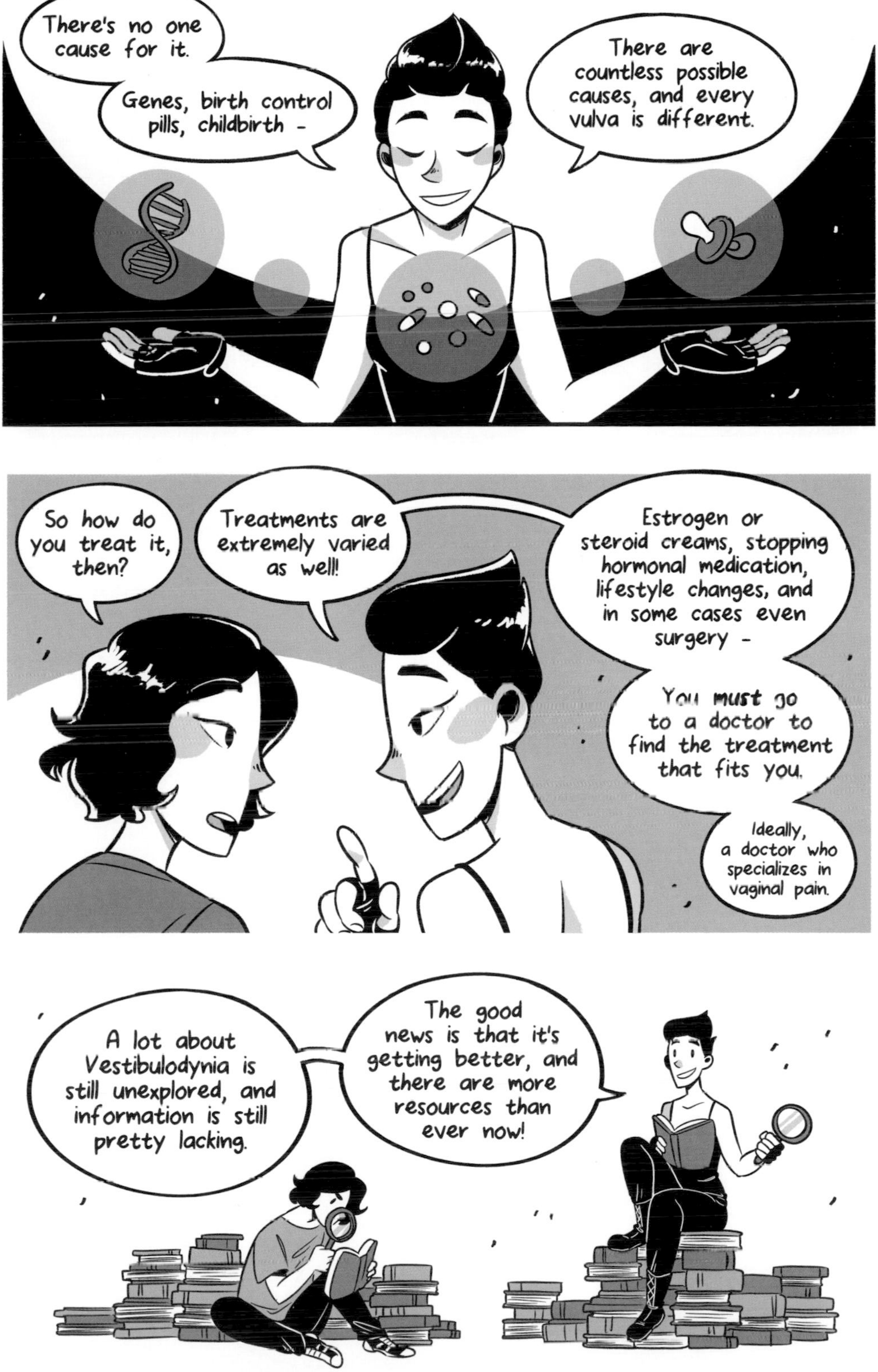
There's no one cause for it.
Genes, birth control pills, childbirth -
There are countless possible causes, and every vulva is different.
So how do you treat it, then?
Treatments are extremely varied as well!
Estrogen or steroid creams, stopping hormonal medication, lifestyle changes, and in some cases even surgery -
You **must** go to a doctor to find the treatment that fits you.
Ideally, a doctor who specializes in vaginal pain.
A lot about Vestibulodynia is still unexplored, and information is still pretty lacking.
The good news is that it's getting better, and there are more resources than ever now!

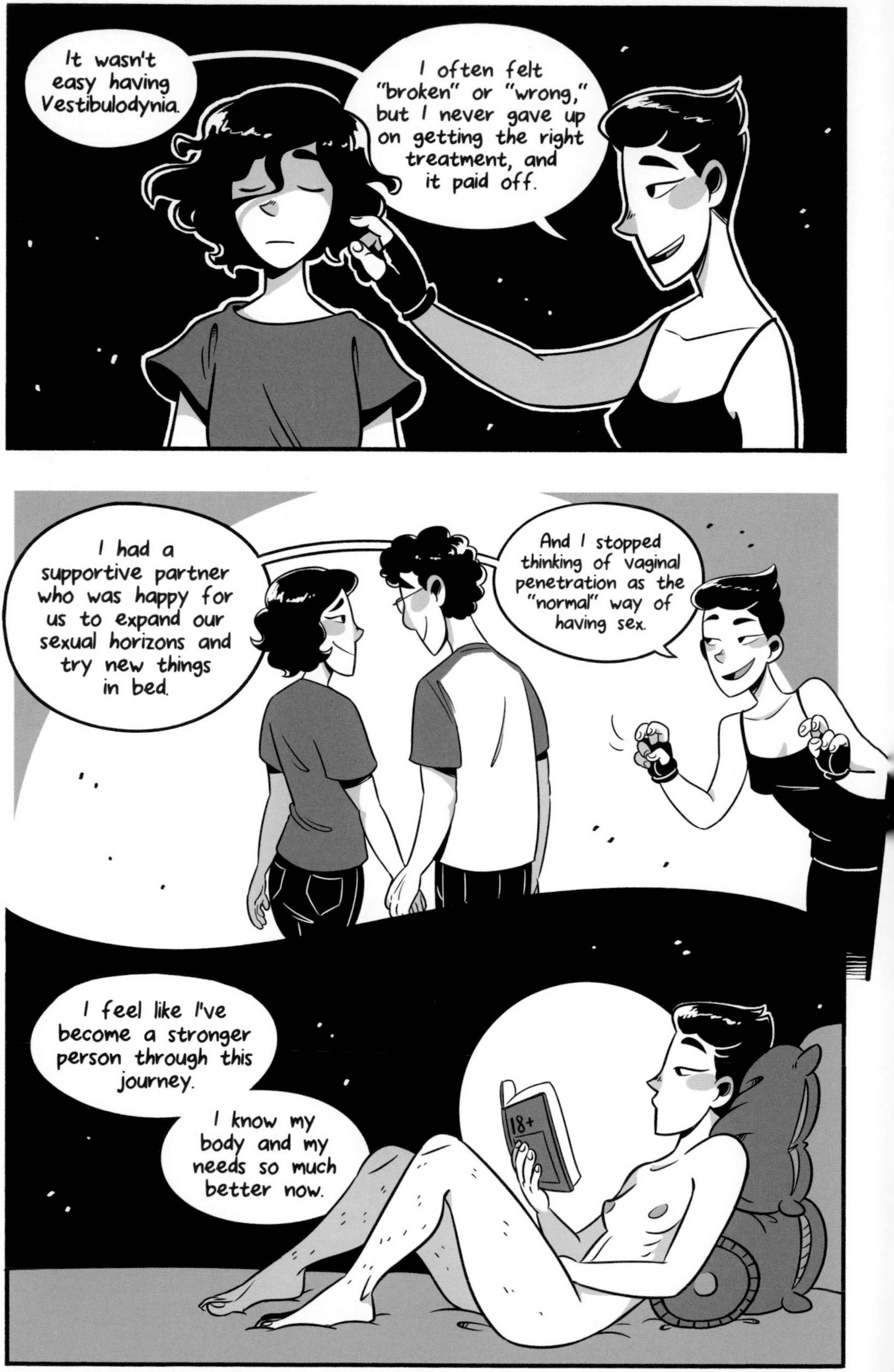

It wasn't easy having Vestibulodynia.
I often felt "broken" or "wrong," but I never gave up on getting the right treatment, and it paid off.
I had a supportive partner who was happy for us to expand our sexual horizons and try new things in bed.
And I stopped thinking of vaginal penetration as the "normal" way of having sex.
I feel like I've become a stronger person through this journey.
I know my body and my needs so much better now.
18+

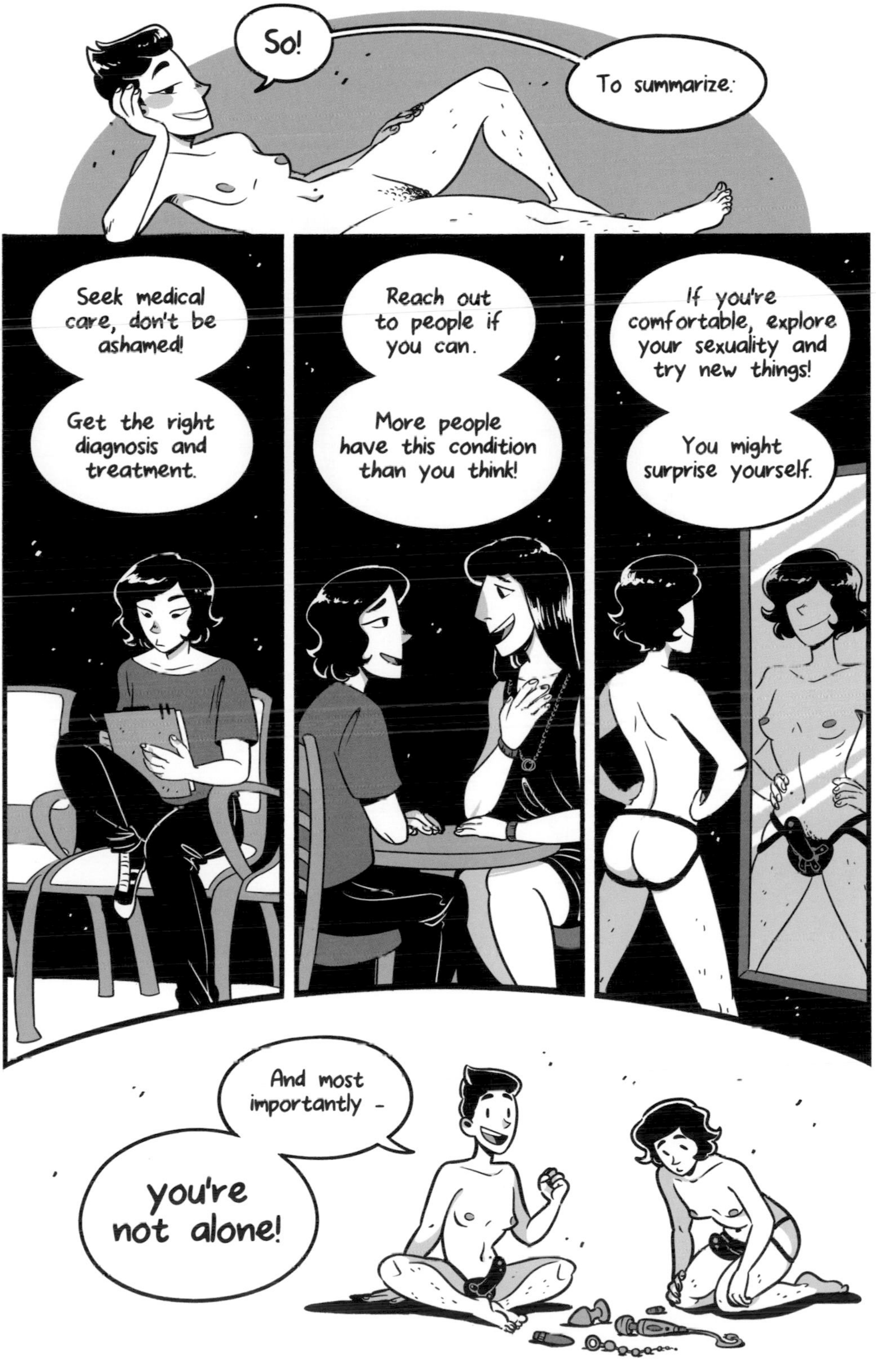

So!
To summarize:
Seek medical care, don't be ashamed!
Get the right diagnosis and treatment.
Reach out to people if you can.
More people have this condition than you think!
If you're comfortable, explore your sexuality and try new things!
You might surprise yourself.
And most importantly -
you're not alone!

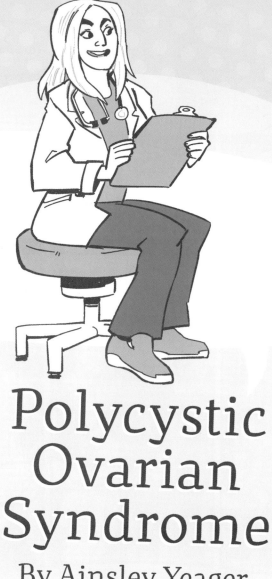

Polycystic Ovarian Syndrome

By Ainsley Yeager
Aainsleyy.com

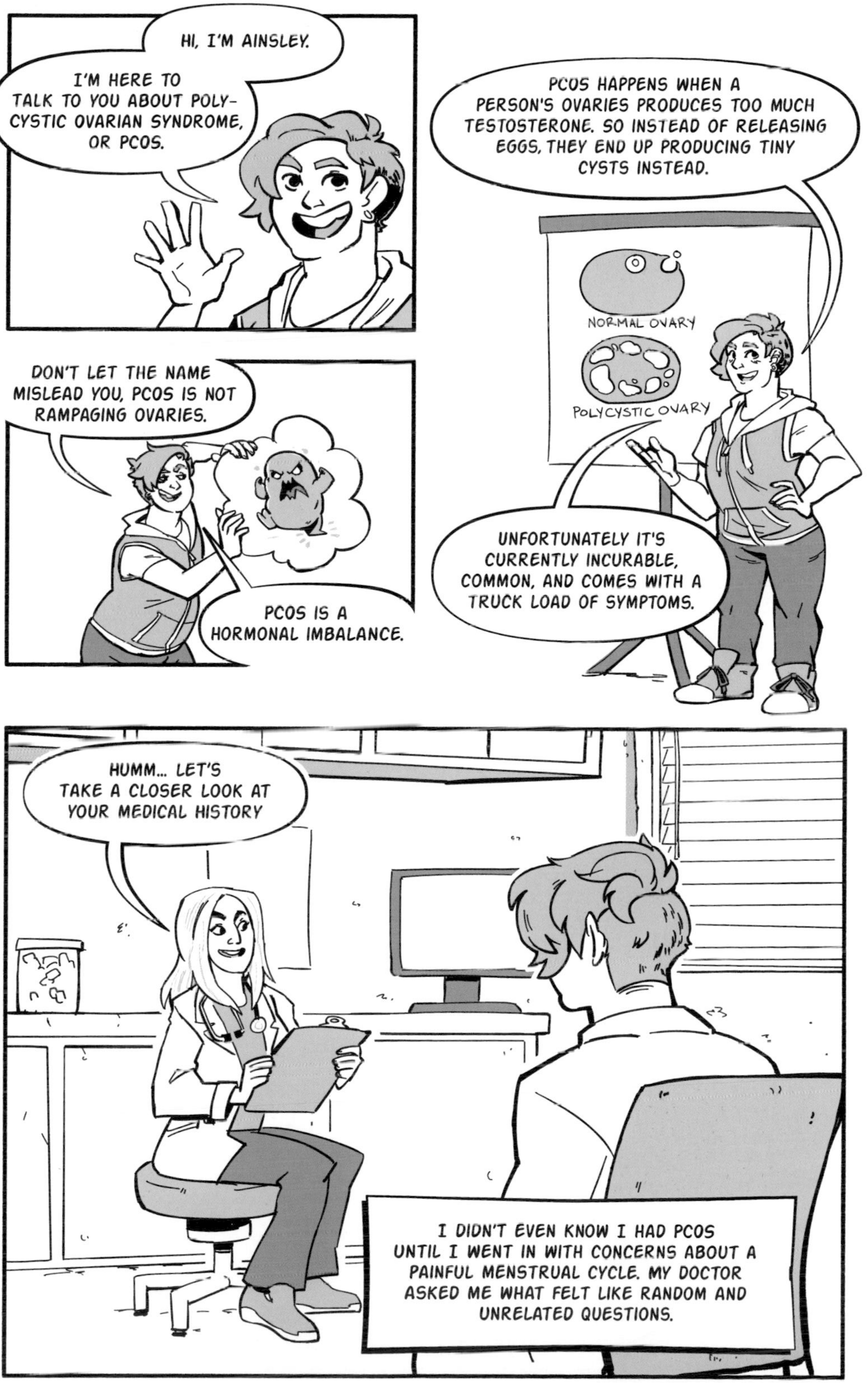
HI, I'M AINSLEY.
I'M HERE TO TALK TO YOU ABOUT POLY-CYSTIC OVARIAN SYNDROME, OR PCOS.
PCOS HAPPENS WHEN A PERSON'S OVARIES PRODUCES TOO MUCH TESTOSTERONE. SO INSTEAD OF RELEASING EGGS, THEY END UP PRODUCING TINY CYSTS INSTEAD.
NORMAL OVARY
POLYCYSTIC OVARY
DON'T LET THE NAME MISLEAD YOU, PCOS IS NOT RAMPAGING OVARIES.
PCOS IS A HORMONAL IMBALANCE.
UNFORTUNATELY IT'S CURRENTLY INCURABLE, COMMON, AND COMES WITH A TRUCK LOAD OF SYMPTOMS.
HUMM... LET'S TAKE A CLOSER LOOK AT YOUR MEDICAL HISTORY
I DIDN'T EVEN KNOW I HAD PCOS UNTIL I WENT IN WITH CONCERNS ABOUT A PAINFUL MENSTRUAL CYCLE. MY DOCTOR ASKED ME WHAT FELT LIKE RANDOM AND UNRELATED QUESTIONS.

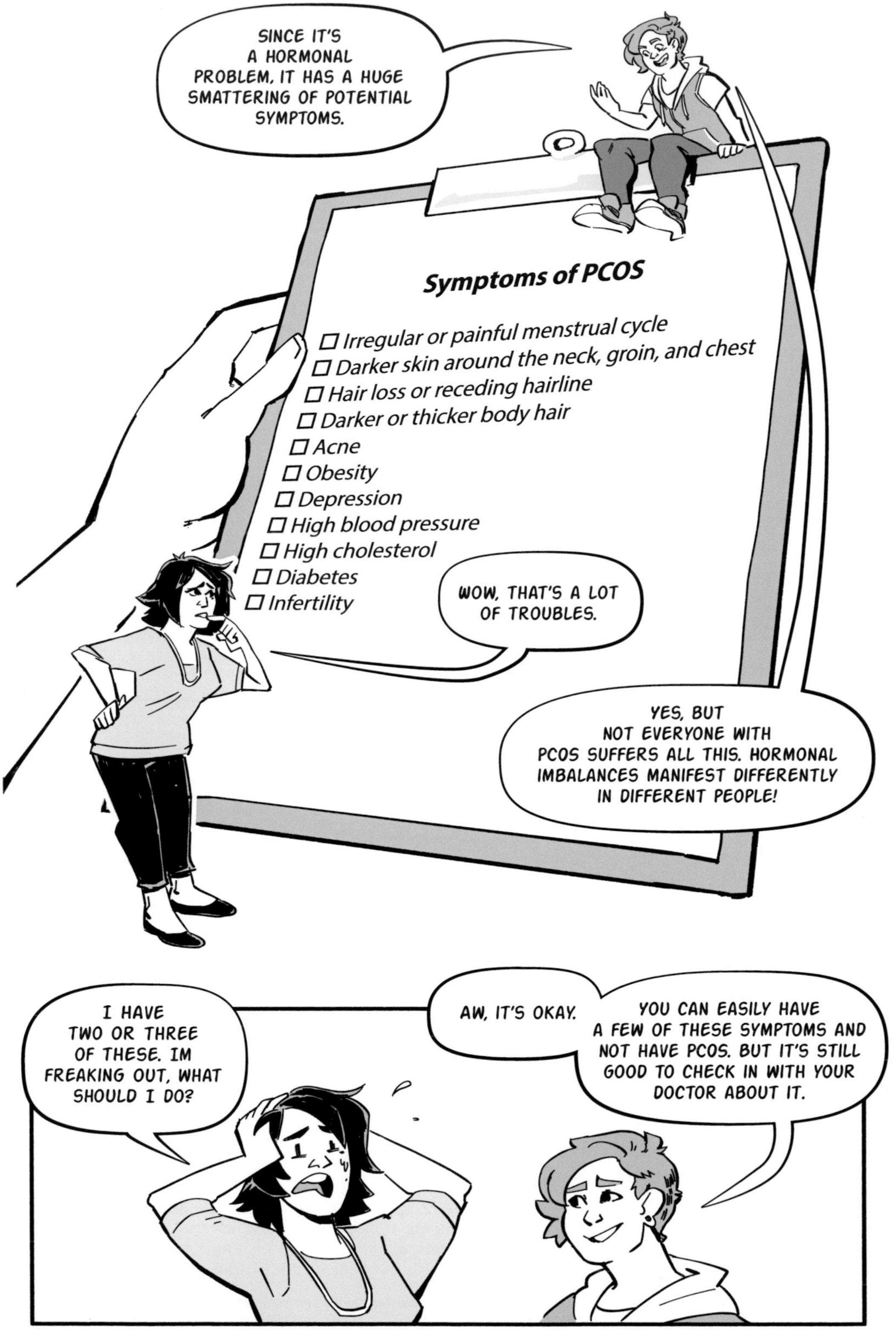
SINCE IT'S A HORMONAL PROBLEM, IT HAS A HUGE SMATTERING OF POTENTIAL SYMPTOMS.
Symptoms of PCOS
☐ Irregular or painful menstrual cycle
☐ Darker skin around the neck, groin, and chest
☐ Hair loss or receding hairline
☐ Darker or thicker body hair
☐ Acne
☐ Obesity
☐ Depression
☐ High blood pressure
☐ High cholesterol
☐ Diabetes
☐ Infertility
WOW, THAT'S A LOT OF TROUBLES.
YES, BUT NOT EVERYONE WITH PCOS SUFFERS ALL THIS. HORMONAL IMBALANCES MANIFEST DIFFERENTLY IN DIFFERENT PEOPLE!
I HAVE TWO OR THREE OF THESE. IM FREAKING OUT, WHAT SHOULD I DO?
AW, IT'S OKAY.
YOU CAN EASILY HAVE A FEW OF THESE SYMPTOMS AND NOT HAVE PCOS. BUT IT'S STILL GOOD TO CHECK IN WITH YOUR DOCTOR ABOUT IT.

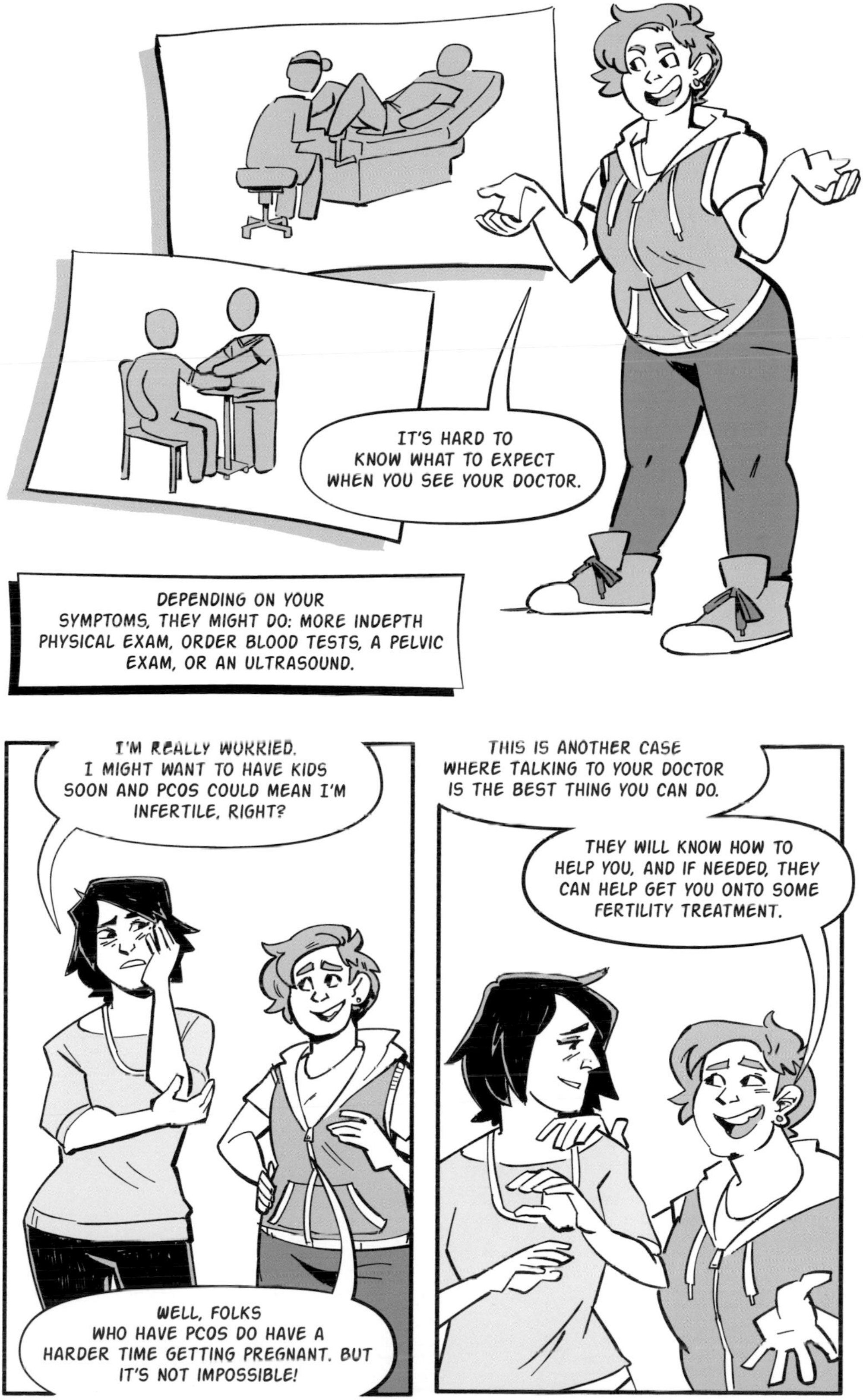
IT'S HARD TO KNOW WHAT TO EXPECT WHEN YOU SEE YOUR DOCTOR.
DEPENDING ON YOUR SYMPTOMS, THEY MIGHT DO: MORE INDEPTH PHYSICAL EXAM, ORDER BLOOD TESTS, A PELVIC EXAM, OR AN ULTRASOUND.
I'M REALLY WORRIED. I MIGHT WANT TO HAVE KIDS SOON AND PCOS COULD MEAN I'M INFERTILE, RIGHT?
WELL, FOLKS WHO HAVE PCOS DO HAVE A HARDER TIME GETTING PREGNANT. BUT IT'S NOT IMPOSSIBLE!
THIS IS ANOTHER CASE WHERE TALKING TO YOUR DOCTOR IS THE BEST THING YOU CAN DO.
THEY WILL KNOW HOW TO HELP YOU, AND IF NEEDED, THEY CAN HELP GET YOU ONTO SOME FERTILITY TREATMENT.

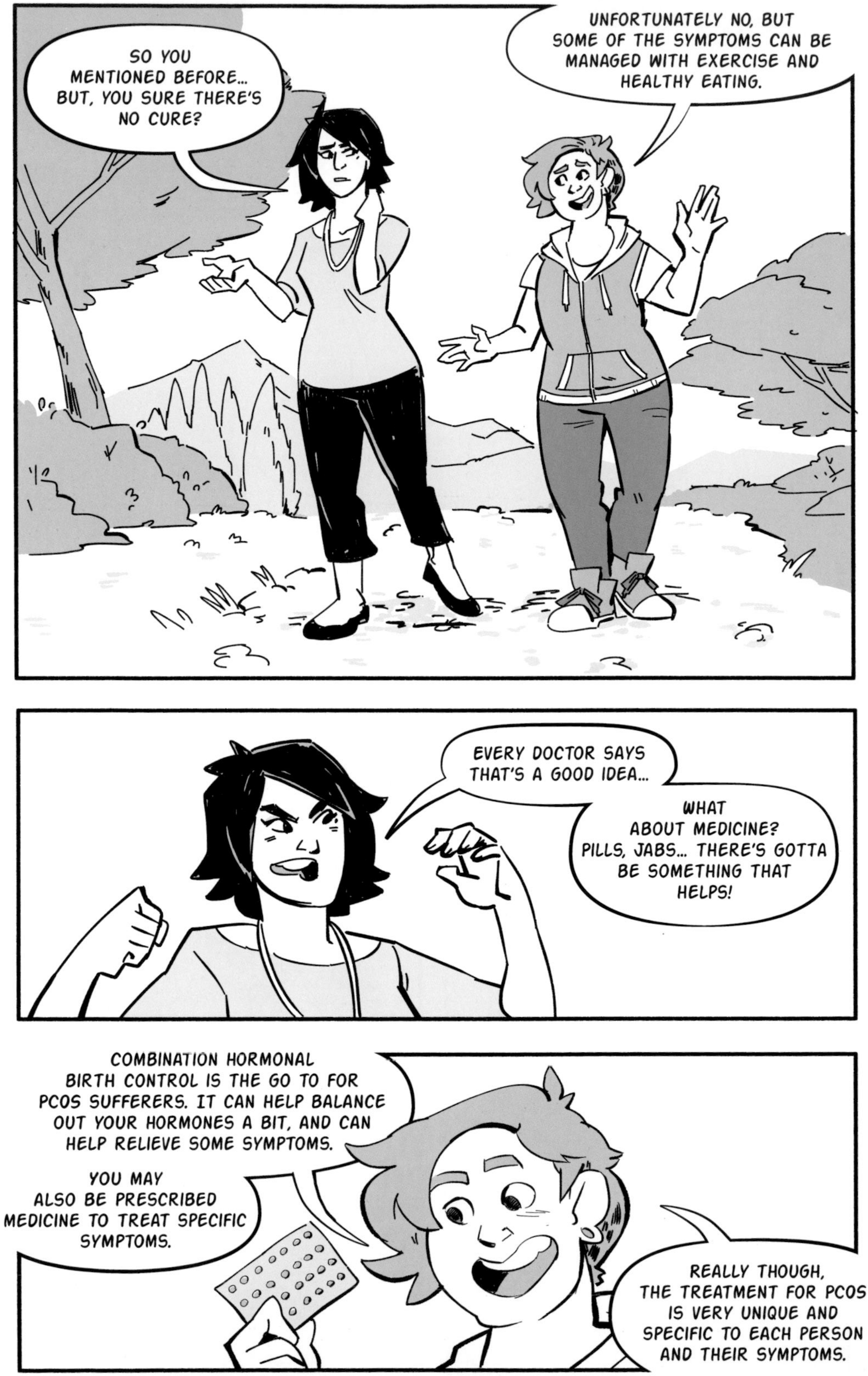
SO YOU MENTIONED BEFORE... BUT, YOU SURE THERE'S NO CURE?
UNFORTUNATELY NO, BUT SOME OF THE SYMPTOMS CAN BE MANAGED WITH EXERCISE AND HEALTHY EATING.
EVERY DOCTOR SAYS THAT'S A GOOD IDEA...
WHAT ABOUT MEDICINE? PILLS, JABS... THERE'S GOTTA BE SOMETHING THAT HELPS!
COMBINATION HORMONAL BIRTH CONTROL IS THE GO TO FOR PCOS SUFFERERS. IT CAN HELP BALANCE OUT YOUR HORMONES A BIT, AND CAN HELP RELIEVE SOME SYMPTOMS.
YOU MAY ALSO BE PRESCRIBED MEDICINE TO TREAT SPECIFIC SYMPTOMS.
REALLY THOUGH, THE TREATMENT FOR PCOS IS VERY UNIQUE AND SPECIFIC TO EACH PERSON AND THEIR SYMPTOMS.

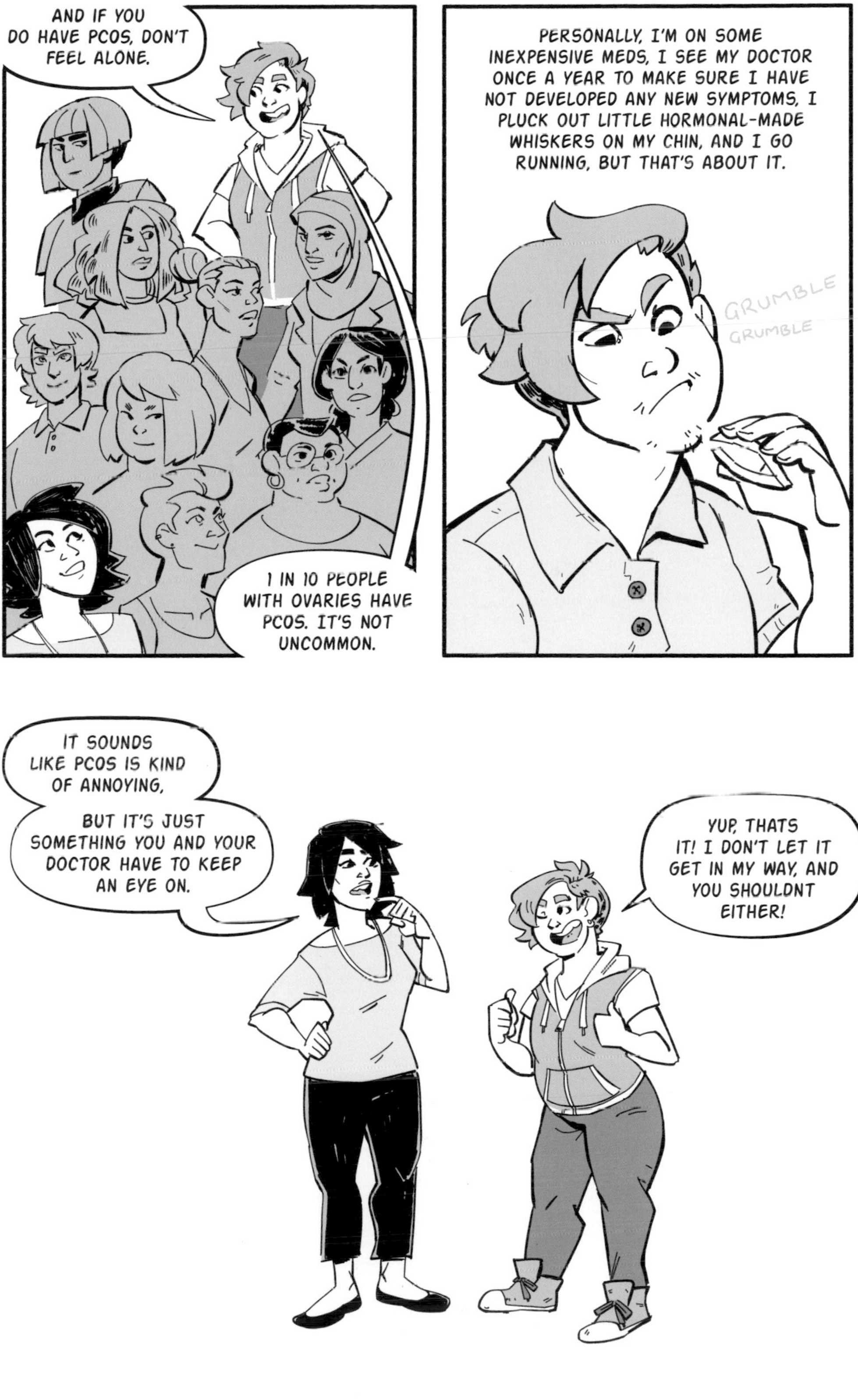
AND IF YOU DO HAVE PCOS, DON'T FEEL ALONE.
1 IN 10 PEOPLE WITH OVARIES HAVE PCOS. IT'S NOT UNCOMMON.
PERSONALLY, I'M ON SOME INEXPENSIVE MEDS, I SEE MY DOCTOR ONCE A YEAR TO MAKE SURE I HAVE NOT DEVELOPED ANY NEW SYMPTOMS, I PLUCK OUT LITTLE HORMONAL-MADE WHISKERS ON MY CHIN, AND I GO RUNNING, BUT THAT'S ABOUT IT.
GRUMBLE
GRUMBLE
IT SOUNDS LIKE PCOS IS KIND OF ANNOYING,
BUT IT'S JUST SOMETHING YOU AND YOUR DOCTOR HAVE TO KEEP AN EYE ON.
YUP, THATS IT! I DON'T LET IT GET IN MY WAY, AND YOU SHOULDNT EITHER!

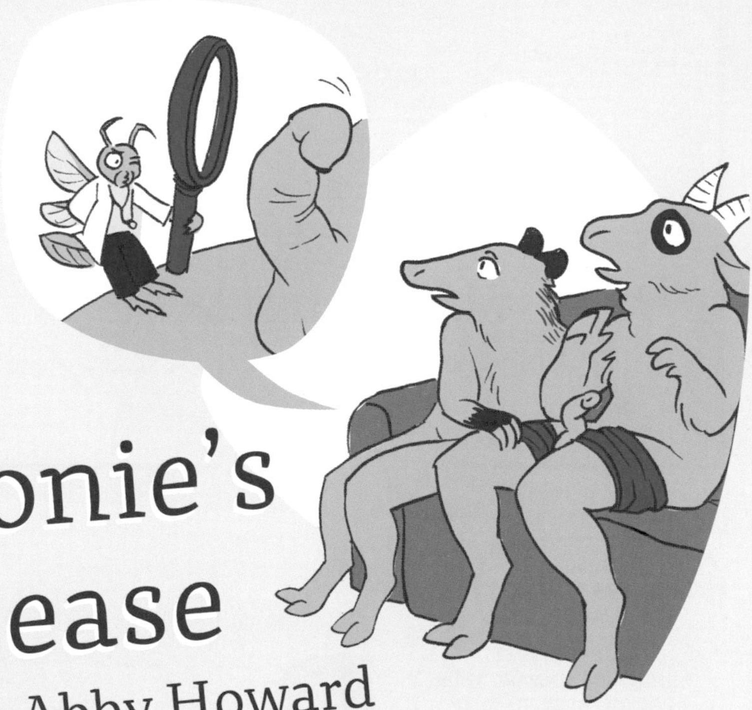

Peyronie's Disease

By Abby Howard
Abbyhowardart.myportfolio.com

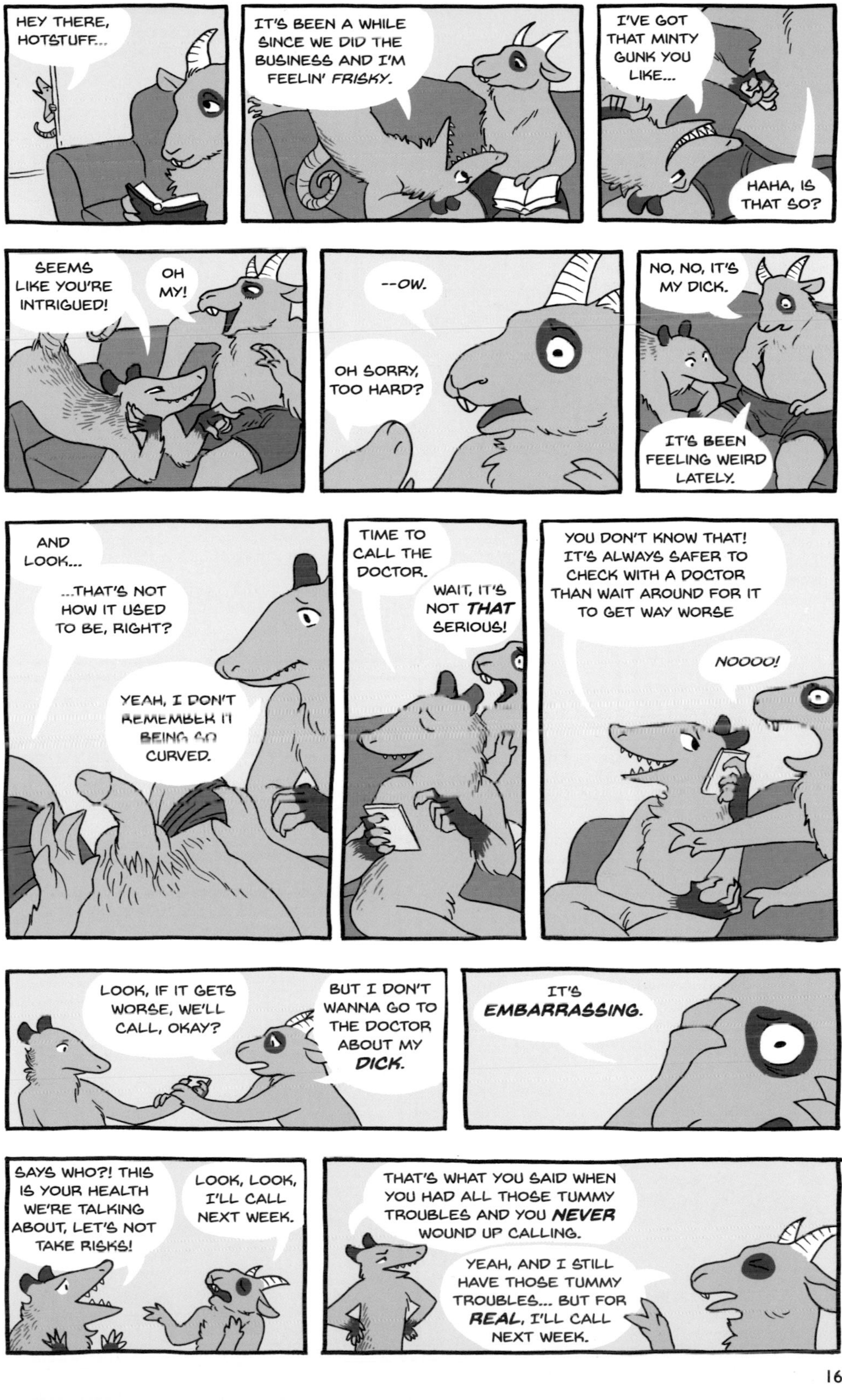
HEY THERE, HOTSTUFF...
IT'S BEEN A WHILE SINCE WE DID THE BUSINESS AND I'M FEELIN' *FRISKY*.
I'VE GOT THAT MINTY GUNK YOU LIKE...
HAHA, IS THAT SO?
SEEMS LIKE YOU'RE INTRIGUED!
OH MY!
--*OW.*
OH SORRY, TOO HARD?
NO, NO, IT'S MY DICK.
IT'S BEEN FEELING WEIRD LATELY.
AND LOOK...
...THAT'S NOT HOW IT USED TO BE, RIGHT?
YEAH, I DON'T REMEMBER IT BEING SO CURVED.
TIME TO CALL THE DOCTOR.
WAIT, IT'S NOT ***THAT*** SERIOUS!
YOU DON'T KNOW THAT! IT'S ALWAYS SAFER TO CHECK WITH A DOCTOR THAN WAIT AROUND FOR IT TO GET WAY WORSE
NOOOO!
LOOK, IF IT GETS WORSE, WE'LL CALL, OKAY?
BUT I DON'T WANNA GO TO THE DOCTOR ABOUT MY ***DICK.***
IT'S ***EMBARRASSING.***
SAYS WHO?! THIS IS YOUR HEALTH WE'RE TALKING ABOUT, LET'S NOT TAKE RISKS!
LOOK, LOOK, I'LL CALL NEXT WEEK.
THAT'S WHAT YOU SAID WHEN YOU HAD ALL THOSE TUMMY TROUBLES AND YOU ***NEVER*** WOUND UP CALLING.
YEAH, AND I STILL HAVE THOSE TUMMY TROUBLES... BUT FOR ***REAL***, I'LL CALL NEXT WEEK.

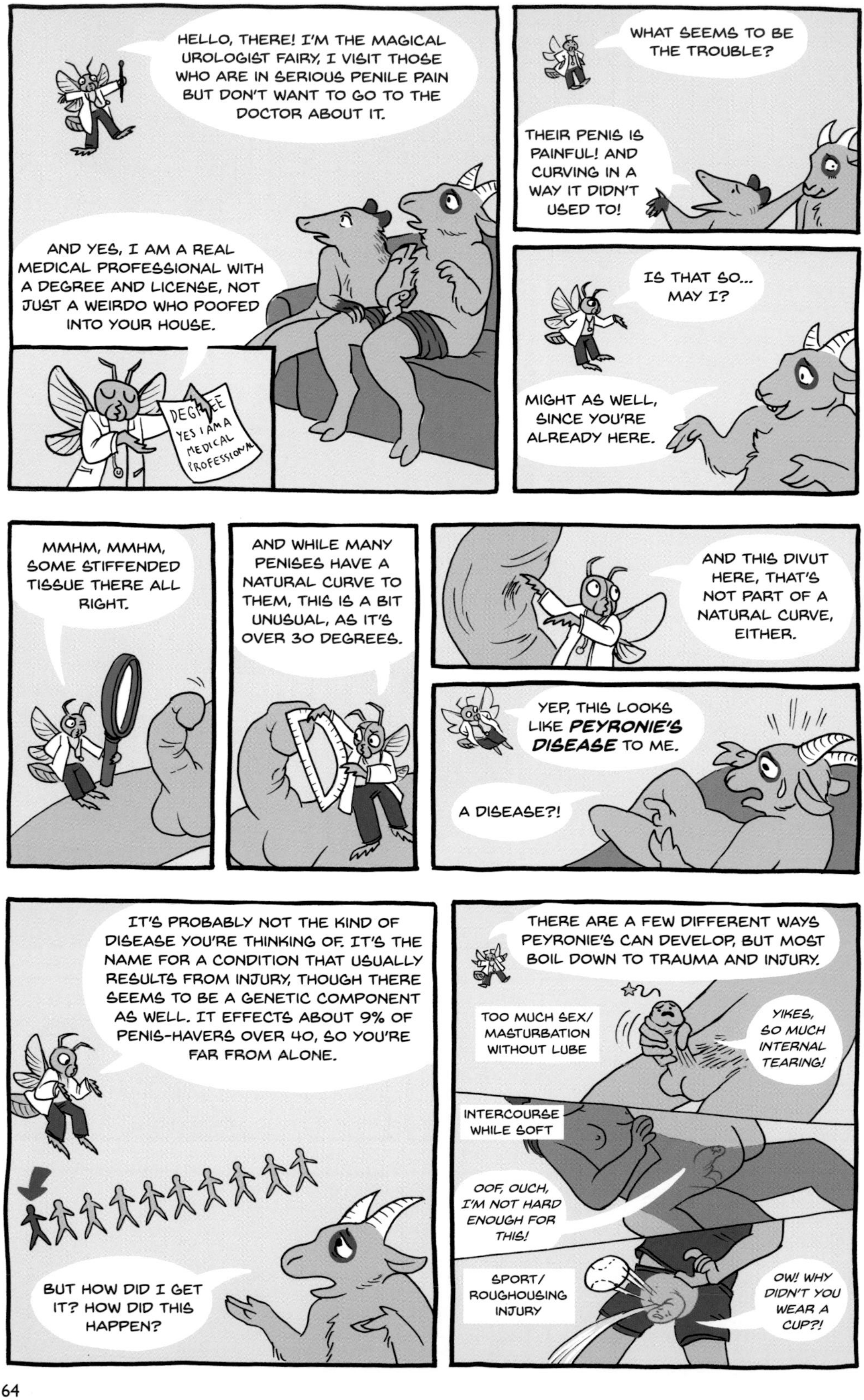
HELLO, THERE! I'M THE MAGICAL UROLOGIST FAIRY, I VISIT THOSE WHO ARE IN SERIOUS PENILE PAIN BUT DON'T WANT TO GO TO THE DOCTOR ABOUT IT.
AND YES, I AM A REAL MEDICAL PROFESSIONAL WITH A DEGREE AND LICENSE, NOT JUST A WEIRDO WHO POOFED INTO YOUR HOUSE.
DEGREE
YES I AM A MEDICAL PROFESSIONAL
WHAT SEEMS TO BE THE TROUBLE?
THEIR PENIS IS PAINFUL! AND CURVING IN A WAY IT DIDN'T USED TO!
IS THAT SO... MAY I?
MIGHT AS WELL, SINCE YOU'RE ALREADY HERE.
MMHM, MMHM, SOME STIFFENDED TISSUE THERE ALL RIGHT.
AND WHILE MANY PENISES HAVE A NATURAL CURVE TO THEM, THIS IS A BIT UNUSUAL, AS IT'S OVER 30 DEGREES.
AND THIS DIVUT HERE, THAT'S NOT PART OF A NATURAL CURVE, EITHER.
YEP, THIS LOOKS LIKE PEYRONIE'S DISEASE TO ME.
A DISEASE?!
IT'S PROBABLY NOT THE KIND OF DISEASE YOU'RE THINKING OF. IT'S THE NAME FOR A CONDITION THAT USUALLY RESULTS FROM INJURY, THOUGH THERE SEEMS TO BE A GENETIC COMPONENT AS WELL. IT EFFECTS ABOUT 9% OF PENIS-HAVERS OVER 40, SO YOU'RE FAR FROM ALONE.
BUT HOW DID I GET IT? HOW DID THIS HAPPEN?
THERE ARE A FEW DIFFERENT WAYS PEYRONIE'S CAN DEVELOP, BUT MOST BOIL DOWN TO TRAUMA AND INJURY.
TOO MUCH SEX/ MASTURBATION WITHOUT LUBE
YIKES, SO MUCH INTERNAL TEARING!
INTERCOURSE WHILE SOFT
OOF, OUCH, I'M NOT HARD ENOUGH FOR THIS!
SPORT/ ROUGHOUSING INJURY
OW! WHY DIDN'T YOU WEAR A CUP?!

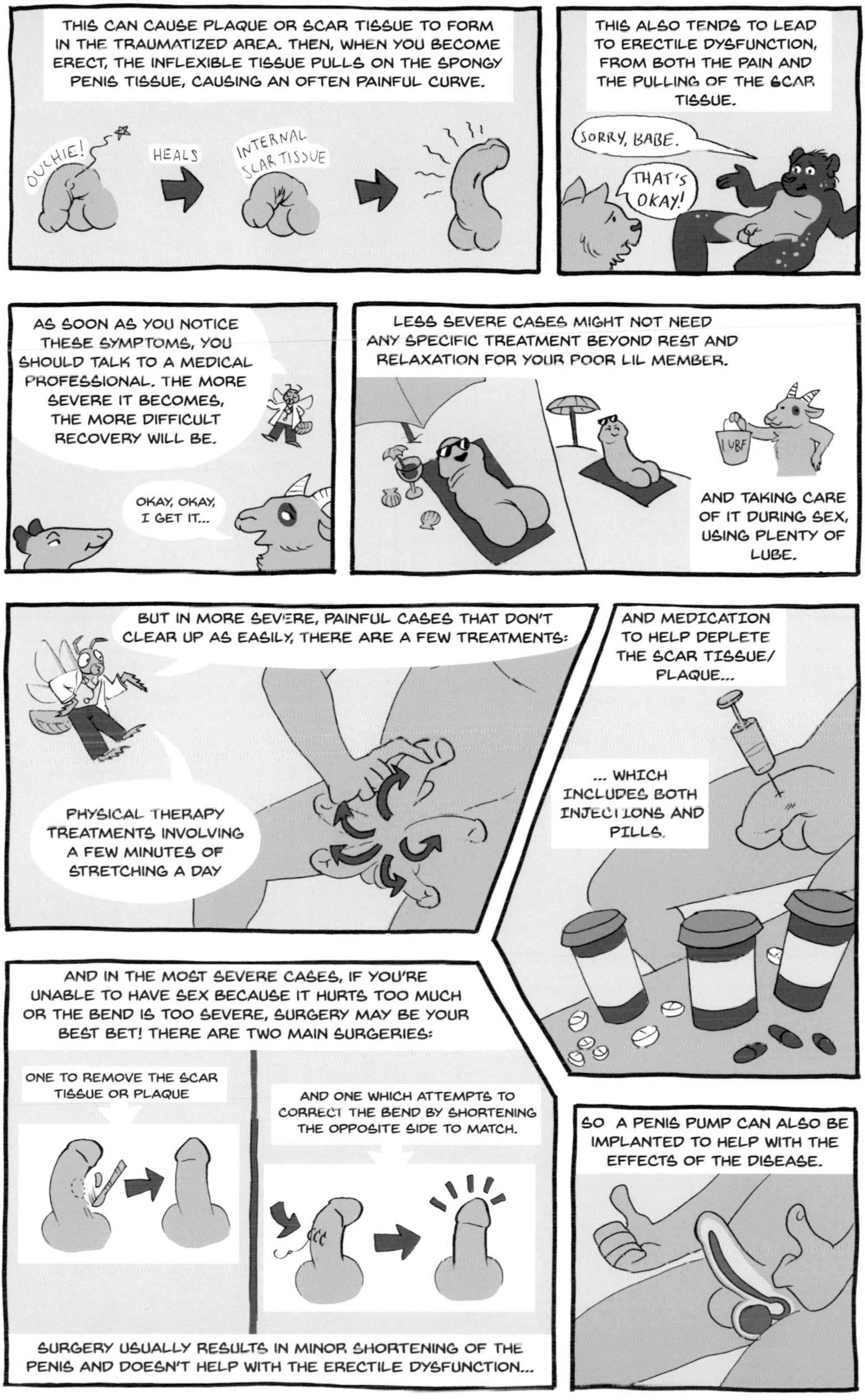
THIS CAN CAUSE PLAQUE OR SCAR TISSUE TO FORM IN THE TRAUMATIZED AREA. THEN, WHEN YOU BECOME ERECT, THE INFLEXIBLE TISSUE PULLS ON THE SPONGY PENIS TISSUE, CAUSING AN OFTEN PAINFUL CURVE.
OUCHIE!
HEALS
INTERNAL SCAR TISSUE
THIS ALSO TENDS TO LEAD TO ERECTILE DYSFUNCTION, FROM BOTH THE PAIN AND THE PULLING OF THE SCAR TISSUE.
SORRY, BABE.
THAT'S OKAY!
AS SOON AS YOU NOTICE THESE SYMPTOMS, YOU SHOULD TALK TO A MEDICAL PROFESSIONAL. THE MORE SEVERE IT BECOMES, THE MORE DIFFICULT RECOVERY WILL BE.
OKAY, OKAY, I GET IT...
LESS SEVERE CASES MIGHT NOT NEED ANY SPECIFIC TREATMENT BEYOND REST AND RELAXATION FOR YOUR POOR LIL MEMBER.
LUBE
AND TAKING CARE OF IT DURING SEX, USING PLENTY OF LUBE.
BUT IN MORE SEVERE, PAINFUL CASES THAT DON'T CLEAR UP AS EASILY, THERE ARE A FEW TREATMENTS:
PHYSICAL THERAPY TREATMENTS INVOLVING A FEW MINUTES OF STRETCHING A DAY
AND MEDICATION TO HELP DEPLETE THE SCAR TISSUE/ PLAQUE...
... WHICH INCLUDES BOTH INJECTIONS AND PILLS.
AND IN THE MOST SEVERE CASES, IF YOU'RE UNABLE TO HAVE SEX BECAUSE IT HURTS TOO MUCH OR THE BEND IS TOO SEVERE, SURGERY MAY BE YOUR BEST BET! THERE ARE TWO MAIN SURGERIES:
ONE TO REMOVE THE SCAR TISSUE OR PLAQUE
AND ONE WHICH ATTEMPTS TO CORRECT THE BEND BY SHORTENING THE OPPOSITE SIDE TO MATCH.
SURGERY USUALLY RESULTS IN MINOR SHORTENING OF THE PENIS AND DOESN'T HELP WITH THE ERECTILE DYSFUNCTION...
SO A PENIS PUMP CAN ALSO BE IMPLANTED TO HELP WITH THE EFFECTS OF THE DISEASE.

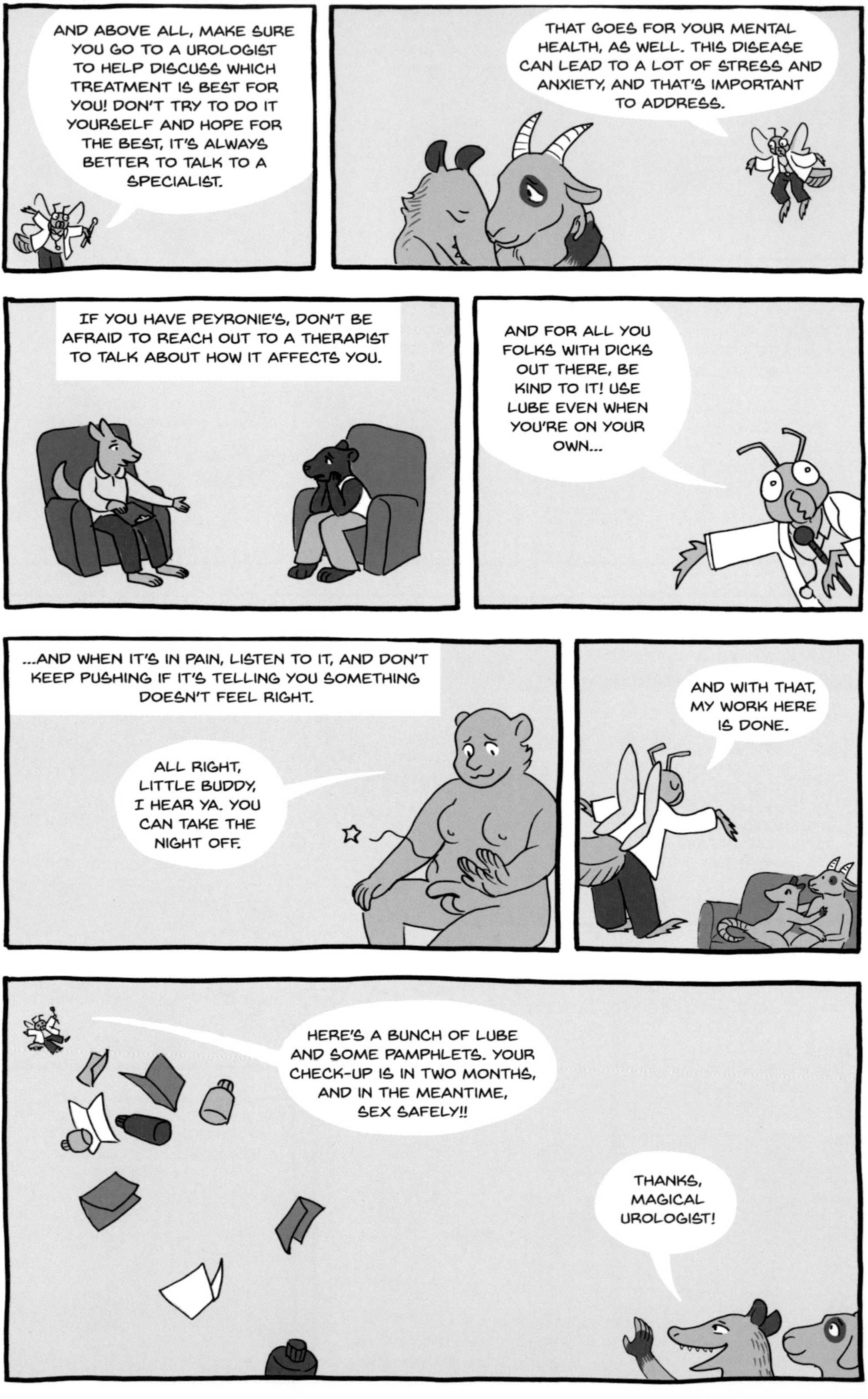
AND ABOVE ALL, MAKE SURE YOU GO TO A UROLOGIST TO HELP DISCUSS WHICH TREATMENT IS BEST FOR YOU! DON'T TRY TO DO IT YOURSELF AND HOPE FOR THE BEST, IT'S ALWAYS BETTER TO TALK TO A SPECIALIST.
THAT GOES FOR YOUR MENTAL HEALTH, AS WELL. THIS DISEASE CAN LEAD TO A LOT OF STRESS AND ANXIETY, AND THAT'S IMPORTANT TO ADDRESS.
IF YOU HAVE PEYRONIE'S, DON'T BE AFRAID TO REACH OUT TO A THERAPIST TO TALK ABOUT HOW IT AFFECTS YOU.
AND FOR ALL YOU FOLKS WITH DICKS OUT THERE, BE KIND TO IT! USE LUBE EVEN WHEN YOU'RE ON YOUR OWN...
...AND WHEN IT'S IN PAIN, LISTEN TO IT, AND DON'T KEEP PUSHING IF IT'S TELLING YOU SOMETHING DOESN'T FEEL RIGHT.
ALL RIGHT, LITTLE BUDDY, I HEAR YA. YOU CAN TAKE THE NIGHT OFF.
AND WITH THAT, MY WORK HERE IS DONE.
HERE'S A BUNCH OF LUBE AND SOME PAMPHLETS. YOUR CHECK-UP IS IN TWO MONTHS, AND IN THE MEANTIME, SEX SAFELY!!
THANKS, MAGICAL UROLOGIST!

SEX

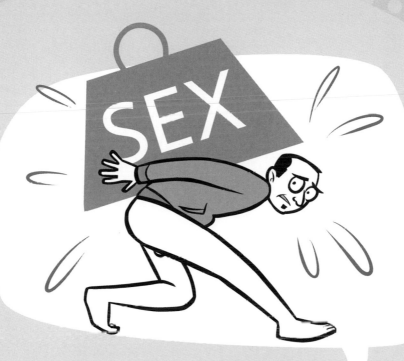

Sexual Dysfunction

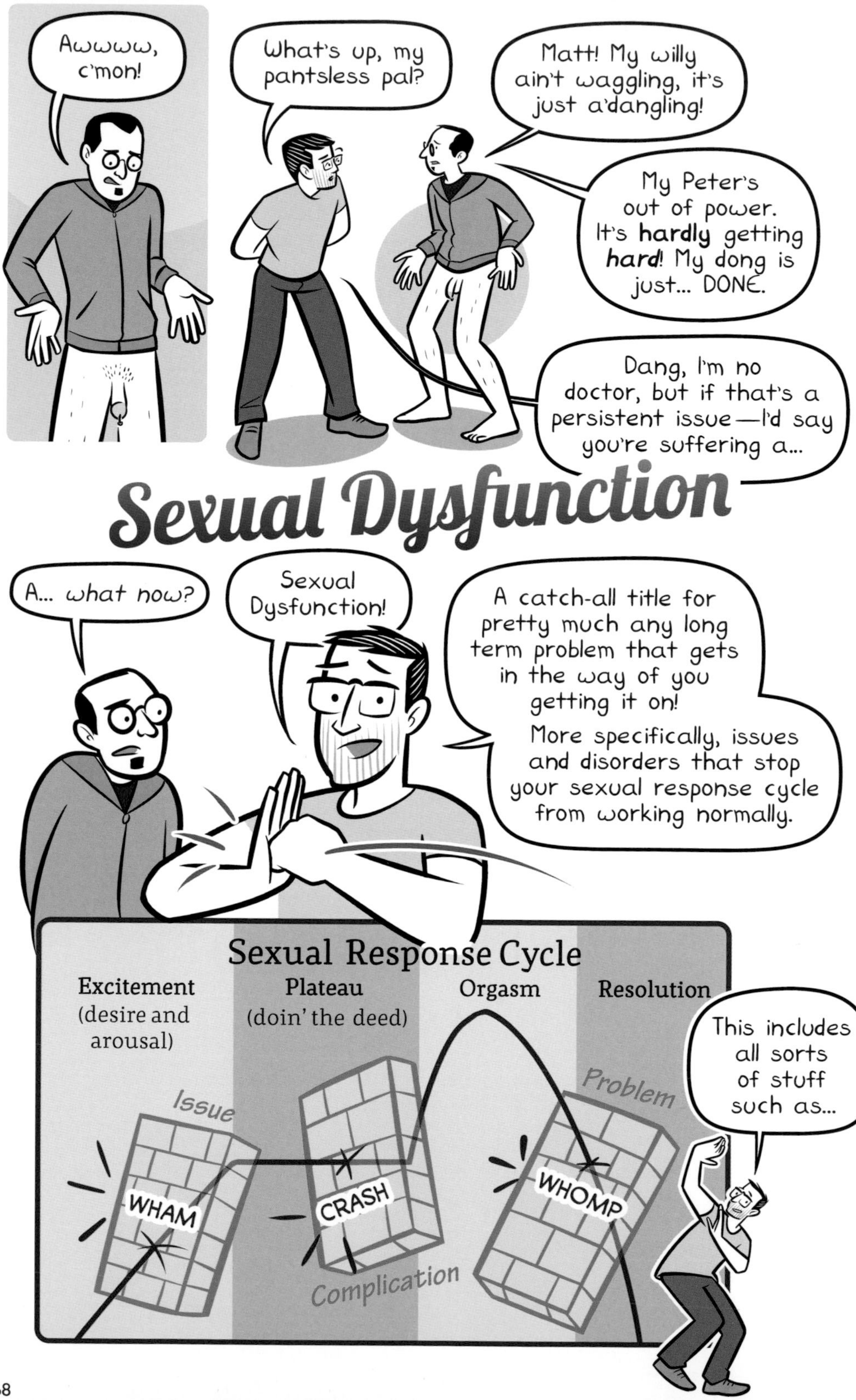
Awwww, c'mon!
What's up, my pantsless pal?
Matt! My willy ain't waggling, it's just a'dangling!
My Peter's out of power. It's **hardly** getting ***hard***! My dong is just... DONE.
Dang, I'm no doctor, but if that's a persistent issue—I'd say you're suffering a...
Sexual Dysfunction
A... what now?
Sexual Dysfunction!
A catch-all title for pretty much any long term problem that gets in the way of you getting it on!
More specifically, issues and disorders that stop your sexual response cycle from working normally.
Sexual Response Cycle
Excitement (desire and arousal)
Plateau (doin' the deed)
Orgasm
Resolution
Issue
WHAM
CRASH
Complication
Problem
WHOMP
This includes all sorts of stuff such as...

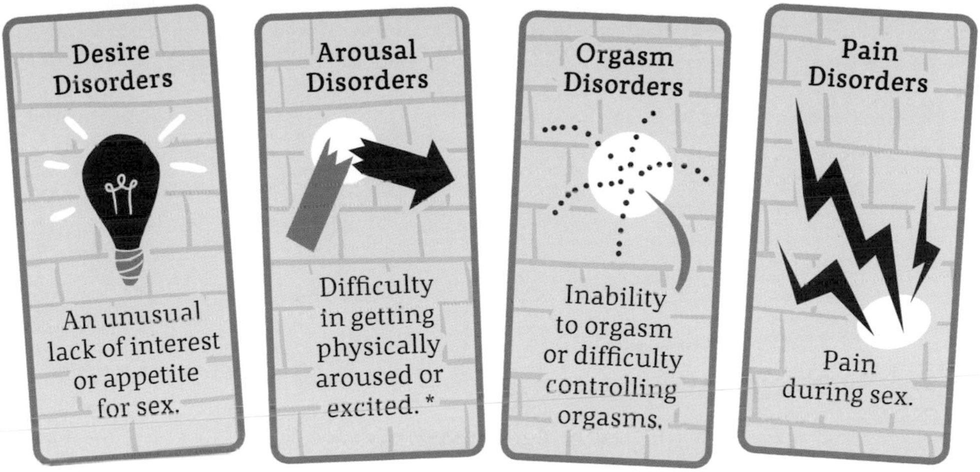
Desire Disorders
An unusual lack of interest or appetite for sex.
Arousal Disorders
Difficulty in getting physically aroused or excited. *
Orgasm Disorders
Inability to orgasm or difficulty controlling orgasms.
Pain Disorders
Pain during sex.

* Stuff like not being able to get hard, wet, or relaxed enough to allow for activity.

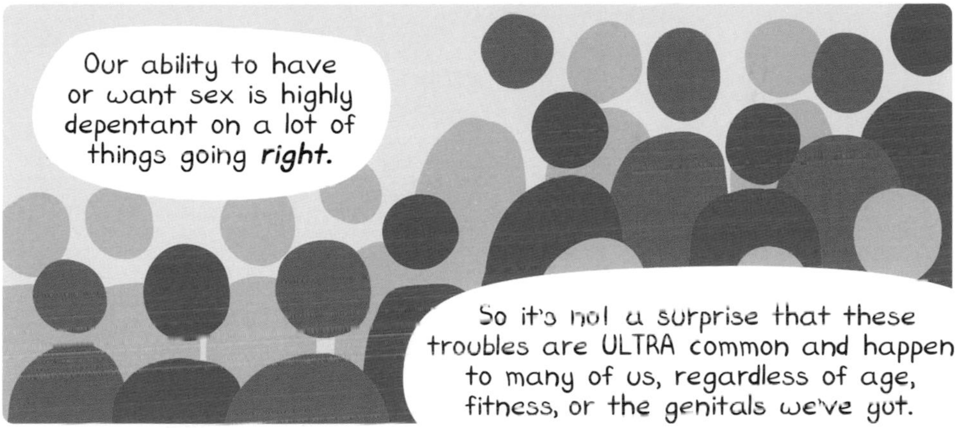
Our ability to have or want sex is highly depentant on a lot of things going *right*.
So it's not a surprise that these troubles are ULTRA common and happen to many of us, regardless of age, fitness, or the genitals we've got.

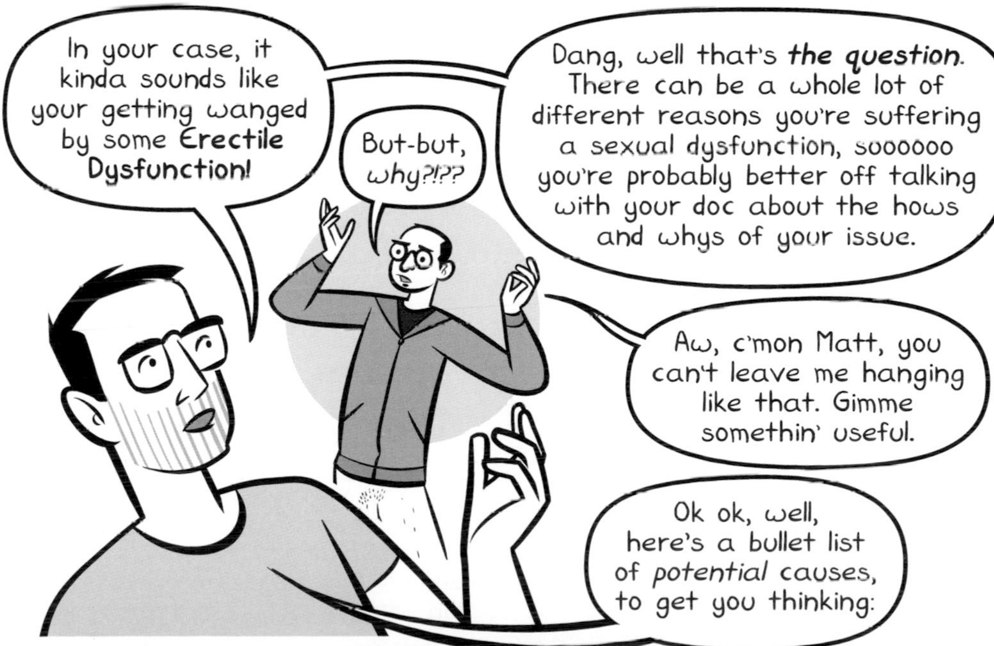
In your case, it kinda sounds like your getting wanged by some **Erectile Dysfunction!**
But-but, *why?!??*
Dang, well that's ***the question***. There can be a whole lot of different reasons you're suffering a sexual dysfunction, soooooo you're probably better off talking with your doc about the hows and whys of your issue.
Aw, c'mon Matt, you can't leave me hanging like that. Gimme somethin' useful.
Ok ok, well, here's a bullet list of *potential* causes, to get you thinking:

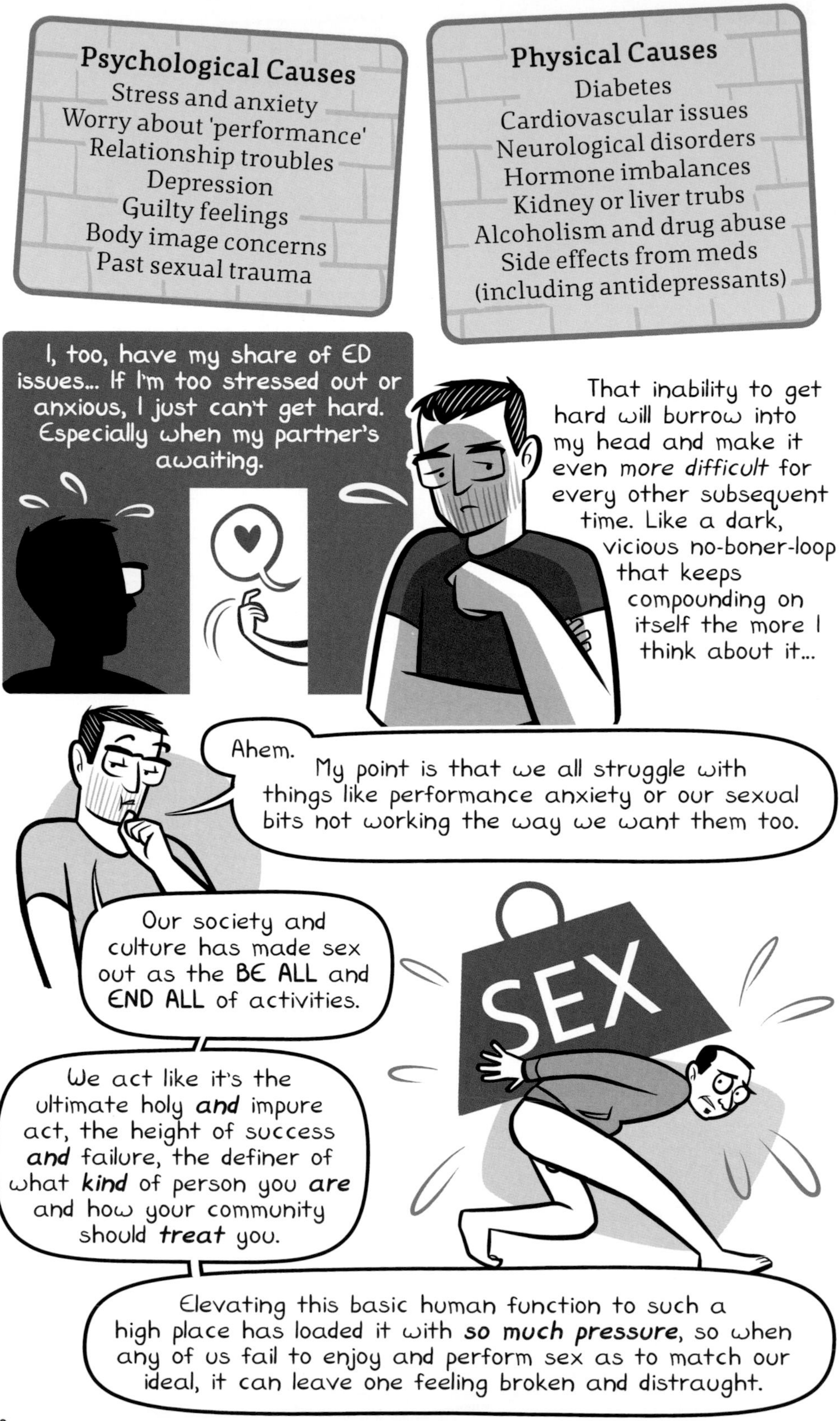
Psychological Causes
Stress and anxiety
Worry about 'performance'
Relationship troubles
Depression
Guilty feelings
Body image concerns
Past sexual trauma
Physical Causes
Diabetes
Cardiovascular issues
Neurological disorders
Hormone imbalances
Kidney or liver trubs
Alcoholism and drug abuse
Side effects from meds
(including antidepressants)
I, too, have my share of ED issues... If I'm too stressed out or anxious, I just can't get hard. Especially when my partner's awaiting.
That inability to get hard will burrow into my head and make it even more *difficult* for every other subsequent time. Like a dark, vicious no-boner-loop that keeps compounding on itself the more I think about it...
Ahem.
My point is that we all struggle with things like performance anxiety or our sexual bits not working the way we want them too.
Our society and culture has made sex out as the **BE ALL** and **END ALL** of activities.
SEX
We act like it's the ultimate holy ***and*** impure act, the height of success ***and*** failure, the definer of what ***kind*** of person you ***are*** and how your community should ***treat*** you.
Elevating this basic human function to such a high place has loaded it with ***so much pressure***, so when any of us fail to enjoy and perform sex as to match our ideal, it can leave one feeling broken and distraught.

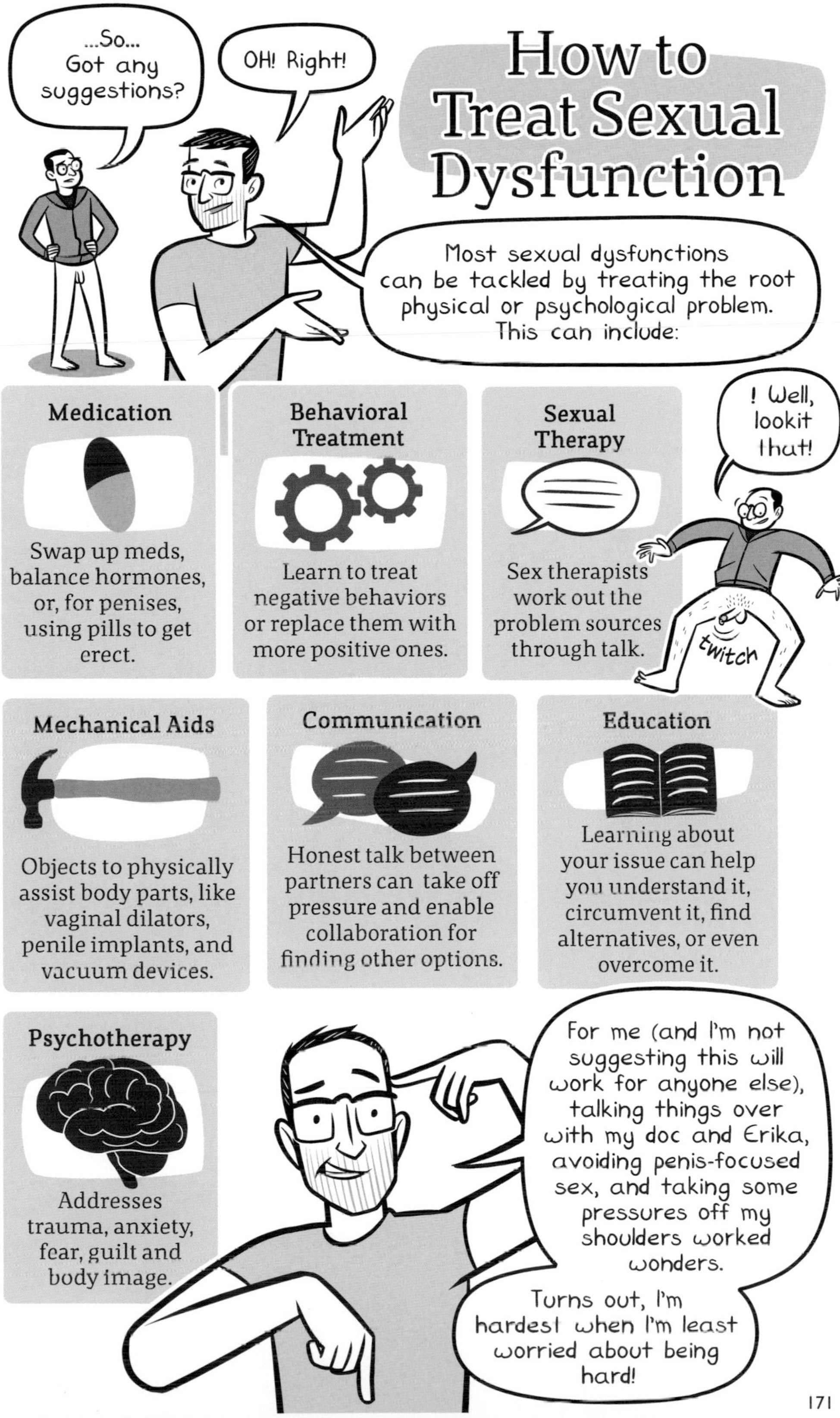
...So...
Got any suggestions?
OH! Right!
How to Treat Sexual Dysfunction
Most sexual dysfunctions can be tackled by treating the root physical or psychological problem. This can include:
Medication
Swap up meds, balance hormones, or, for penises, using pills to get erect.
Behavioral Treatment
Learn to treat negative behaviors or replace them with more positive ones.
Sexual Therapy
Sex therapists work out the problem sources through talk.
! Well, lookit that!
twitch
Mechanical Aids
Objects to physically assist body parts, like vaginal dilators, penile implants, and vacuum devices.
Communication
Honest talk between partners can take off pressure and enable collaboration for finding other options.
Education
Learning about your issue can help you understand it, circumvent it, find alternatives, or even overcome it.
Psychotherapy
Addresses trauma, anxiety, fear, guilt and body image.
For me (and I'm not suggesting this will work for anyone else), talking things over with my doc and Erika, avoiding penis-focused sex, and taking some pressures off my shoulders worked wonders.
Turns out, I'm hardest when I'm least worried about being hard!

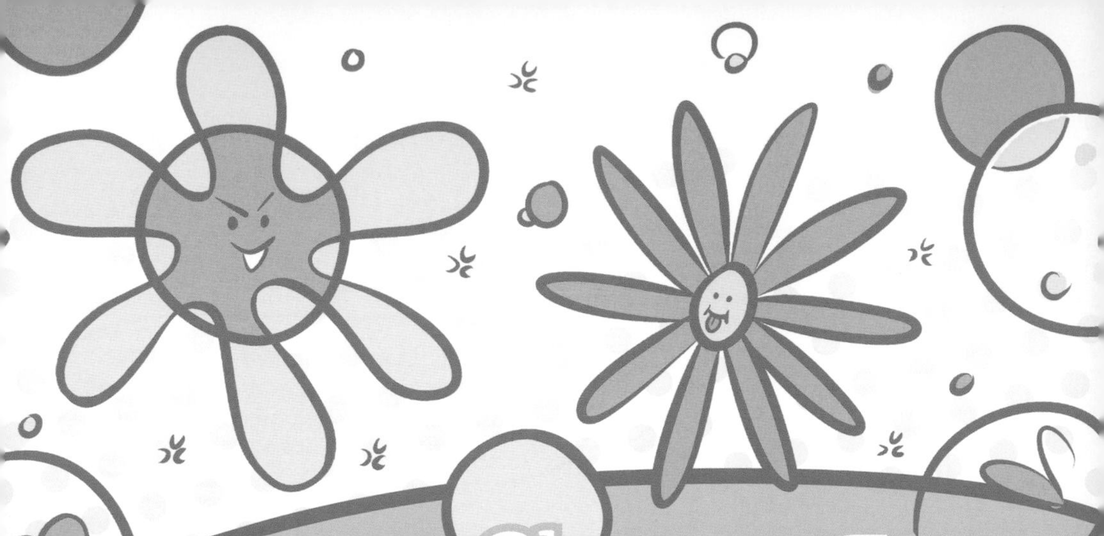

Chapter Five

Let's Look at STIs

Sexually Transmitted Infections and Diseases, STIs and STDs, they're the hobgoblins of sex — spooking us all and keeping us terrified of any kind of genital or fluid contact. Well, this chapter is here to tell you that the majority of them? Are NO BIG DEAL.

Sounds bonkers, right? But it's true! There are A LOT of infections you can get and pass through sex (and don't get us wrong, they do suck), but we live in the future! There are cures and tools for almost all of them, and even ways to cope with and survive the truly bad ones. If you're reading this and fretting about that burning sensation, or worried over a broken condom, we're here to tell you it'll be OK. This stuff happens to ALL of us. Book yourself an appointment to see the doc and listen to them. If you *have* caught something, it doesn't mean you're dirty or bad or wrong — it just means you're human.

But, ah, don't go tossing your condoms away — *that's* bonkers! Take the precautions you can, because it's still better to prevent getting something than *having to get rid of something.* Get regular STI tests, see your doctor when things feel funny, and generally use boundaries and common sense.

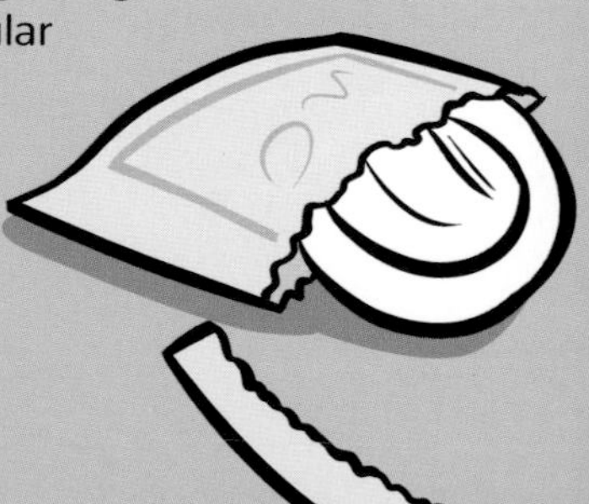

Like with basically everything in your body, knowing more about what's going gives you the tools to manage it and makes it way less scary.

We've got you and you've got this.

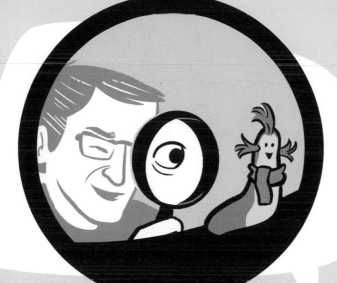

STI Testing

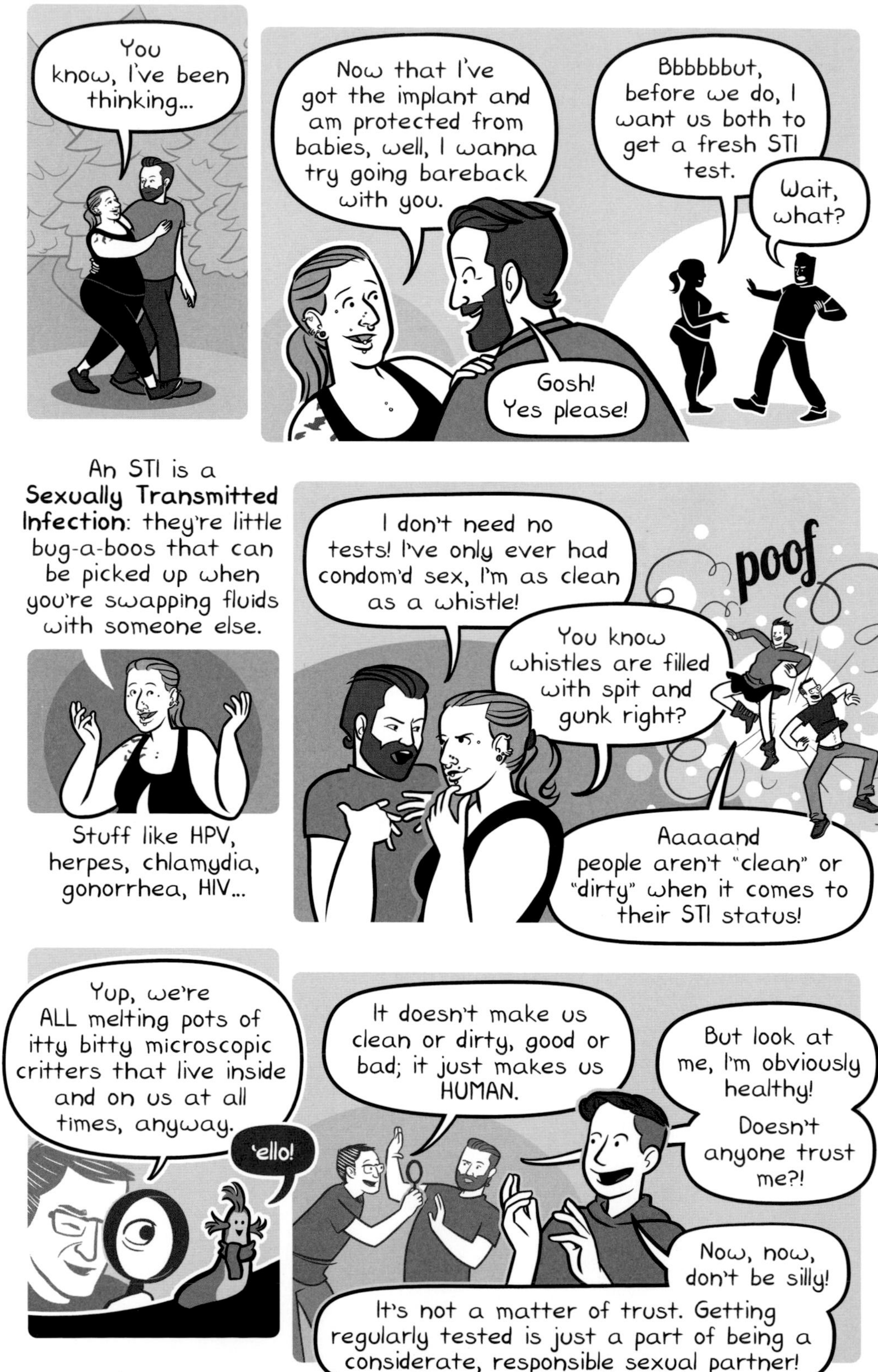
You know, I've been thinking...
Now that I've got the implant and am protected from babies, well, I wanna try going bareback with you.
Gosh! Yes please!
Bbbbbbut, before we do, I want us both to get a fresh STI test.
Wait, what?
An STI is a **Sexually Transmitted Infection**: they're little bug-a-boos that can be picked up when you're swapping fluids with someone else.
Stuff like HPV, herpes, chlamydia, gonorrhea, HIV...
I don't need no tests! I've only ever had condom'd sex, I'm as clean as a whistle!
poof
You know whistles are filled with spit and gunk right?
Aaaaand people aren't "clean" or "dirty" when it comes to their STI status!
Yup, we're ALL melting pots of itty bitty microscopic critters that live inside and on us at all times, anyway.
'ello!
It doesn't make us clean or dirty, good or bad; it just makes us HUMAN.
But look at me, I'm obviously healthy!
Doesn't anyone trust me?!
Now, now, don't be silly!
It's not a matter of trust. Getting regularly tested is just a part of being a considerate, responsible sexual partner!

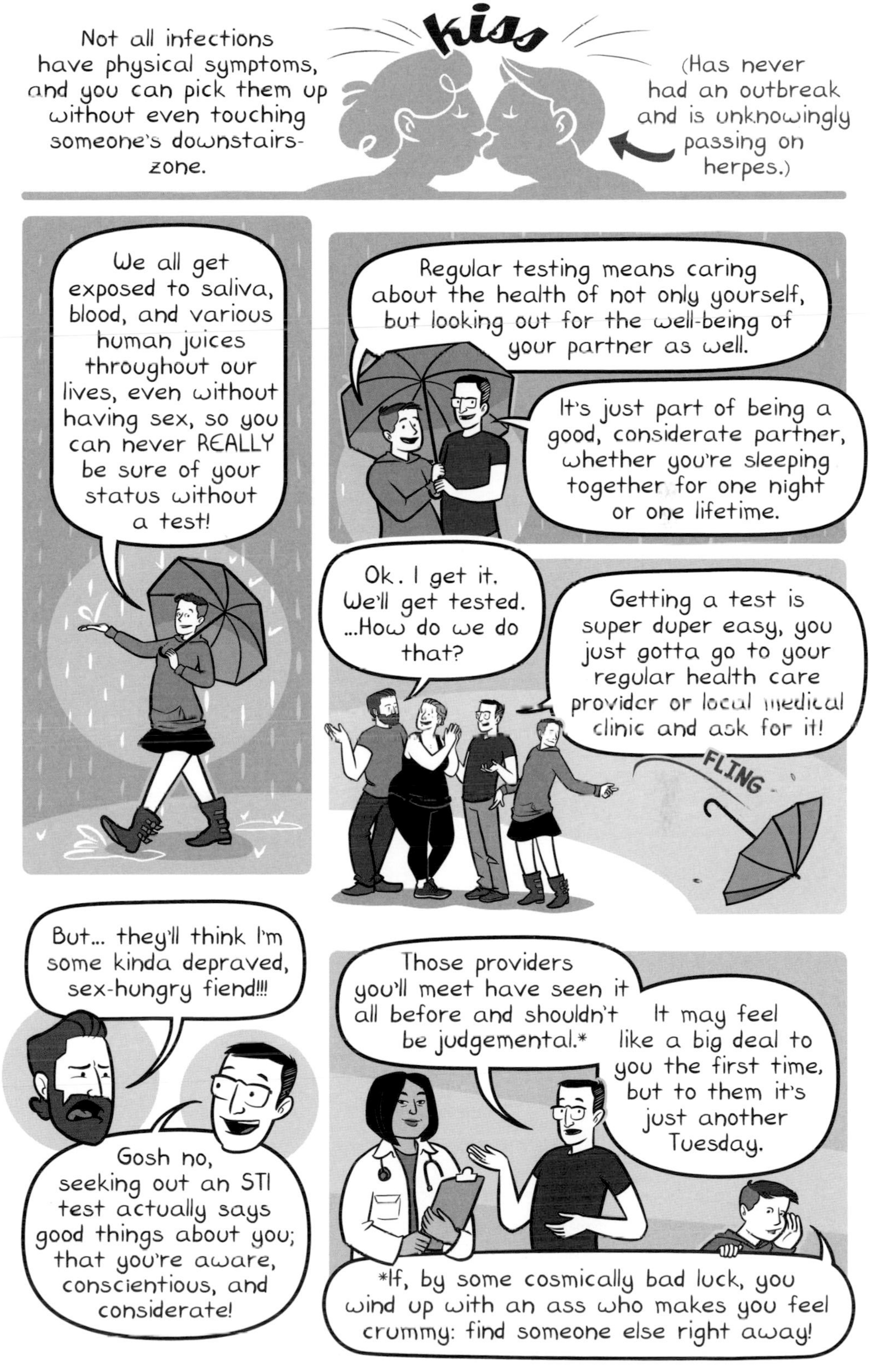
Not all infections have physical symptoms, and you can pick them up without even touching someone's downstairs-zone.
kiss
(Has never had an outbreak and is unknowingly passing on herpes.)
We all get exposed to saliva, blood, and various human juices throughout our lives, even without having sex, so you can never REALLY be sure of your status without a test!
Regular testing means caring about the health of not only yourself, but looking out for the well-being of your partner as well.
It's just part of being a good, considerate partner, whether you're sleeping together for one night or one lifetime.
Ok. I get it. We'll get tested. ...How do we do that?
Getting a test is super duper easy, you just gotta go to your regular health care provider or local medical clinic and ask for it!
FLING
But... they'll think I'm some kinda depraved, sex-hungry fiend!!!
Gosh no, seeking out an STI test actually says good things about you; that you're aware, conscientious, and considerate!
Those providers you'll meet have seen it all before and shouldn't be judgemental.*
It may feel like a big deal to you the first time, but to them it's just another Tuesday.
*If, by some cosmically bad luck, you wind up with an ass who makes you feel crummy: find someone else right away!

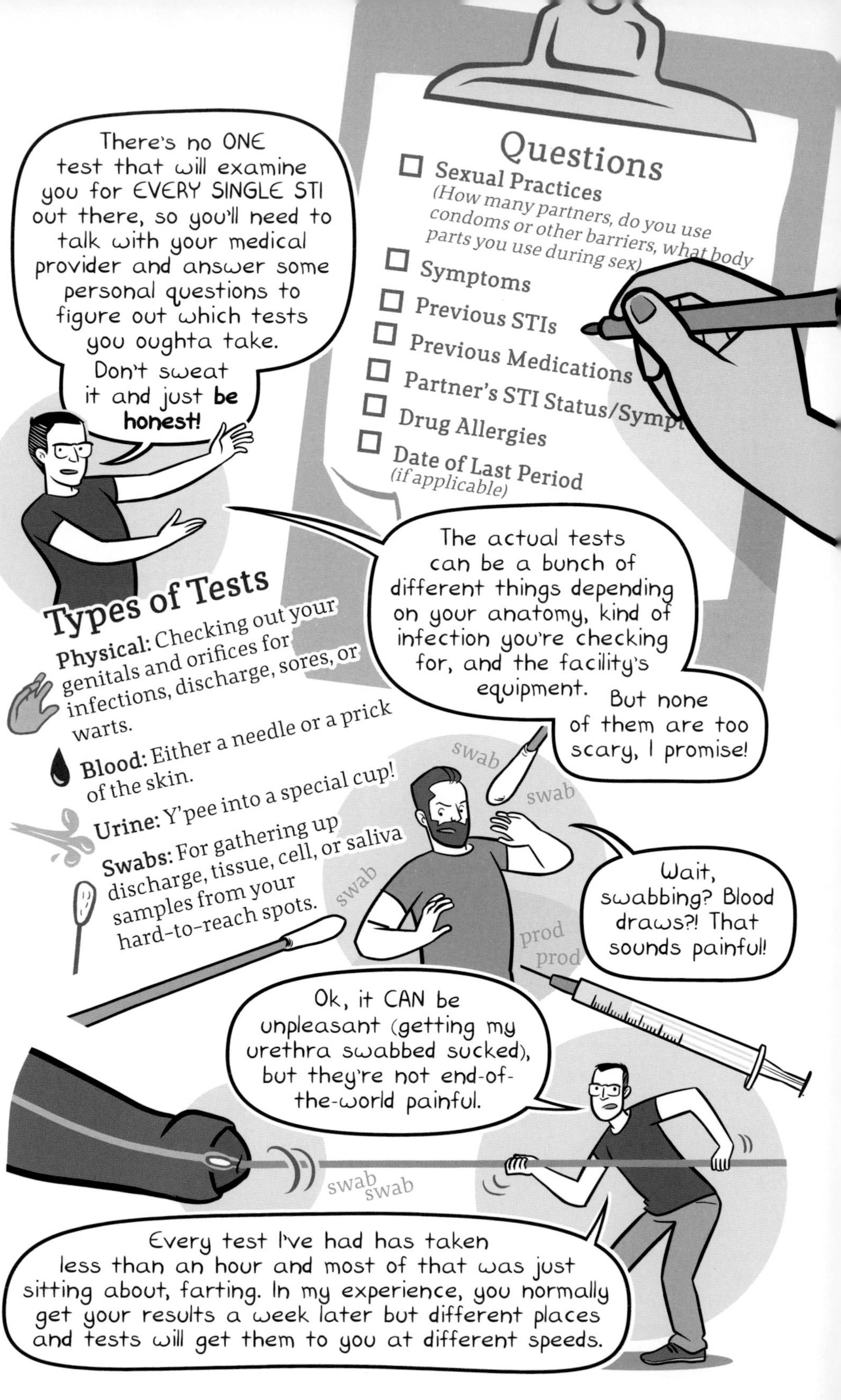
There's no ONE test that will examine you for EVERY SINGLE STI out there, so you'll need to talk with your medical provider and answer some personal questions to figure out which tests you oughta take.
Don't sweat it and just **be honest!**
Questions
Sexual Practices
(How many partners, do you use condoms or other barriers, what body parts you use during sex)
Symptoms
Previous STIs
Previous Medications
Partner's STI Status/Sympt
Drug Allergies
Date of Last Period
(if applicable)
The actual tests can be a bunch of different things depending on your anatomy, kind of infection you're checking for, and the facility's equipment.
But none of them are too scary, I promise!
Types of Tests
Physical: Checking out your genitals and orifices for infections, discharge, sores, or warts.
Blood: Either a needle or a prick of the skin.
Urine: Y'pee into a special cup!
Swabs: For gathering up discharge, tissue, cell, or saliva samples from your hard-to-reach spots.
swab
swab
swab
Wait, swabbing? Blood draws?! That sounds painful!
prod
prod
Ok, it CAN be unpleasant (getting my urethra swabbed sucked), but they're not end-of-the-world painful.
swab
swab
Every test I've had has taken less than an hour and most of that was just sitting about, farting. In my experience, you normally get your results a week later but different places and tests will get them to you at different speeds.

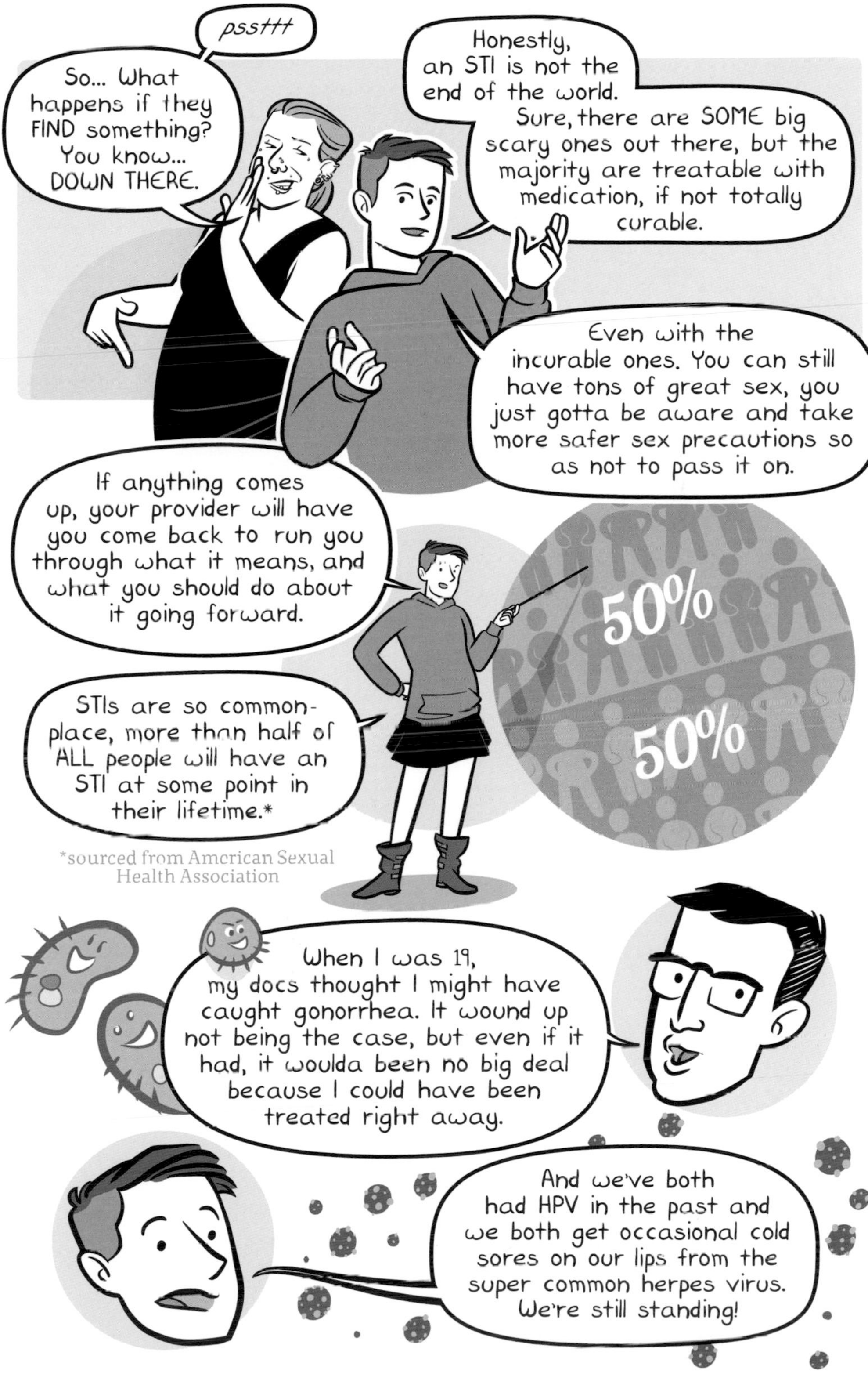
psstt
So... What happens if they FIND something? You know... DOWN THERE.
Honestly, an STI is not the end of the world.
Sure, there are SOME big scary ones out there, but the majority are treatable with medication, if not totally curable.
Even with the incurable ones. You can still have tons of great sex, you just gotta be aware and take more safer sex precautions so as not to pass it on.
If anything comes up, your provider will have you come back to run you through what it means, and what you should do about it going forward.
50%
50%
STIs are so common-place, more than half of ALL people will have an STI at some point in their lifetime.*
*sourced from American Sexual Health Association
When I was 19, my docs thought I might have caught gonorrhea. It wound up not being the case, but even if it had, it woulda been no big deal because I could have been treated right away.
And we've both had HPV in the past and we both get occasional cold sores on our lips from the super common herpes virus. We're still standing!

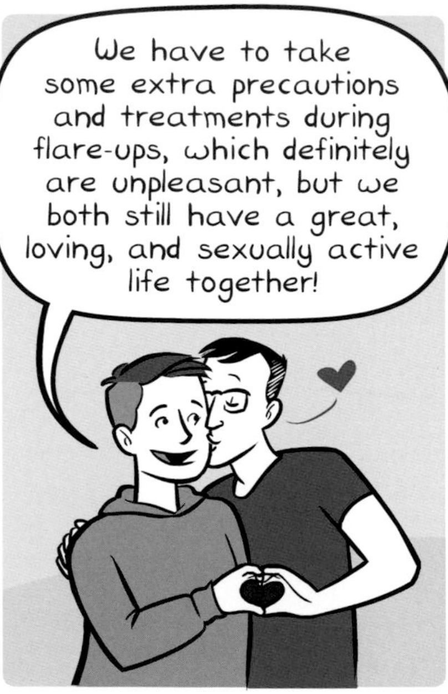

We have to take some extra precautions and treatments during flare-ups, which definitely are unpleasant, but we both still have a great, loving, and sexually active life together!

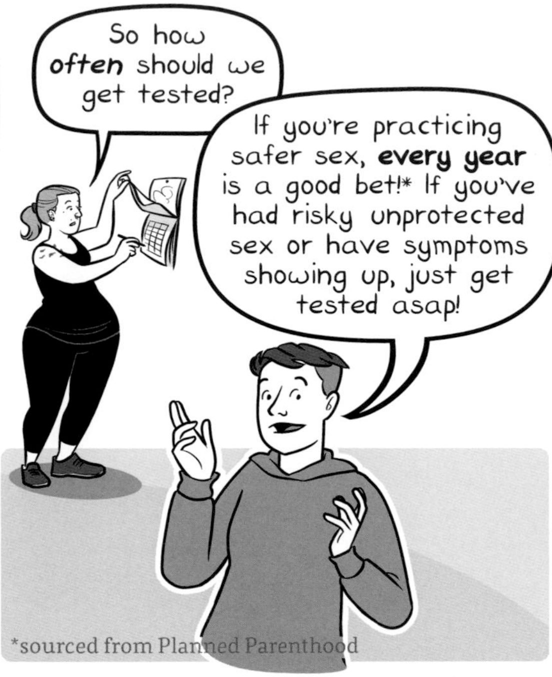

So how **often** should we get tested?
If you're practicing safer sex, **every year** is a good bet!* If you've had risky unprotected sex or have symptoms showing up, just get tested asap!
*sourced from Planned Parenthood

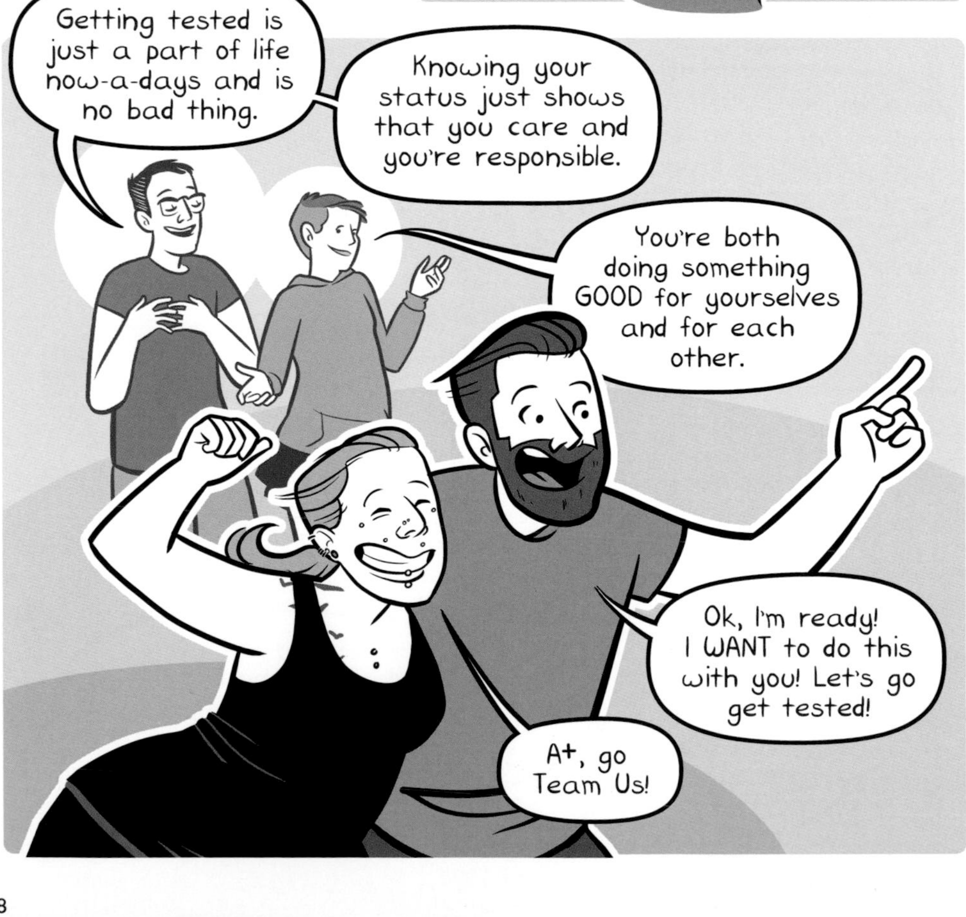

Getting tested is just a part of life now-a-days and is no bad thing.
Knowing your status just shows that you care and you're responsible.
You're both doing something GOOD for yourselves and for each other.
Ok, I'm ready! I WANT to do this with you! Let's go get tested!
A+, go Team Us!

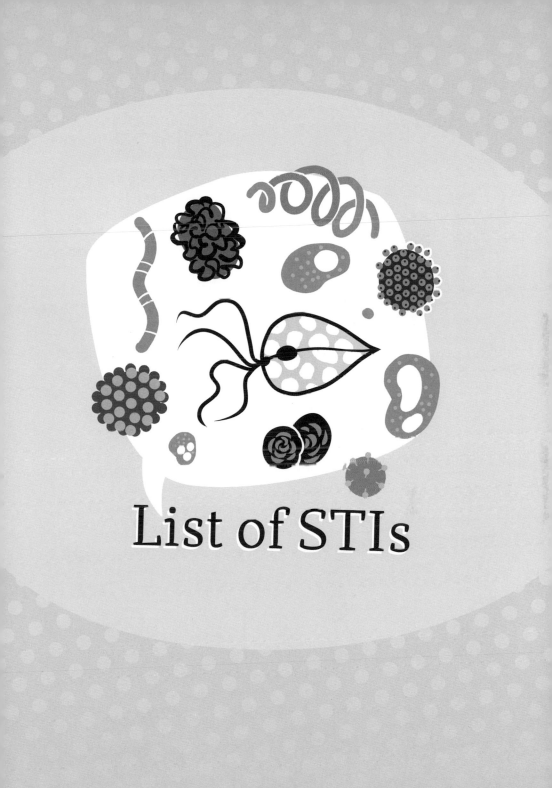

List of STIs

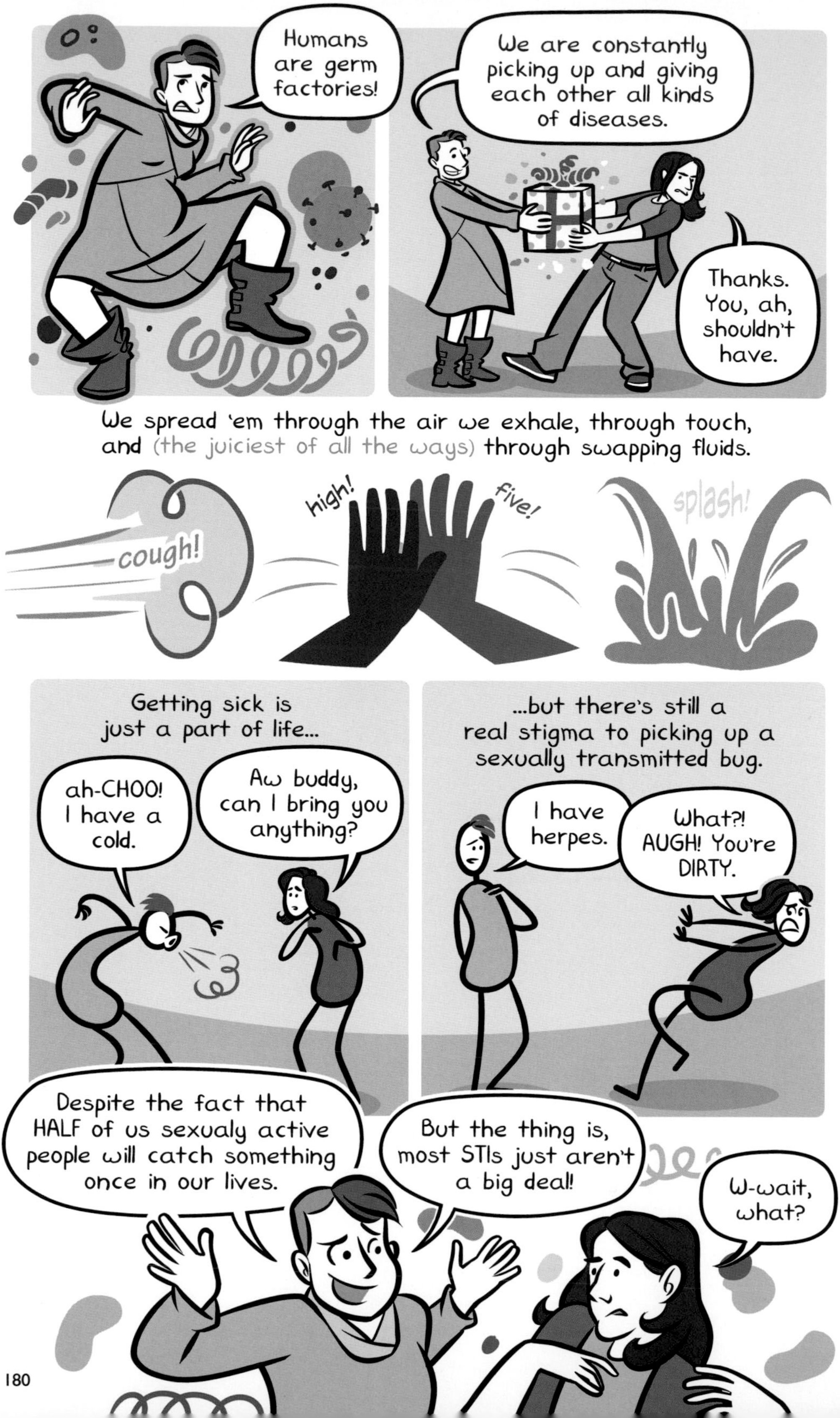
Humans are germ factories!
We are constantly picking up and giving each other all kinds of diseases.
Thanks. You, ah, shouldn't have.
We spread 'em through the air we exhale, through touch, and (the juiciest of all the ways) through swapping fluids.
cough!
high!
five!
splash!
Getting sick is just a part of life...
ah-CHOO! I have a cold.
Aw buddy, can I bring you anything?
...but there's still a real stigma to picking up a sexually transmitted bug.
I have herpes.
What?! AUGH! You're DIRTY.
Despite the fact that HALF of us sexualy active people will catch something once in our lives.
But the thing is, most STIs just aren't a big deal!
W-wait, what?

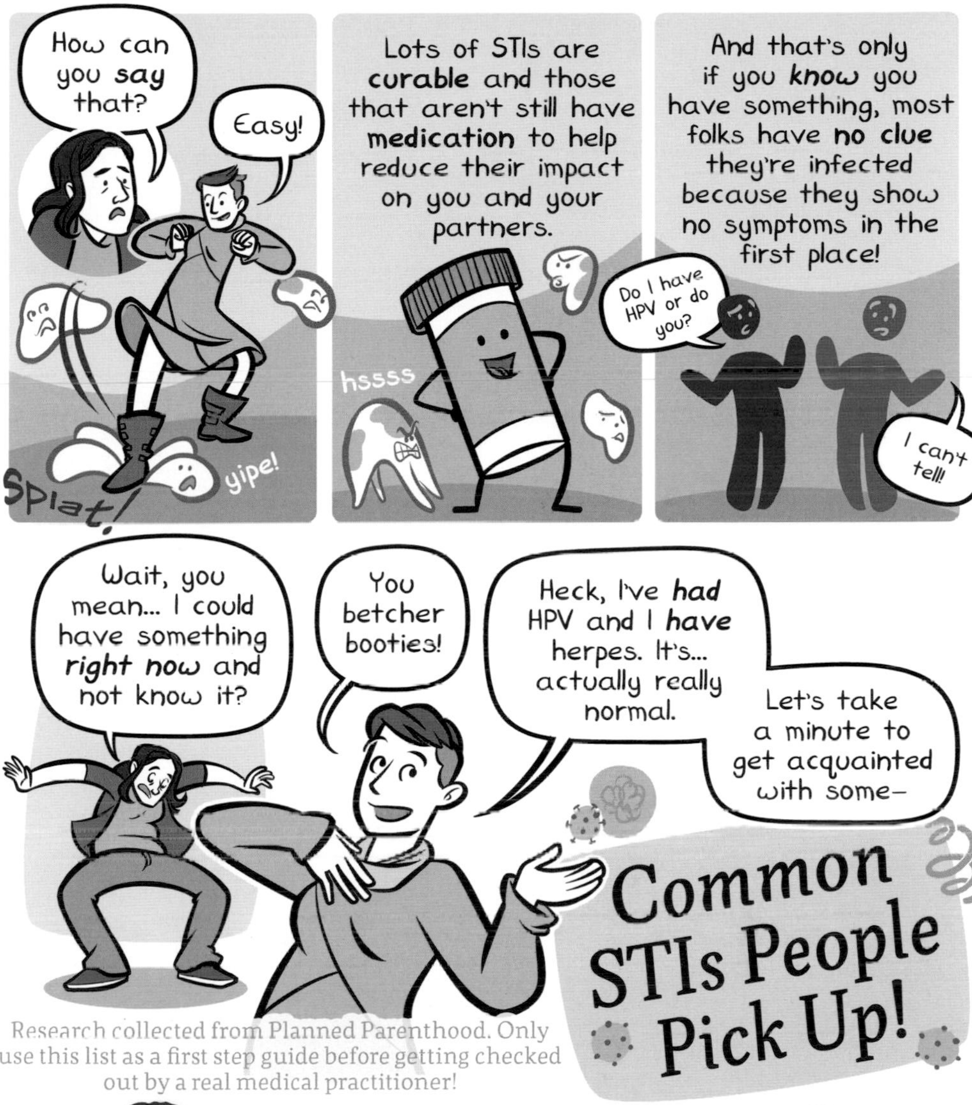
How can you **say** that?
Easy!
Splat!
yipe!
Lots of STIs are **curable** and those that aren't still have **medication** to help reduce their impact on you and your partners.
hssss
And that's only if you **know** you have something, most folks have **no clue** they're infected because they show no symptoms in the first place!
Do I have HPV or do you?
I can't tell!
Wait, you mean... I could have something **right now** and not know it?
You betcher booties!
Heck, I've **had** HPV and I **have** herpes. It's... actually really normal.
Let's take a minute to get acquainted with some–

Common STIs People Pick Up!

Research collected from Planned Parenthood. Only use this list as a first step guide before getting checked out by a real medical practitioner!

Chlamydia

- Bacterial
- Super common! 3 million Americans get it every year.
- Passed through most forms of sex, anything that exchanges sexual fluids.
- Can infect any of your soft, damp and delicate zones, like genitals, anus, eyes and throats!
- Can lead to major health trubs and infertility if left untreated.
- Treated with antibiotics

Sneaky and almost **symptomless**, but you might have:

- Pain when peeing
- Painful sex
- Tummy pain
- Abnormal vaginal or penial or anus discharge
- Bleeding between periods
- Painful testicles
- Sore or bloody butt hole

Difficulty Level: No big deal as long as it's treated!

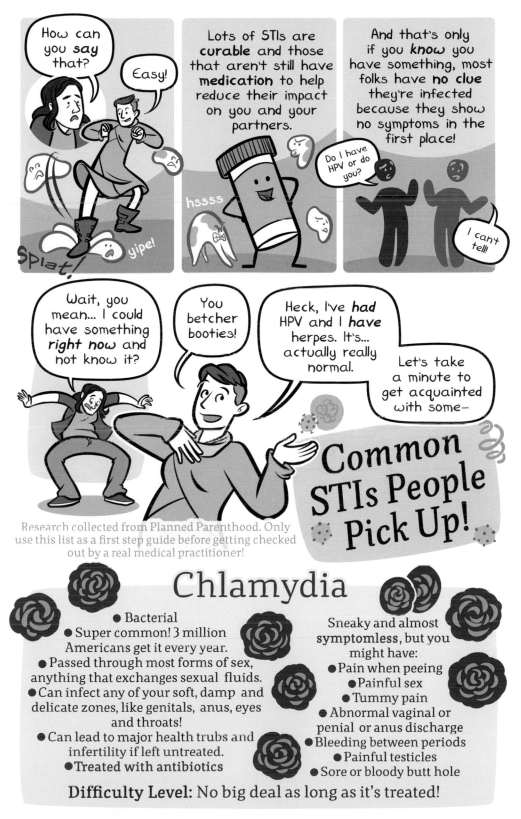

Gonorrhea

AKA: *The Clap* or *Drip*

- Bacterial
- Super common! 1–2 million Americans get it every year!
- Transferred by sexual fluids, so most forms of sex.
- Can infect any of your soft, damp and delicate zones, including genitals, anus, eyes, and throat.
- Can lead to major health trubs and infertility if left untreated.
- Treated with antibiotics

Most of the times it's symptomless, but you might get:
- Pain when peeing
- Painful sex
- Abnormal vaginal or penial or anus discharge
- Bleeding between periods
- Painful testicles
- Pain when you poop
- An itchy butt hole

Difficulty Level: Easy-peasy, just get treated.

HPV

AKA: *Human Papillomavirus*

- Virus
- The most common sexually transmitted virus out there, most who engage in sex will get it.
- Transmits through our soft moist zones contacting each other such as vulvas, vaginas, penises, anuses and mouths.
- Pretty much symptomless, but you might get some warts (that can be removed)

- Some of the more aggressive HPVs can cause cancer and people with cervixes are especially vulnerable.
- No cure, but our bodies usually fight it off after a little while; or there are medical treatments for resulting symptoms. Regular pap smears are key and there are vaccines for children that can immunize them to some of the worst strains.

Difficulty Level: Stressful, but usually harmless. The bad results can typically be treated with medical procedures.

HIV and AIDs

- HIV is a virus that infects and attacks your immune system and can cause AIDs, the point when your immune system is so busted that you're in the danger zone.
- Rare, about 1 million total Americans have HIV
- Transferred by sexual fluids, blood, and breast milk. To debunk a myth, you CAN'T get it from kissing or holding hands or anything like that.

- HIV is symptomless (although you may feel like you have a cold the first few weeks after infection) until your white blood cell count gets too low (maybe years and years after infection) and you start suffering from AIDs, which has just about every symptom under the sun.
- Can lead to major health issues and death.
- No cure, but with medication, it's not the death sentence it was 40 years ago.

Difficulty: Hard, but survivable. Caught early, HIV can be kept in check with antivirals and even reduced to the point where its undetectable and untransmittable in a person. There are also great pre-exposure meds out there called PrEP that drastically help in reducing the chance of catching it; they are worth exploring if you're having sexy fun in a higher-risk community.

Herpes AKA: *HSV-1 & 2*

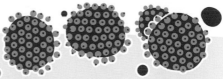

- Virus
- *ULTRA common! More than half* of Americans have it.
- You pick it up through skin-to-skin contact with an infected zone, especially during an outbreak, but you're lowkey infectious to others all the time. To debunk a myth: it won't live long outside the body so you *CAN'T get it from holding hands, coughing, sneezing or sitting on a toilet.*
- Can infect any of the soft, damp and delicate zones, genitals to anus, eyes and throats.
- Isn't apparent *until* you experience an outbreak, when the virus shows up as big sores that heal after a week.
- Rarely gets worse than that.
- **No cure,** but there are **prescriptions that help** reduce outbreak times.

👍 **Difficulty Level:** Uncomfortable AF during outbreaks, but the rest of the time? You can't even tell you have anything.

Scabies

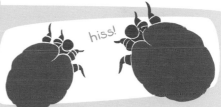

hiss!

- TINY burrowing parasites.
- Infects your skin.
- About 200,000 cases a year.
- You pick it up through skin to skin contact, like when your conoodling with your infected boo.
- Just some crazy itchy red bumps on your skin that sometimes follows a line.
- **You'll need prescribed meds to get rid of these nasties,** and you'll have to sanitize your bedding, clothes and towels! Blarf!

Difficulty Level:
One of our old roommates got this from a long and gross Greyhound bus trip. He didn't much like it, but, I mean, it went away with a bit of time and medication, no biggie.

Hepatitis B

- Virus
- Not that common nowadays thanks to child vaccinations! Only about a million Americans are carriers.
- You pick it up through genital fluids, urine, and blood.
- Infects your liver.

You probably won't get any symptoms, but if you do, here's a list:
Feeling flu-ish
Tired
Painful tummy zone
Loss of appetite, nausea and vomiting
Painful joints
Headaches
Fever
Hives
Dark colored pee
Weird looking poop
Yellowing skin.

- Can lead to liver disease
- There ARE other kinds of Hepatitis, but B is the most commonly associated with sexual transfer.
- **NO CURE,** but 9/10 people **fight it off after 4-8 weeks,** like a really bad cold. Plus you can be vaccinated against it!

Difficulty Level:
Sucks, but chances are you'll crush it.

Molluscum Contagiosum

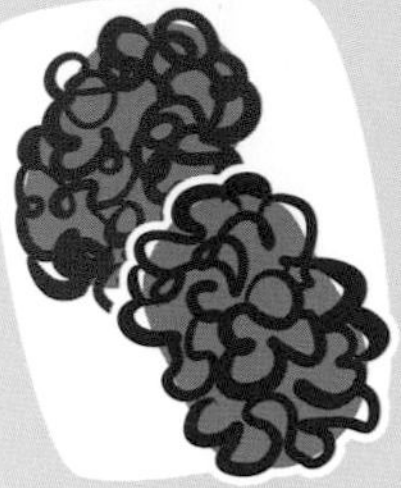

- Skin Virus
- About 200,000 cases a year
- You pick it up through contact, usually during some good-time sexytimes rubbin'.
- Just some hard itchy little bumps on your skin.
- **NO CURE** but it'll **go away on its own within 6-12 months**. Some **prescription topical treatments** can help, and there are options if bumps don't go away with time.

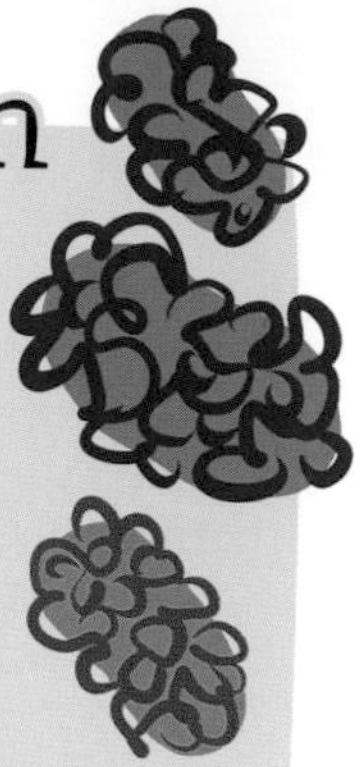

Difficulty Level: You'll want to avoid having sexy times with others while your body clears it out, which is a bummer, but it's **temporary**.

Pubic Lice AKA: *crabs*

- Parasites
- Infects your coarse hair.
- You pick it up through contact, they'll clamber from pubes to pubes!
- Really common, millions and millions get 'em every year.
- Visually obvious little critters, you can *see* them and their eggs! While they are there you might suffer:
  - Some real bad itching
  - Agitated skin
  - Feverish and feeling run-down

- **Tons of cures** out there: gels, shampoos, liquids, foams. Most of it available over the counter too, but there's strong stuff available via prescription as well. They'll hang out in your clothes too, so you're gonna have to wash them on the hottest setting.

Difficulty Level: Nobody likes the idea of lice. But, whatevs, you can handle this with some treatment.

Syphilis

- Bacterial
- About 200,000 cases a year
- Picked up through sexual contact, when soft moist zones meet a syphilis sore, such as all sets of genitals, anuses and sometimes mouths.
- Can lead to a lot of issues *if* it's left alone long enough. Can even *kill you* if it gets super bad, but we're talking like *10-20 years after infection.*
- **Easily treated early on with antibiotics**, but *left untreated* it gets harder and harder to deal with.

Stages:
Usually **starts with** a sore lump that's highly contagious and easy to mistake for a pimple or ingrown hair, which lasts for 3-6 weeks.

Then it might develop into a rash that'll show up on your body, that'll last 2-6 weeks and might come and go for up to 2 years.

Finally it chills out and enters its late stage, where its pretty symptomless, but potentially dangerous.

 Difficulty Level: Look for a weird lump and then GET THEE TO THE DOCTOR and they'll sort this shit right out.

Trichomoniasis

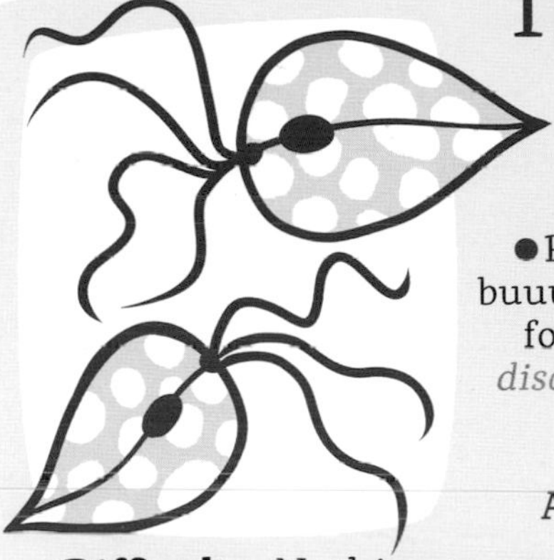

- Microscopic Parasites
- The most common STI out there.
- Transferred by sexual fluids meeting your genitals.
- Pretty darn **symptomless** for all genitals, buuuut can lead to **vaginitis** for vagina-having folks, which can SUPER suck (*Bad vaginal discharge, itchy vagina, genital swelling, pain during sex*)
- Super easy to diagnose and treat. **Antibiotics destroy these tiny villains.**

Difficulty: Nothing to sweat about, once you take your meds!

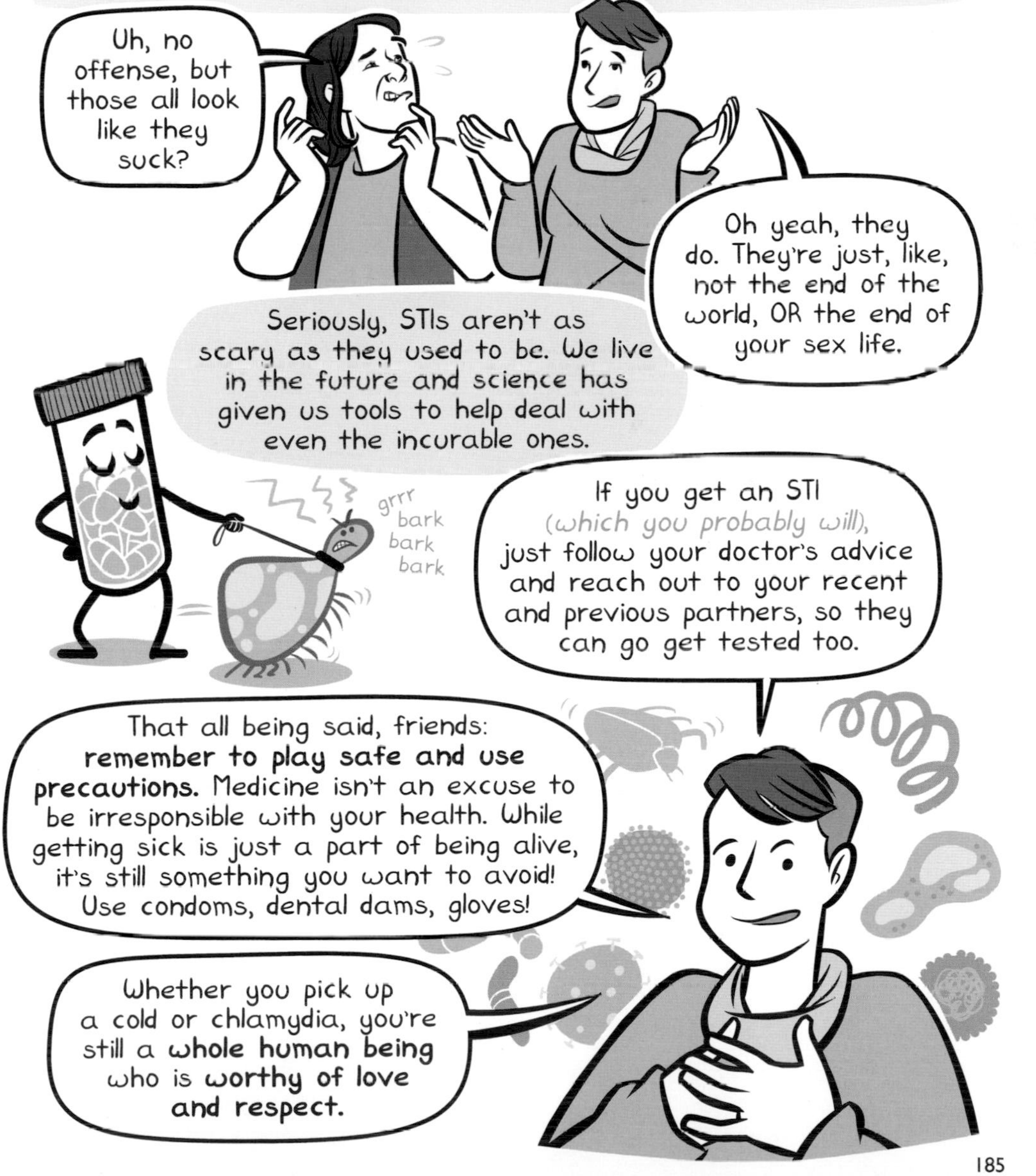
Uh, no offense, but those all look like they suck?
Oh yeah, they do. They're just, like, not the end of the world, OR the end of your sex life.
Seriously, STIs aren't as scary as they used to be. We live in the future and science has given us tools to help deal with even the incurable ones.
grrr bark bark bark
If you get an STI (which you probably will), just follow your doctor's advice and reach out to your recent and previous partners, so they can go get tested too.
That all being said, friends: **remember to play safe and use precautions.** Medicine isn't an excuse to be irresponsible with your health. While getting sick is just a part of being alive, it's still something you want to avoid! Use condoms, dental dams, gloves!
Whether you pick up a cold or chlamydia, you're still a **whole human being** who is **worthy of love and respect.**

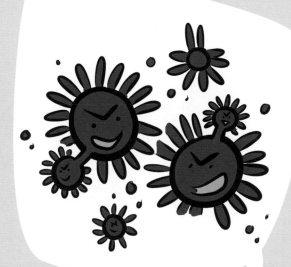

A Closer Look At
Herpes

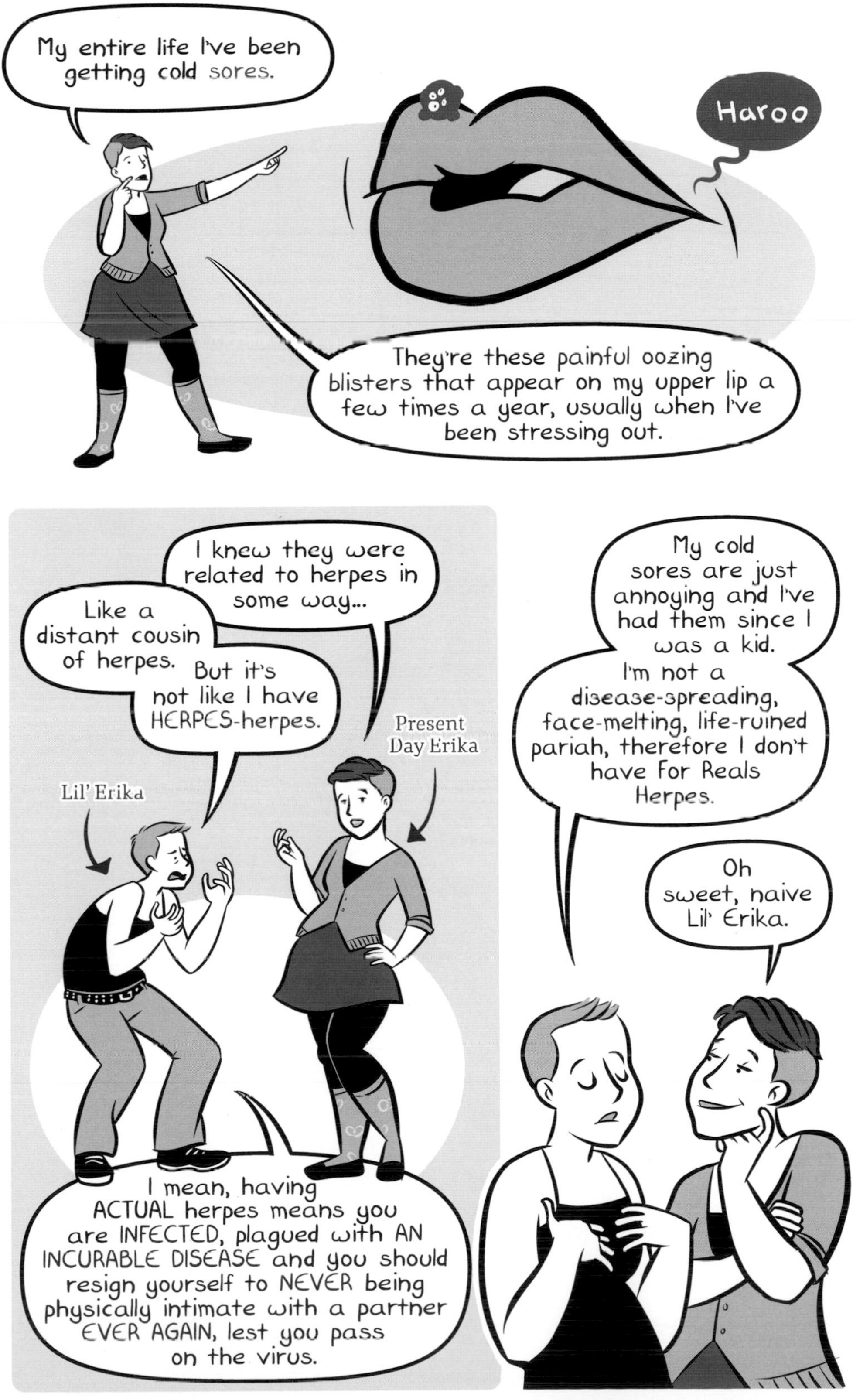

My entire life I've been getting cold sores.
Haroo
They're these painful oozing blisters that appear on my upper lip a few times a year, usually when I've been stressing out.
I knew they were related to herpes in some way...
Like a distant cousin of herpes.
But it's not like I have HERPES-herpes.
Present Day Erika
Lil' Erika
I mean, having ACTUAL herpes means you are INFECTED, plagued with AN INCURABLE DISEASE and you should resign yourself to NEVER being physically intimate with a partner EVER AGAIN, lest you pass on the virus.
My cold sores are just annoying and I've had them since I was a kid.
I'm not a disease-spreading, face-melting, life-ruined pariah, therefore I don't have For Reals Herpes.
Oh sweet, naive Lil' Erika.

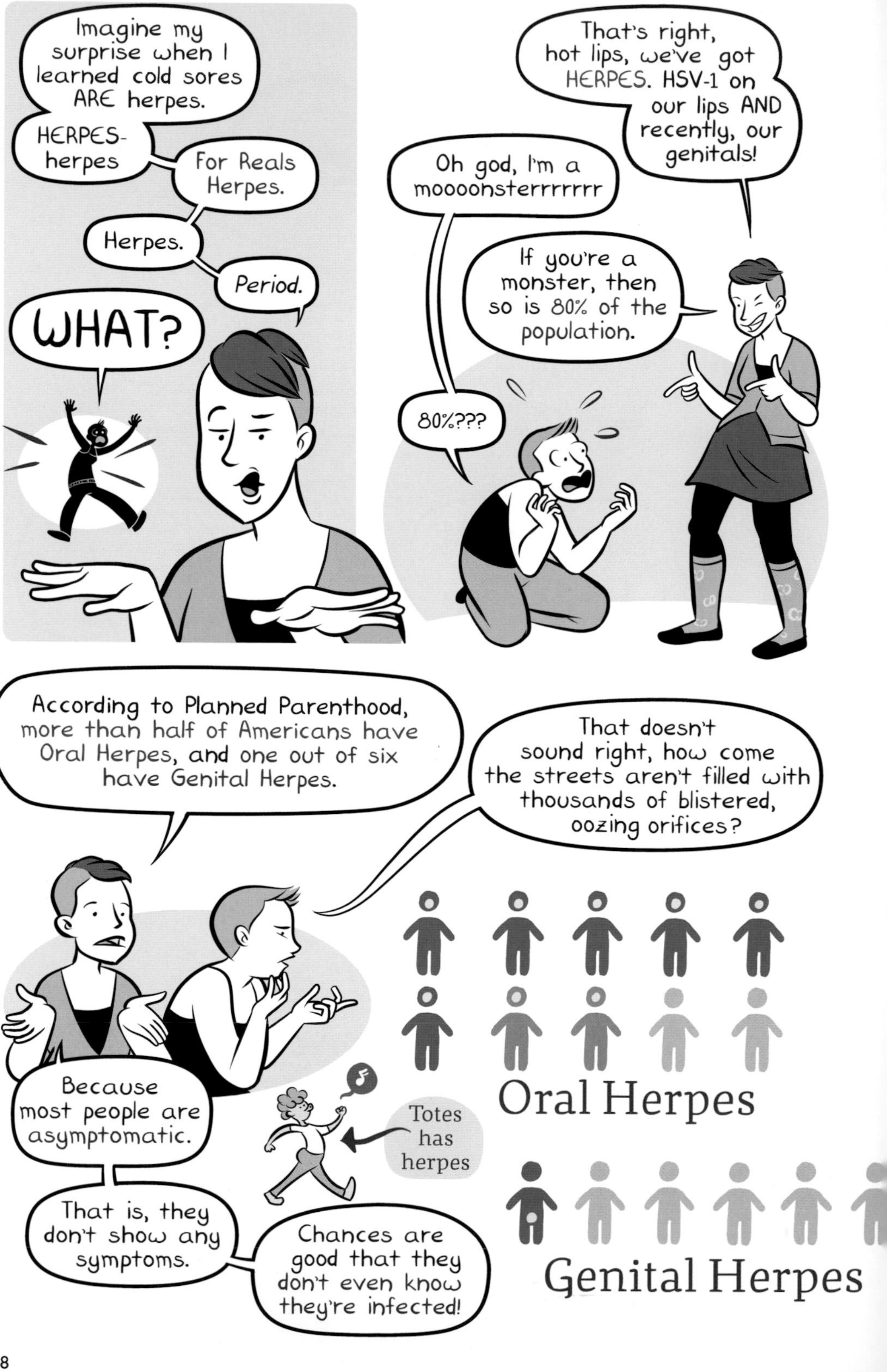
Imagine my surprise when I learned cold sores ARE herpes.
HERPES-herpes
For Reals Herpes.
Herpes.
Period.
WHAT?
That's right, hot lips, we've got HERPES. HSV-1 on our lips AND recently, our genitals!
Oh god, I'm a moooonsterrrrrrr
If you're a monster, then so is 80% of the population.
80%???
According to Planned Parenthood, more than half of Americans have Oral Herpes, and one out of six have Genital Herpes.
That doesn't sound right, how come the streets aren't filled with thousands of blistered, oozing orifices?
Because most people are asymptomatic.
That is, they don't show any symptoms.
Chances are good that they don't even know they're infected!
Totes has herpes
Oral Herpes
Genital Herpes

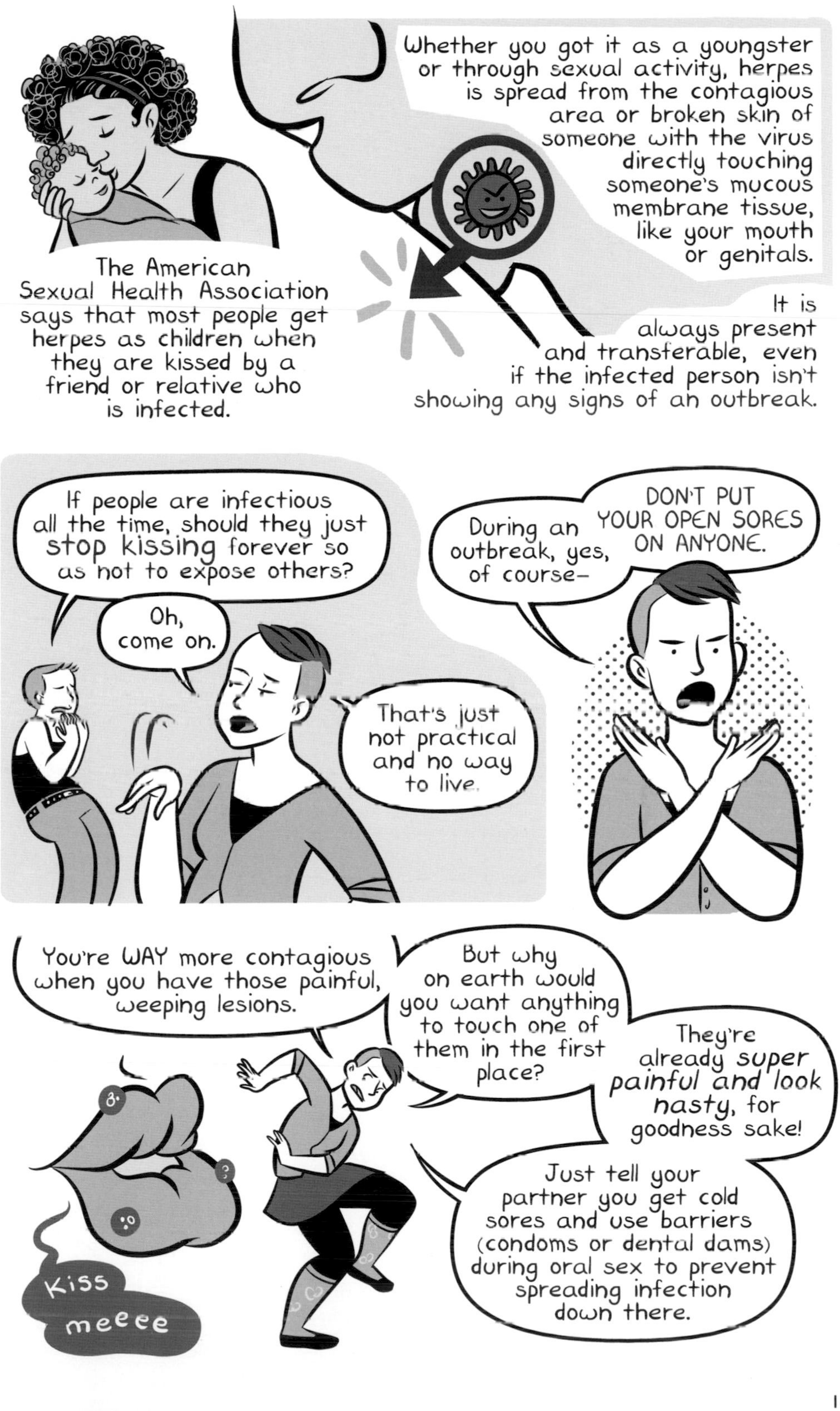
The American Sexual Health Association says that most people get herpes as children when they are kissed by a friend or relative who is infected.
Whether you got it as a youngster or through sexual activity, herpes is spread from the contagious area or broken skin of someone with the virus directly touching someone's mucous membrane tissue, like your mouth or genitals.
It is always present and transferable, even if the infected person isn't showing any signs of an outbreak.
If people are infectious all the time, should they just stop kissing forever so as not to expose others?
Oh, come on.
That's just not practical and no way to live.
During an outbreak, yes, of course–
DON'T PUT YOUR OPEN SORES ON ANYONE.
You're WAY more contagious when you have those painful, weeping lesions.
But why on earth would you want anything to touch one of them in the first place?
They're already *super painful and look nasty*, for goodness sake!
Just tell your partner you get cold sores and use barriers (condoms or dental dams) during oral sex to prevent spreading infection down there.
Kiss meeee

The Life and Times of a Herpes Outbreak:

Remission.
Honk-
-shoo
No symptoms, though still contagious, while the virus lives in your sensory nerve ganglia.
Prodromal
Day 0–1
Tingling/itching sensations and reddening skin begin a few hours or days before physical symptoms appear.
hmm
Start treatment, if you have some!
Inflammation
Day 1
The virus begins reproducing and infecting cells at the end of the nerve.
The healthy cells begin swelling and the skin around them becomes reddened.
Pre-sore
Day 2–3
Aw, crap
A hard, little, painful bump(s) appears on the skin.
Open lesion
Day 4
Augh, the worst part!
The bump(s) break open & create an open, weeping, super painful sore. This fluid is HIGHLY contagious with active viral particles.
Crusting
Day 5–8
A yellow or brown-ish crust develops.
It will crack open regularly from movement, releasing more contagious fluid from within the lesion.
Healing
Day 9–14
As the virus retreats back to dormancy, new skin grows beneath the scab.
Good job!
... so ... sleepy...
It may still be irritated, itchy, and painful.
Post-scab
Day 12–14
As the destroyed cells regenerate, some redness may linger at the site of the outbreak, and the virus can still shed, even at this stage of recovery.
Okay, so I've heard there's different kinds of herpes.
Explain.

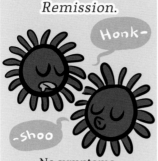

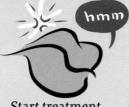

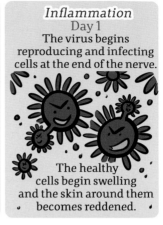

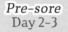

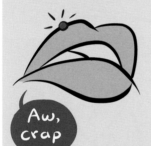

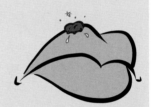

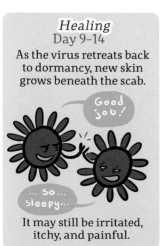

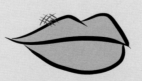

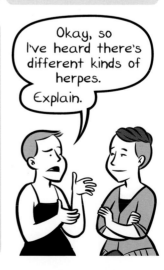

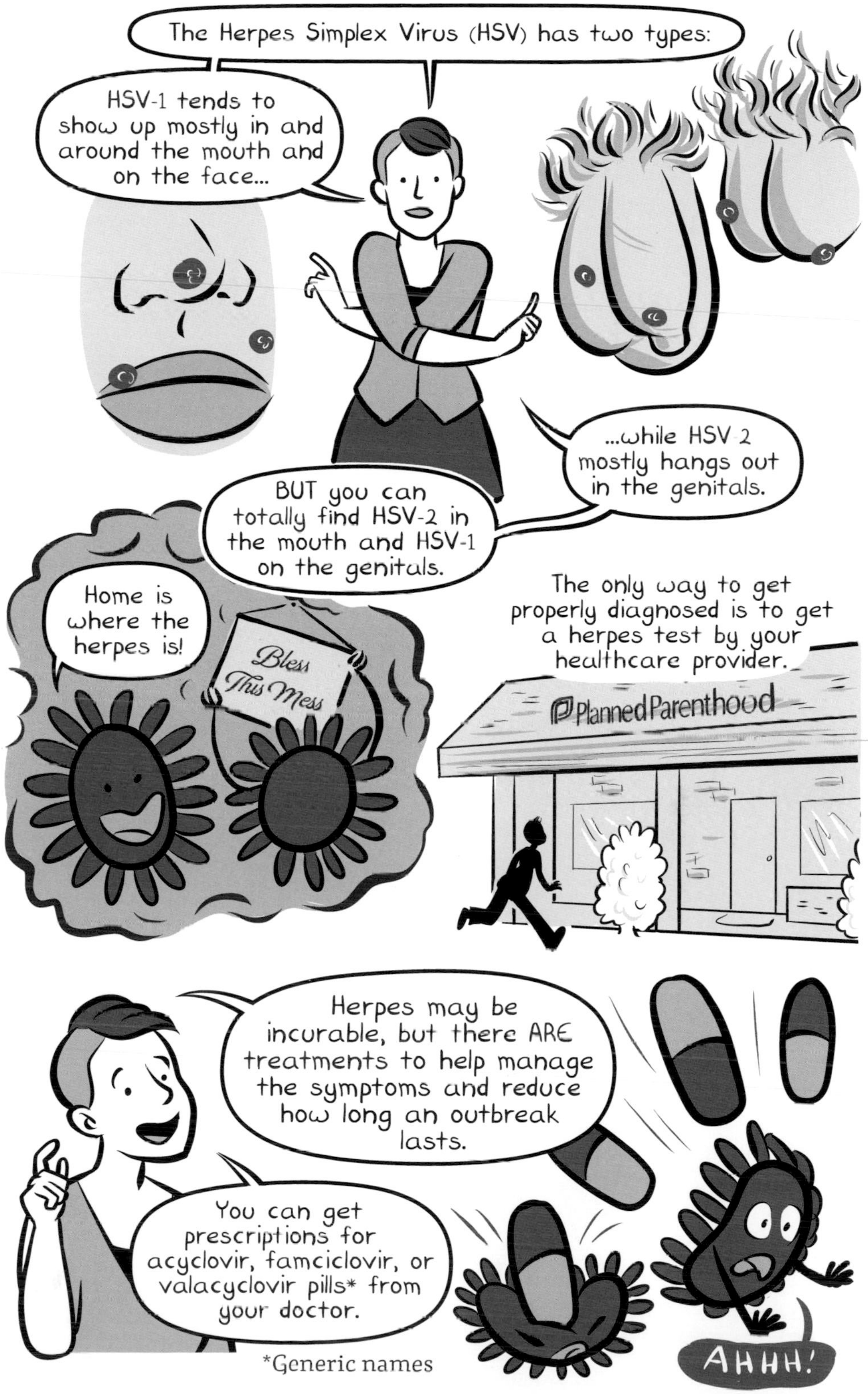
The Herpes Simplex Virus (HSV) has two types:
HSV-1 tends to show up mostly in and around the mouth and on the face...
...while HSV-2 mostly hangs out in the genitals.
BUT you can totally find HSV-2 in the mouth and HSV-1 on the genitals.
Home is where the herpes is!
Bless This Mess
The only way to get properly diagnosed is to get a herpes test by your healthcare provider.
Planned Parenthood
Herpes may be incurable, but there ARE treatments to help manage the symptoms and reduce how long an outbreak lasts.
You can get prescriptions for acyclovir, famciclovir, or valacyclovir pills* from your doctor.
*Generic names
AHHH!

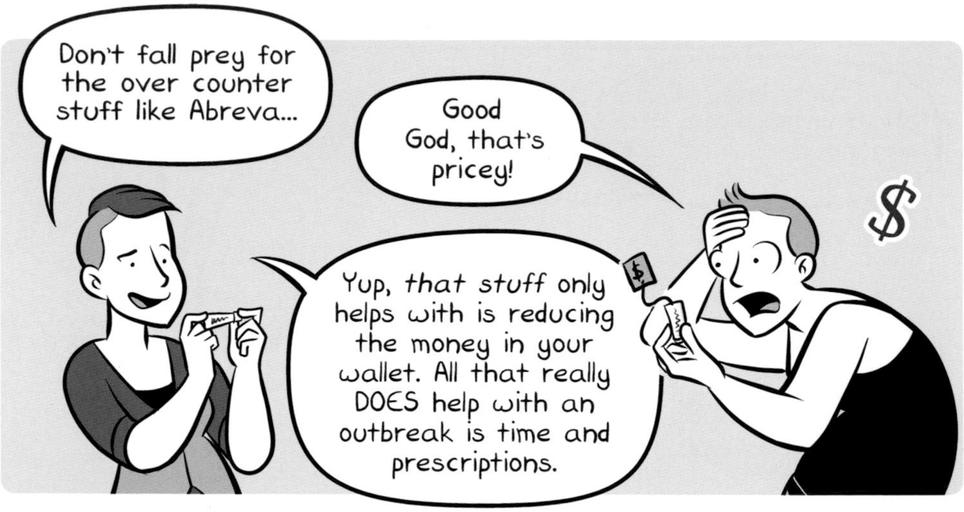
Don't fall prey for the over counter stuff like Abreva...
Good God, that's pricey!
$
Yup, *that stuff* only helps with is reducing the money in your wallet. All that really DOES help with an outbreak is time and prescriptions.

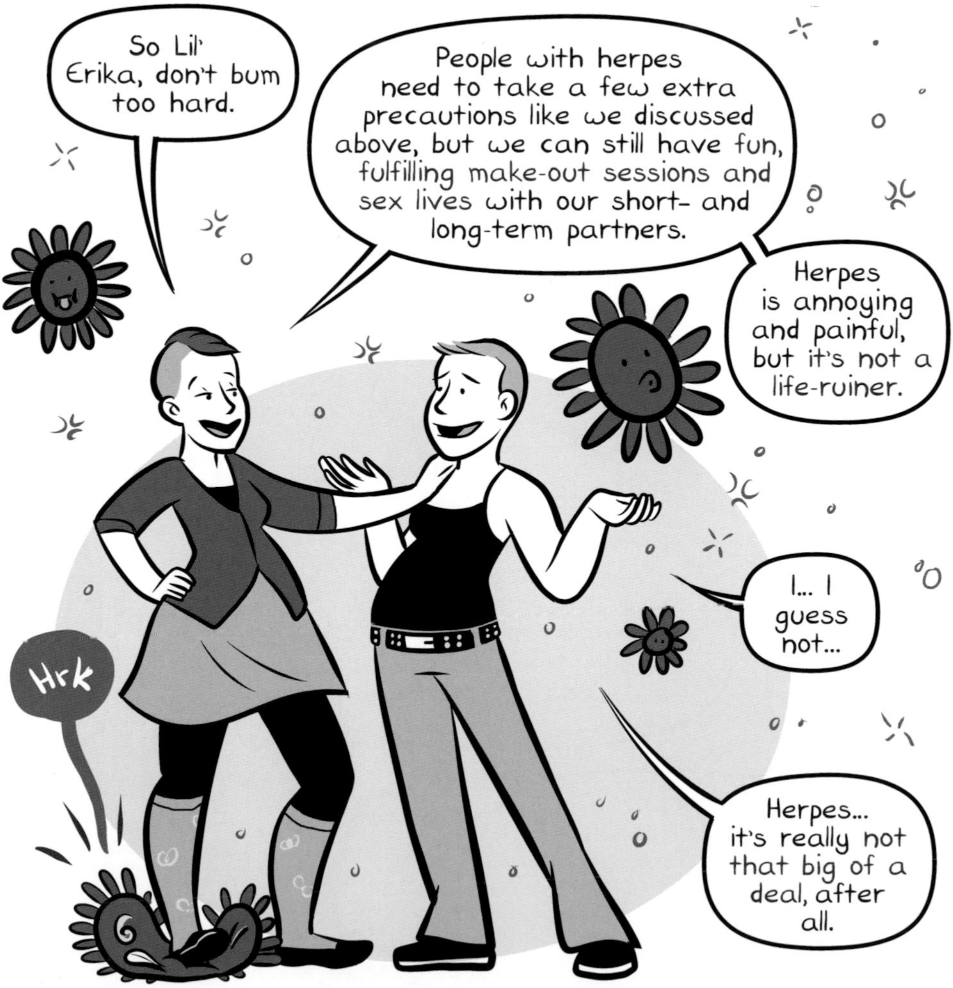
So Lil' Erika, don't bum too hard.
People with herpes need to take a few extra precautions like we discussed above, but we can still have fun, fulfilling make-out sessions and sex lives with our short- and long-term partners.
Herpes is annoying and painful, but it's not a life-ruiner.
I... I guess not...
Hrk
Herpes... it's really not that big of a deal, after all.

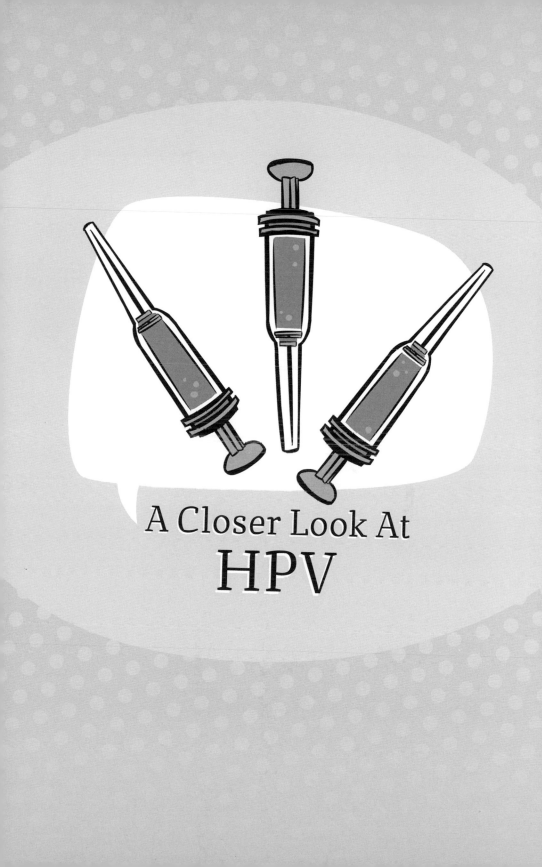

A Closer Look At
HPV

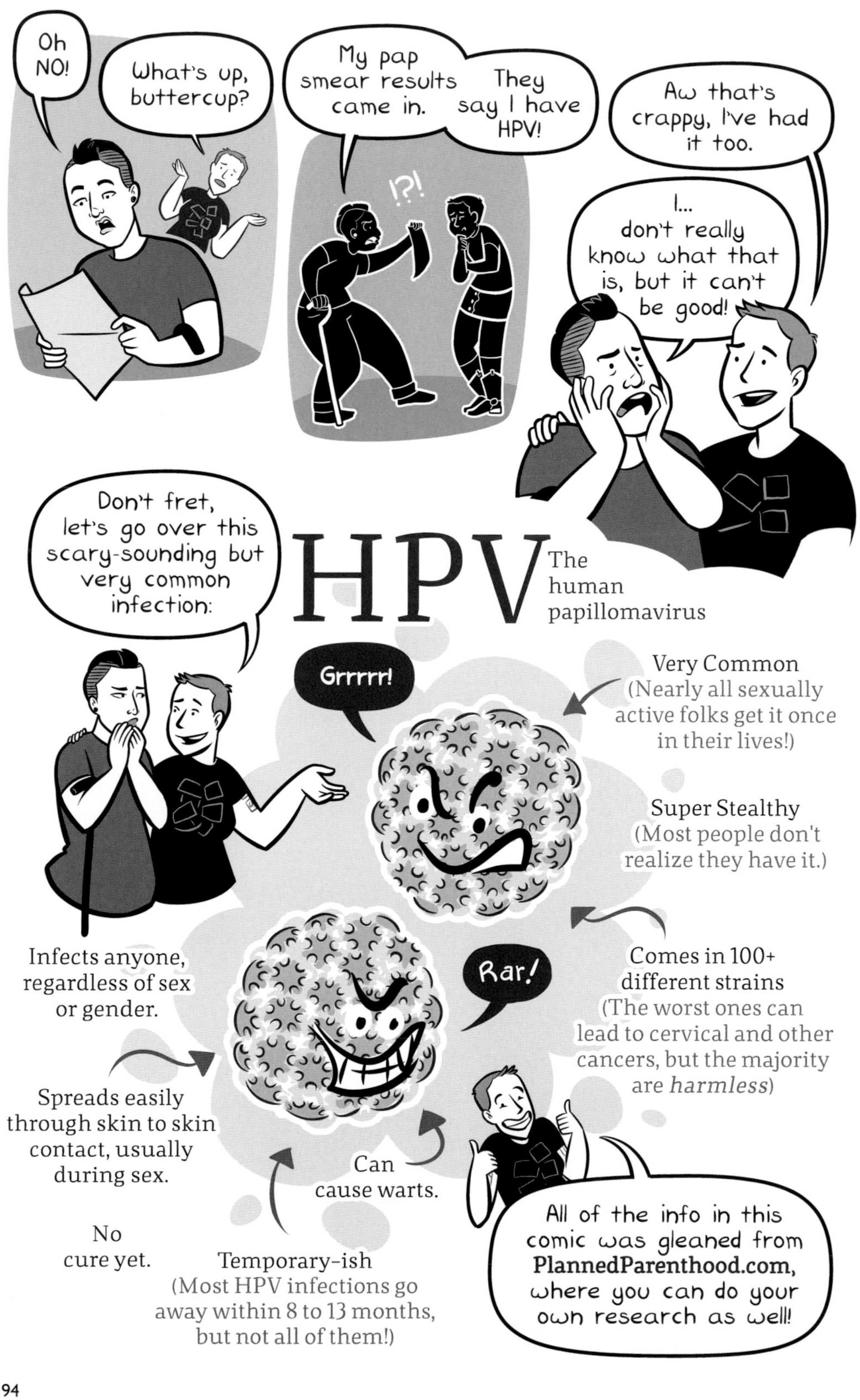
Oh NO!
What's up, buttercup?
My pap smear results came in.
They say I have HPV!
!?!
Aw that's crappy, I've had it too.
I... don't really know what that is, but it can't be good!
Don't fret, let's go over this scary-sounding but very common infection:
HPV
The human papillomavirus
Grrrrr!
Very Common
(Nearly all sexually active folks get it once in their lives!)
Super Stealthy
(Most people don't realize they have it.)
Comes in 100+ different strains
(The worst ones can lead to cervical and other cancers, but the majority are *harmless*)
Rar!
Infects anyone, regardless of sex or gender.
Spreads easily through skin to skin contact, usually during sex.
Can cause warts.
No cure yet.
Temporary-ish
(Most HPV infections go away within 8 to 13 months, but not all of them!)
All of the info in this comic was gleaned from **PlannedParenthood.com,** where you can do your own research as well!

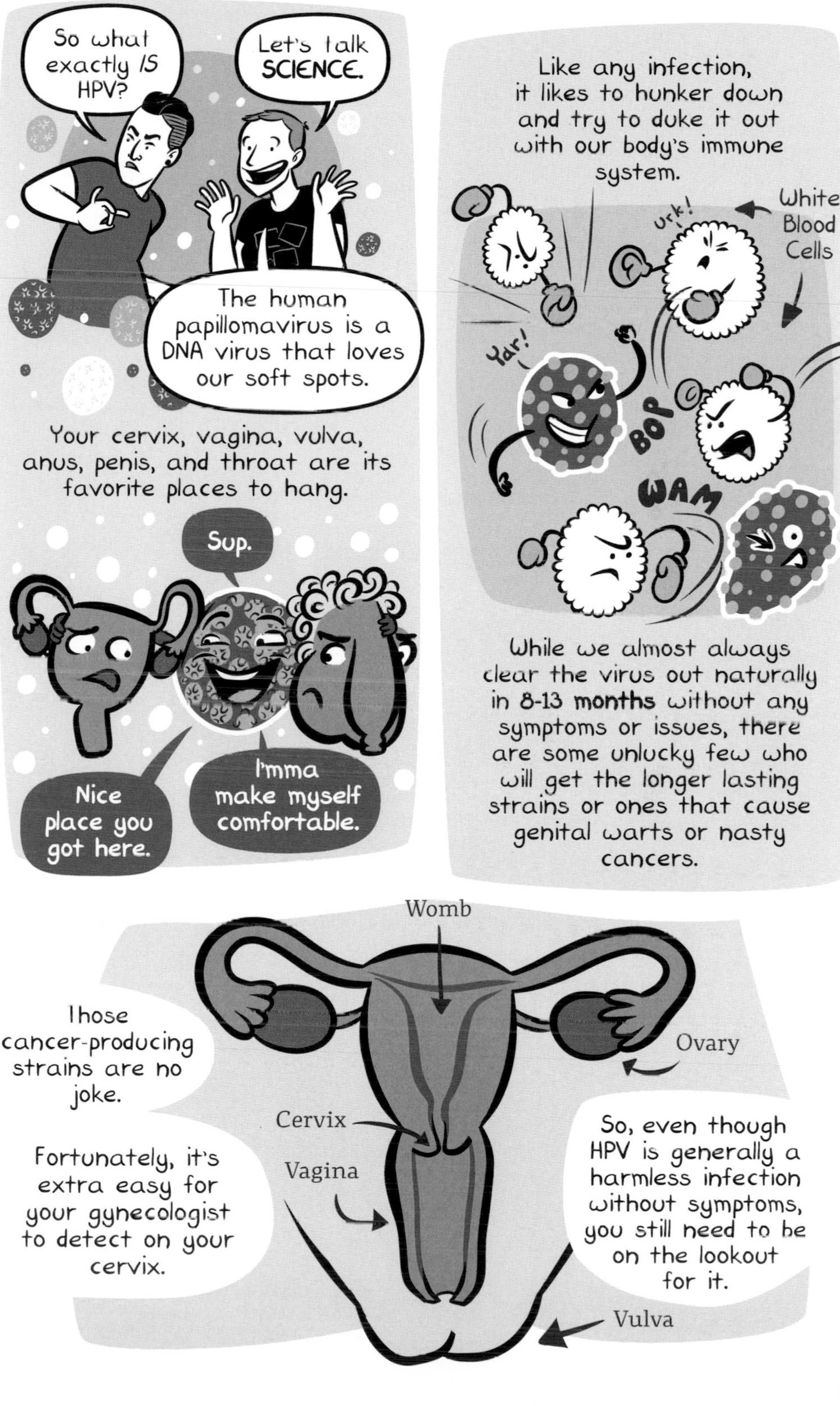
So what exactly IS HPV?
Let's talk SCIENCE.
The human papillomavirus is a DNA virus that loves our soft spots.
Your cervix, vagina, vulva, anus, penis, and throat are its favorite places to hang.
Sup.
Nice place you got here.
I'mma make myself comfortable.
Like any infection, it likes to hunker down and try to duke it out with our body's immune system.
White Blood Cells
Urk!
Yar!
BOP
WAM
While we almost always clear the virus out naturally in **8-13 months** without any symptoms or issues, there are some unlucky few who will get the longer lasting strains or ones that cause genital warts or nasty cancers.
Womb
Ovary
Cervix
Vagina
Vulva
Those cancer-producing strains are no joke.
Fortunately, it's extra easy for your gynecologist to detect on your cervix.
So, even though HPV is generally a harmless infection without symptoms, you still need to be on the lookout for it.

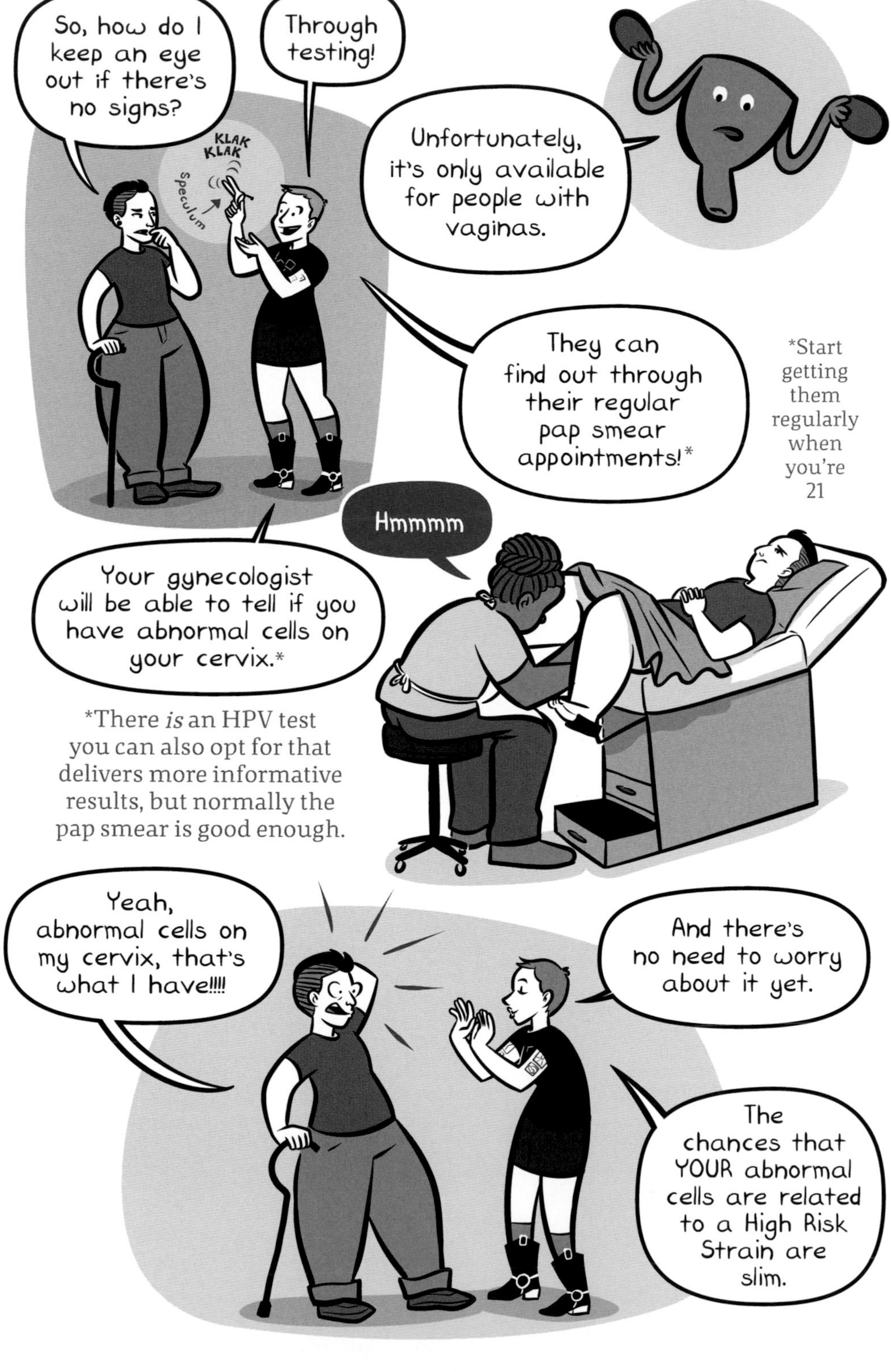
So, how do I keep an eye out if there's no signs?
Through testing!
KLAK KLAK
Speculum
Unfortunately, it's only available for people with vaginas.
They can find out through their regular pap smear appointments!*
*Start getting them regularly when you're 21
Hmmmm
Your gynecologist will be able to tell if you have abnormal cells on your cervix.*
*There *is* an HPV test you can also opt for that delivers more informative results, but normally the pap smear is good enough.
Yeah, abnormal cells on my cervix, that's what I have!!!!
And there's no need to worry about it yet.
The chances that YOUR abnormal cells are related to a High Risk Strain are slim.

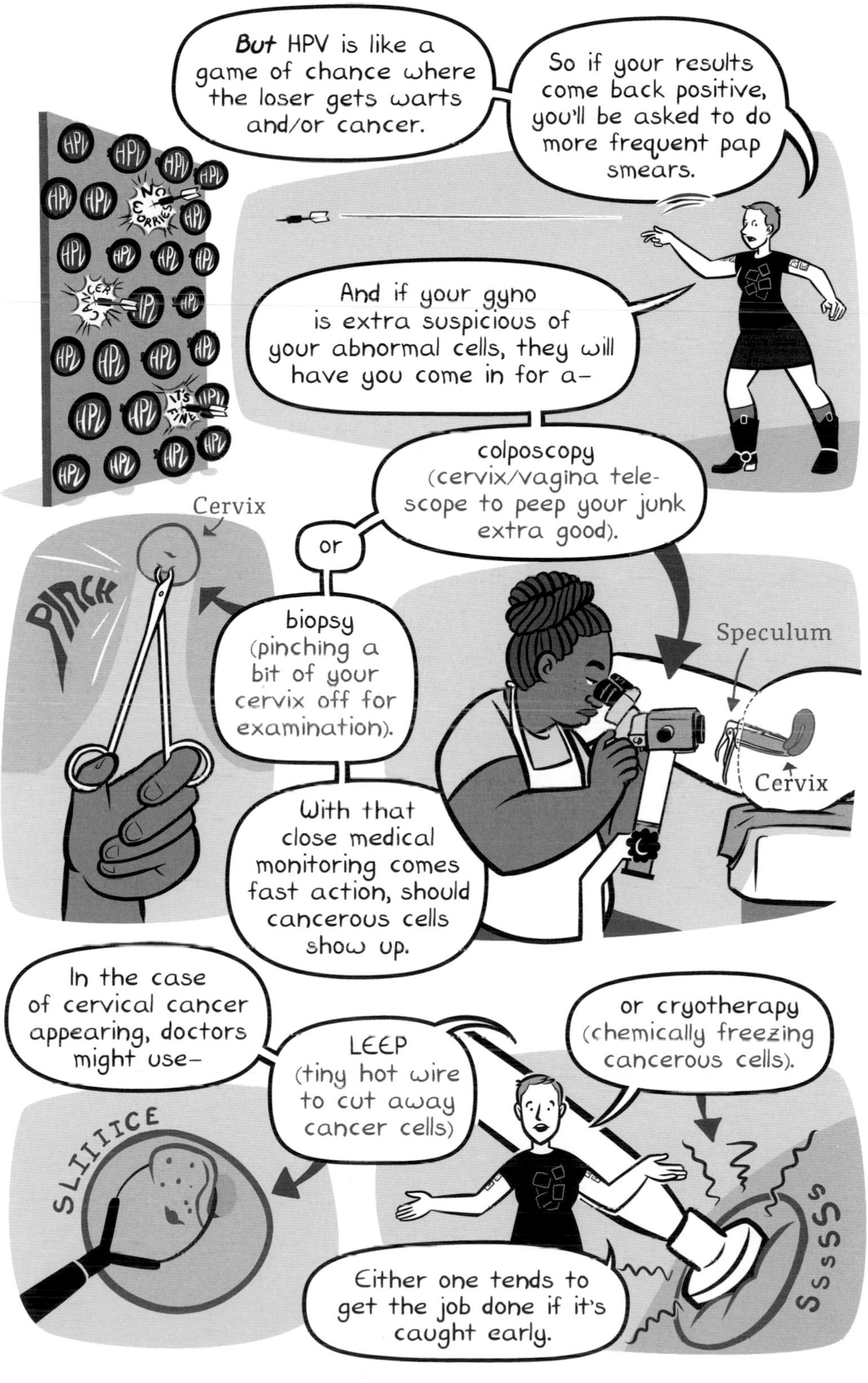

But HPV is like a game of chance where the loser gets warts and/or cancer.
So if your results come back positive, you'll be asked to do more frequent pap smears.
HPV
NO WORRIES
CANCER
IT'S FINE
And if your gyno is extra suspicious of your abnormal cells, they will have you come in for a–
colposcopy (cervix/vagina tele-scope to peep your junk extra good).
or
biopsy (pinching a bit of your cervix off for examination).
Cervix
PINCH
Speculum
Cervix
With that close medical monitoring comes fast action, should cancerous cells show up.
In the case of cervical cancer appearing, doctors might use–
LEEP (tiny hot wire to cut away cancer cells)
or cryotherapy (chemically freezing cancerous cells).
SLIIIICE
Either one tends to get the job done if it's caught early.
Ssssss

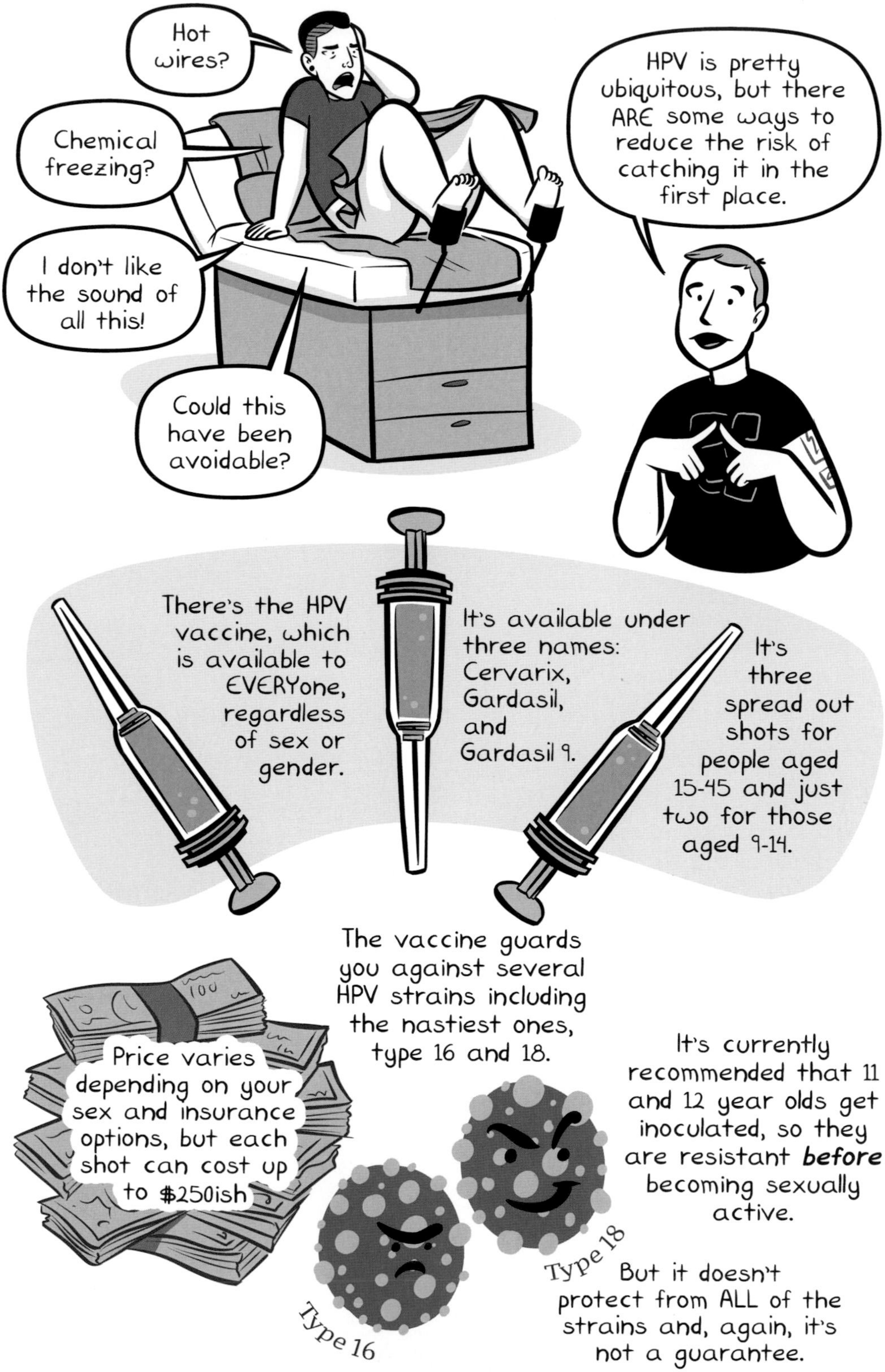
Hot wires?
Chemical freezing?
I don't like the sound of all this!
Could this have been avoidable?
HPV is pretty ubiquitous, but there ARE some ways to reduce the risk of catching it in the first place.
There's the HPV vaccine, which is available to EVERYone, regardless of sex or gender.
It's available under three names: Cervarix, Gardasil, and Gardasil 9.
It's three spread out shots for people aged 15-45 and just two for those aged 9-14.
The vaccine guards you against several HPV strains including the nastiest ones, type 16 and 18.
Price varies depending on your sex and insurance options, but each shot can cost up to $250ish
It's currently recommended that 11 and 12 year olds get inoculated, so they are resistant ***before*** becoming sexually active.
Type 18
Type 16
But it doesn't protect from ALL of the strains and, again, it's not a guarantee.

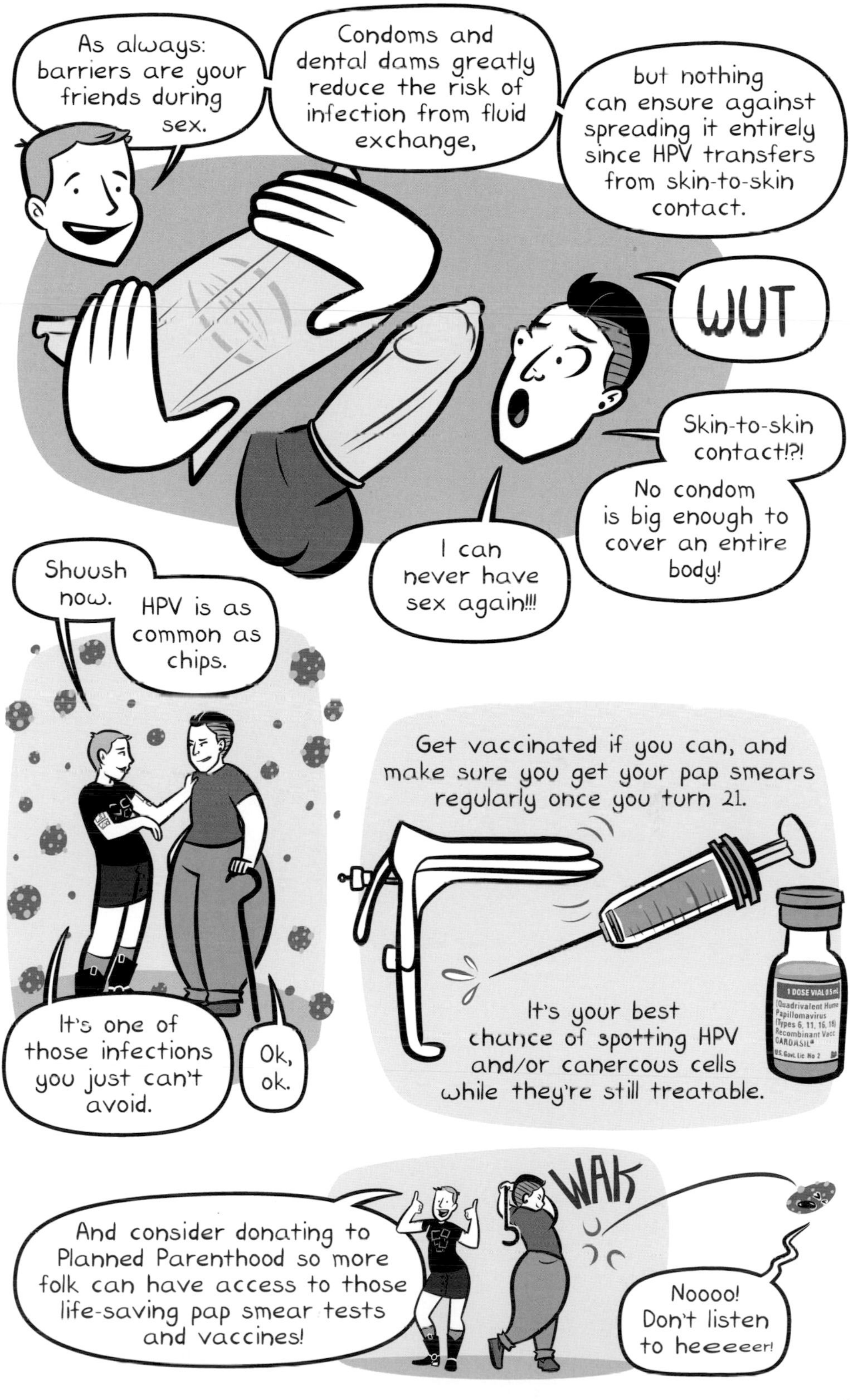
As always: barriers are your friends during sex.
Condoms and dental dams greatly reduce the risk of infection from fluid exchange,
but nothing can ensure against spreading it entirely since HPV transfers from skin-to-skin contact.
WUT
Skin-to-skin contact!?!
No condom is big enough to cover an entire body!
I can never have sex again!!!
Shuush now.
HPV is as common as chips.
It's one of those infections you just can't avoid.
Ok, ok.
Get vaccinated if you can, and make sure you get your pap smears regularly once you turn 21.
It's your best chance of spotting HPV and/or canercous cells while they're still treatable.
And consider donating to Planned Parenthood so more folk can have access to those life-saving pap smear tests and vaccines!
WAK
Noooo! Don't listen to heeeeer!

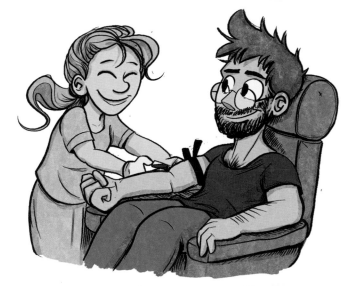

A Closer Look At
HIV, AIDS
& PrEP

By Silver
SilverIllustrations.com

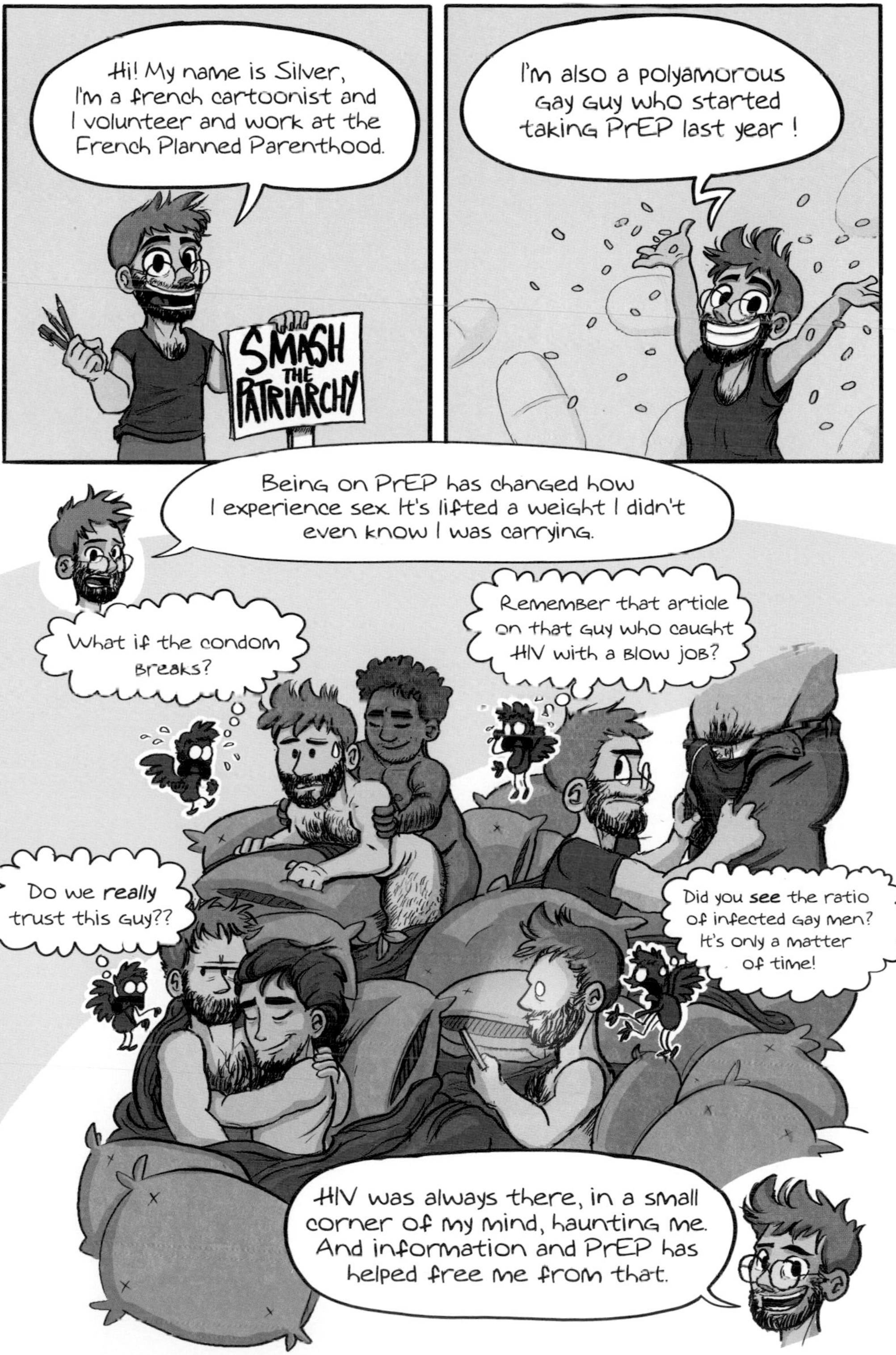
Hi! My name is Silver, I'm a french cartoonist and I volunteer and work at the French Planned Parenthood.
SMASH THE PATRIARCHY
I'm also a polyamorous gay guy who started taking PrEP last year !
Being on PrEP has changed how I experience sex. It's lifted a weight I didn't even know I was carrying.
What if the condom breaks?
Remember that article on that guy who caught HIV with a blow job?
Do we **really** trust this guy??
Did you **see** the ratio of infected gay men? It's only a matter of time!
HIV was always there, in a small corner of my mind, haunting me. And information and PrEP has helped free me from that.

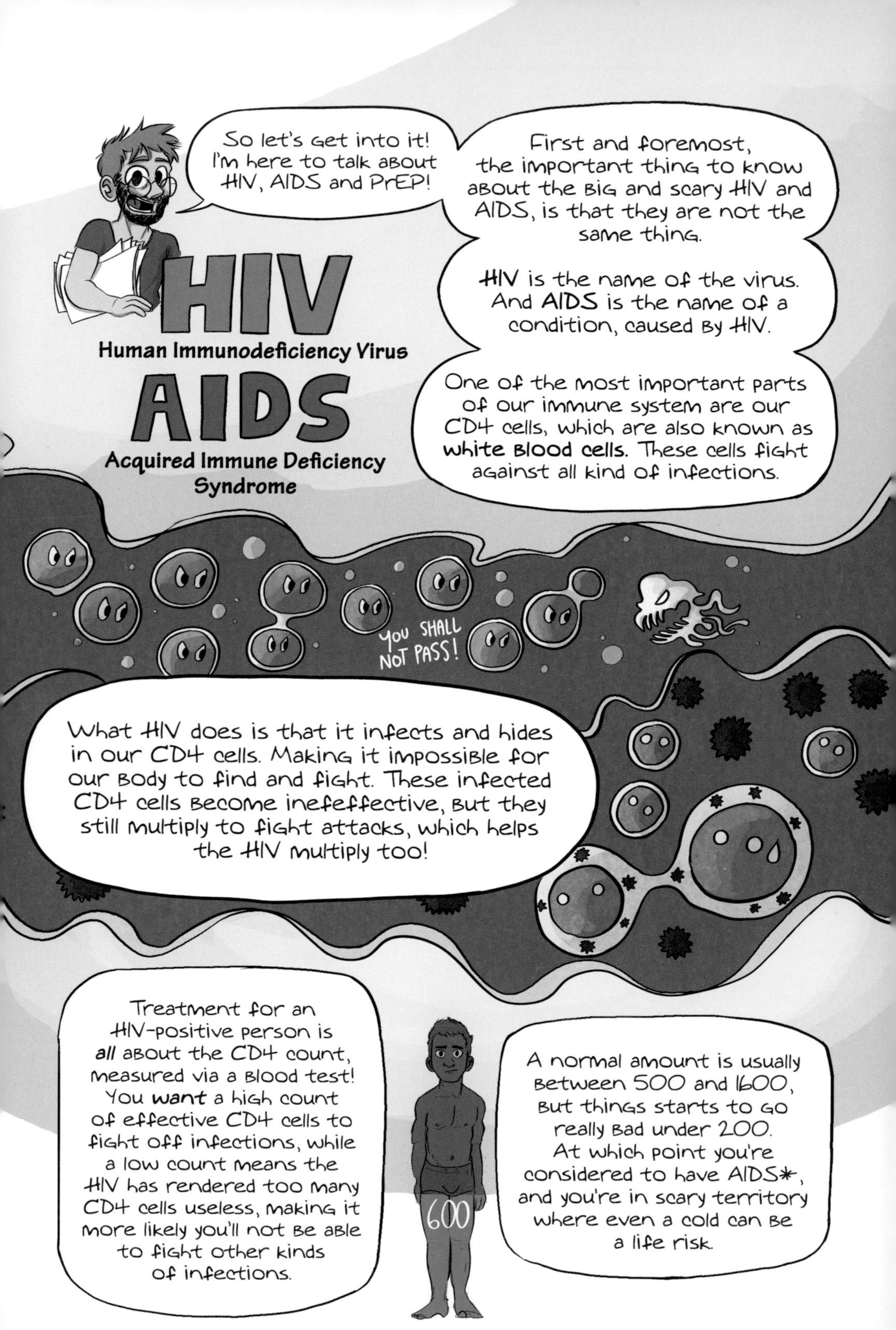
So let's get into it! I'm here to talk about HIV, AIDS and PrEP!
First and foremost, the important thing to know about the big and scary HIV and AIDS, is that they are not the same thing.
HIV is the name of the virus. And **AIDS** is the name of a condition, caused by HIV.
HIV
Human Immunodeficiency Virus
AIDS
Acquired Immune Deficiency Syndrome
One of the most important parts of our immune system are our CD4 cells, which are also known as **white blood cells**. These cells fight against all kind of infections.
YOU SHALL NOT PASS!
What HIV does is that it infects and hides in our CD4 cells. Making it impossible for our body to find and fight. These infected CD4 cells become inefeffective, but they still multiply to fight attacks, which helps the HIV multiply too!
Treatment for an HIV-positive person is *all* about the CD4 count, measured via a blood test! You **want** a high count of effective CD4 cells to fight off infections, while a low count means the HIV has rendered too many CD4 cells useless, making it more likely you'll not be able to fight other kinds of infections.
600
A normal amount is usually between 500 and 1600, but things starts to go really bad under 200. At which point you're considered to have AIDS*, and you're in scary territory where even a cold can be a life risk.

*According to the US Centers for Disease Control.

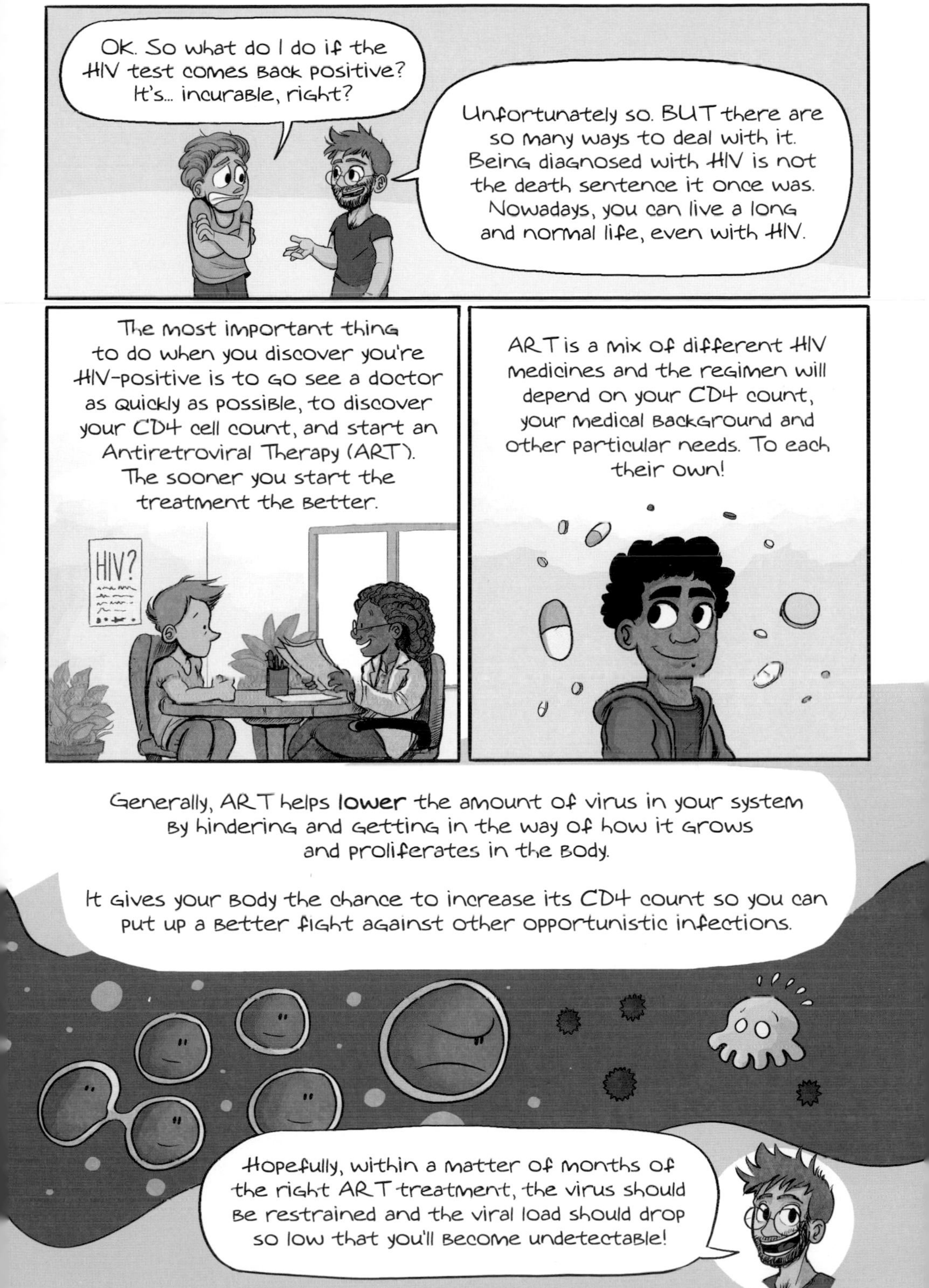
OK. So what do I do if the HIV test comes back positive? It's... incurable, right?
Unfortunately so. BUT there are so many ways to deal with it. Being diagnosed with HIV is not the death sentence it once was. Nowadays, you can live a long and normal life, even with HIV.
The most important thing to do when you discover you're HIV-positive is to go see a doctor as quickly as possible, to discover your CD4 cell count, and start an Antiretroviral Therapy (ART). The sooner you start the treatment the better.
HIV?
ART is a mix of different HIV medicines and the regimen will depend on your CD4 count, your medical background and other particular needs. To each their own!
Generally, ART helps **lower** the amount of virus in your system by hindering and getting in the way of how it grows and proliferates in the body.
It gives your body the chance to increase its CD4 count so you can put up a better fight against other opportunistic infections.
Hopefully, within a matter of months of the right ART treatment, the virus should be restrained and the viral load should drop so low that you'll become undetectable!

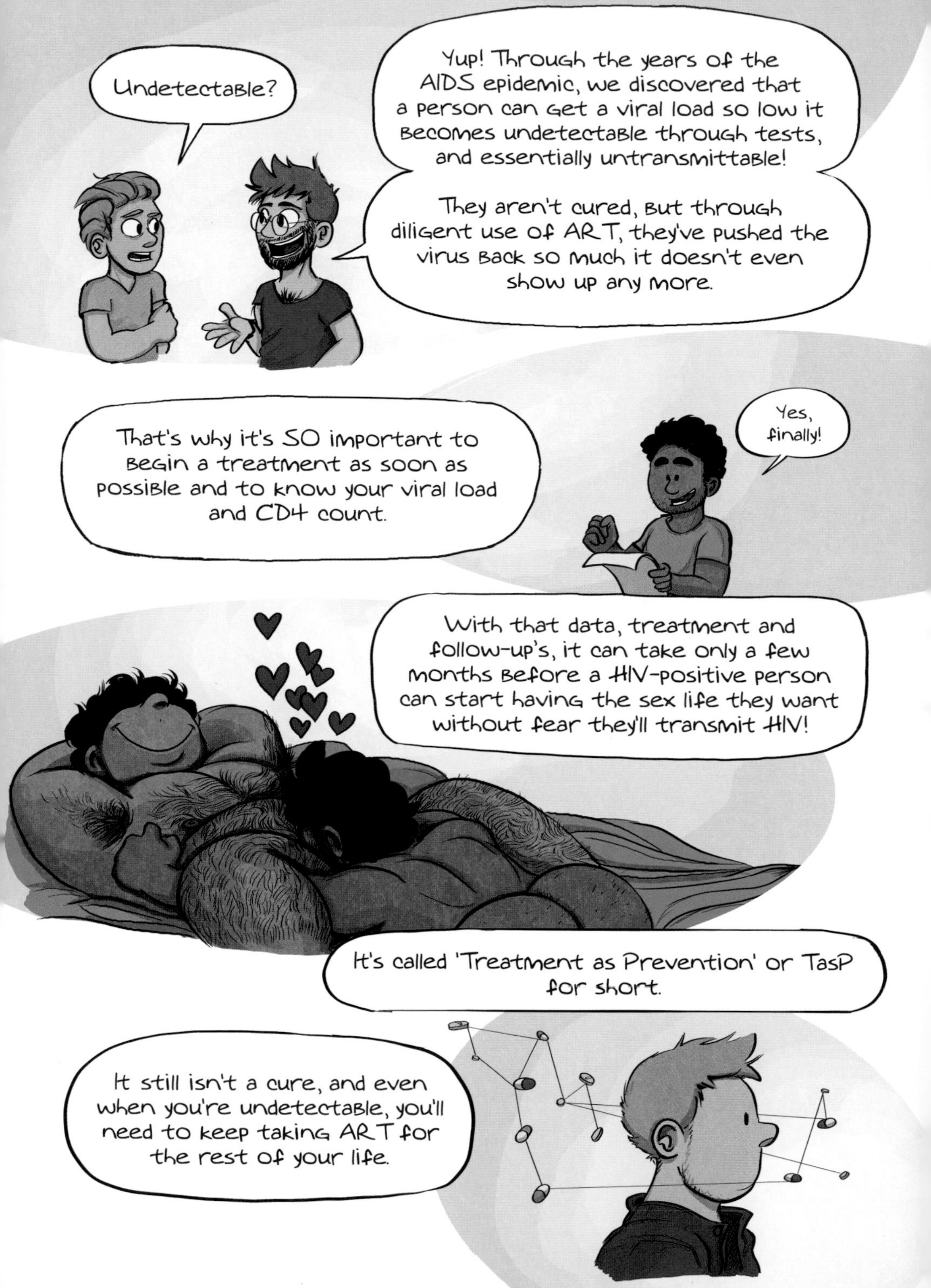
Undetectable?
Yup! Through the years of the AIDS epidemic, we discovered that a person can get a viral load so low it becomes undetectable through tests, and essentially untransmittable!
They aren't cured, but through diligent use of ART, they've pushed the virus back so much it doesn't even show up any more.
That's why it's SO important to begin a treatment as soon as possible and to know your viral load and CD4 count.
Yes, finally!
With that data, treatment and follow-up's, it can take only a few months before a HIV-positive person can start having the sex life they want without fear they'll transmit HIV!
It's called 'Treatment as Prevention' or TasP for short.
It still isn't a cure, and even when you're undetectable, you'll need to keep taking ART for the rest of your life.

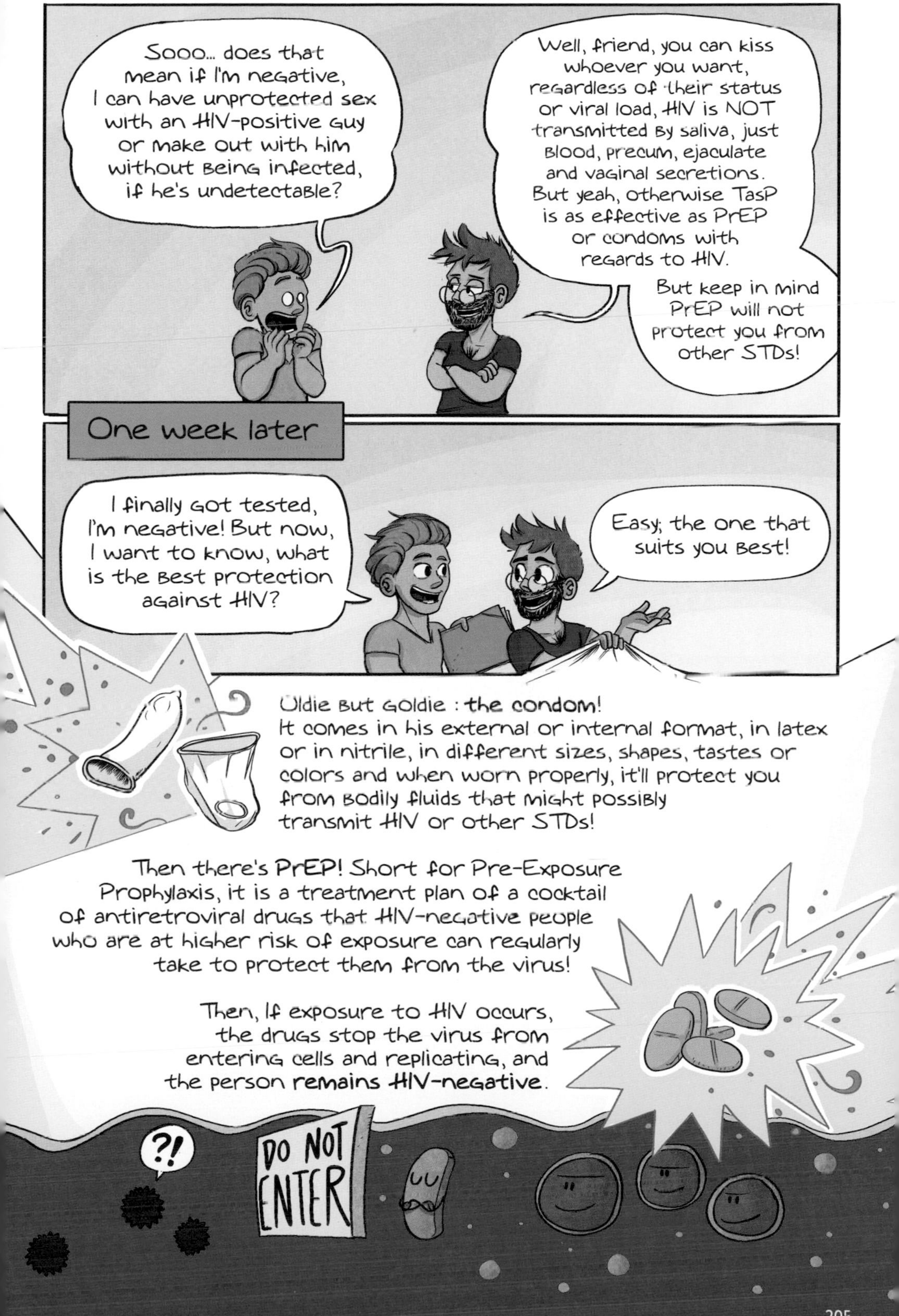
Sooo... does that mean if I'm negative, I can have unprotected sex with an HIV-positive guy or make out with him without being infected, if he's undetectable?
Well, friend, you can kiss whoever you want, regardless of their status or viral load, HIV is NOT transmitted by saliva, just blood, precum, ejaculate and vaginal secretions. But yeah, otherwise TasP is as effective as PrEP or condoms with regards to HIV.
But keep in mind PrEP will not protect you from other STDs!
One week later
I finally got tested, I'm negative! But now, I want to know, what is the best protection against HIV?
Easy; the one that suits you best!
Oldie but Goldie : **the condom**!
It comes in his external or internal format, in latex or in nitrile, in different sizes, shapes, tastes or colors and when worn properly, it'll protect you from bodily fluids that might possibly transmit HIV or other STDs!
Then there's **PrEP**! Short for Pre-Exposure Prophylaxis, it is a treatment plan of a cocktail of antiretroviral drugs that HIV-negative people who are at higher risk of exposure can regularly take to protect them from the virus!
Then, If exposure to HIV occurs, the drugs stop the virus from entering cells and replicating, and the person **remains HIV-negative**.
?!
DO NOT ENTER

Right now (2018) in the United States, you have to take PrEP on a daily basis (in some other countries, you can choose to take PrEP « On demand »).

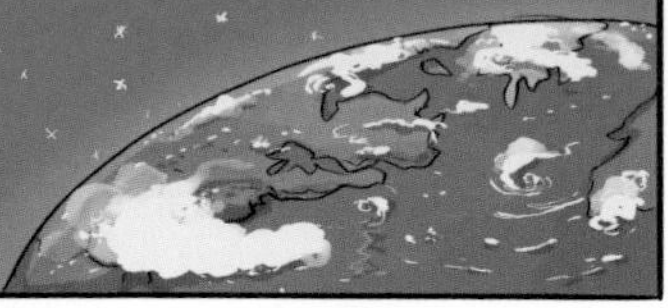

To begin the treatment, you have to go to a doctor, nurse, or to your local Planned Parenthood to talk with them about your sex life, medical history and then take some HIV/STD tests to see if you're negative before starting the treatment. After a few days on PrEP (usually 7 days), you should be covered!

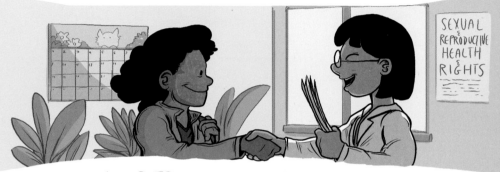

SEXUAL & REPRODUCTIVE HEALTH & RIGHTS

Also, PrEP **always** comes with a mandatory medical follow up every 3 months so you can get tested for other STDs and check on your sexual health in general!

The use of PrEP changes according to the country you live in. Some countries like France have universal healthcare so PrEP is totally free, and in other like the United States, it will depend on your insurance.

Good to know: there are also organizations that can help you pay for PrEP if you have no insurance!

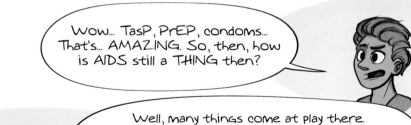

Wow... TasP, PrEP, condoms... That's... AMAZING. So, then, how is AIDS still a THING then?

Well, many things come at play there. There's a huge lack of funding, so the people and organizations fighting against the virus can't do their work. As a result, a lot of people accross the world don't have access to information, tests and therapy.

So we end up with people who are not tested nor taking a treatment. And it's the 'not knowing' that's the most dangerous thing; an HIV-positive person who doesn't know their status can be highly contagious.

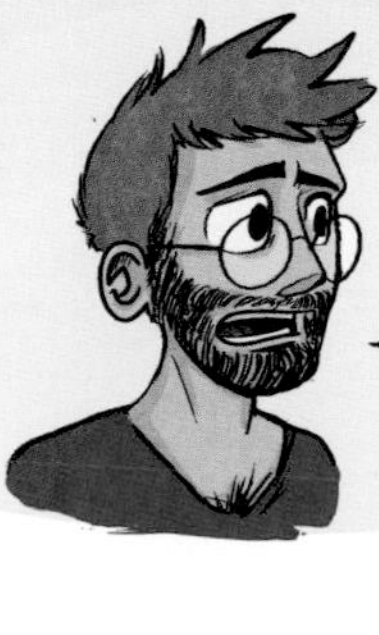

In conclusion, what I've learned these past years is that one of the best ways to fight HIV is to know as much as possible about it.

It is so important to know your status, so get tested.

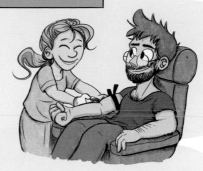

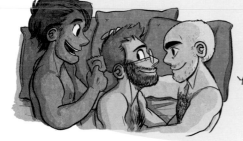

You have to feel free to talk about it with your partners and choose the protection that is best for you.

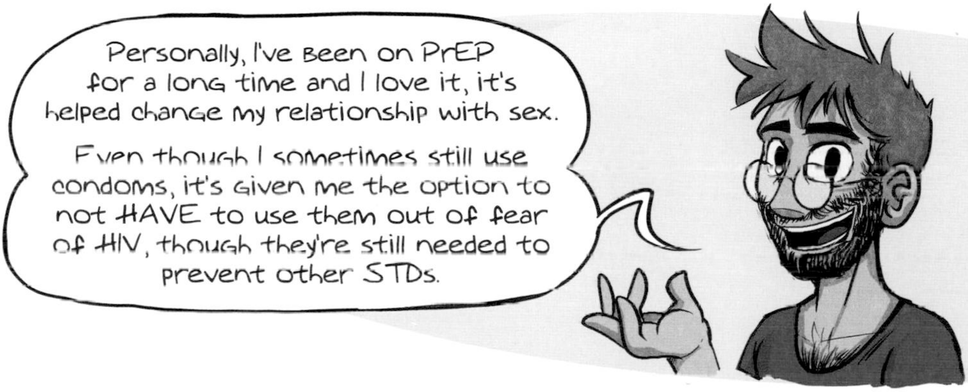

Personally, I've been on PrEP for a long time and I love it, it's helped change my relationship with sex.

Even though I sometimes still use condoms, it's given me the option to not HAVE to use them out of fear of HIV, though they're still needed to prevent other STDs.

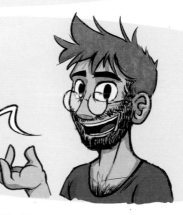

The fight against HIV/AIDS is far from over yet, especially for lower-income populations. But we don't have to live in the constant fear of it. We have great tools like condoms, PrEP, or TasP and the treatments have never been more efficient.

Together we're gonna fight this thing.

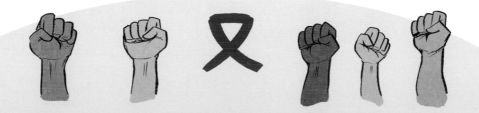

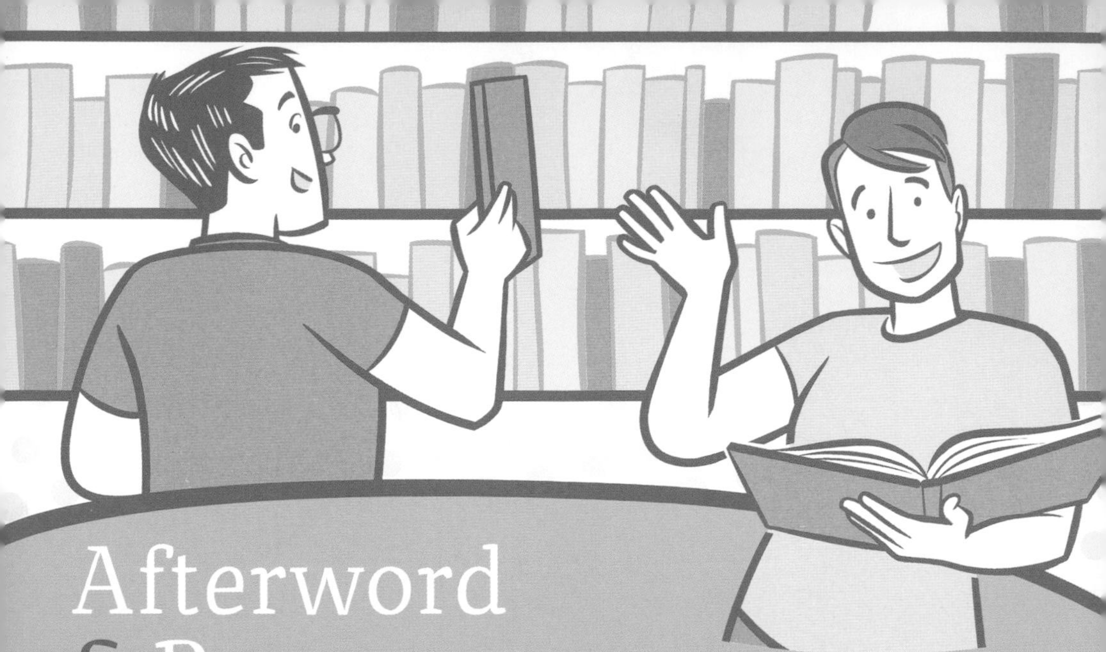

Afterword & Resources

It's sad to say but, with time, this book will age. Information will fall out of date, new medical treatments will become available, and our knowledge of the body will improve. Maybe you're reading this in the hover-board-future and you're wondering why there isn't a chapter about those new Space-STIs everyone's catching now.

We built this book over the course of six years as part of our webcomic, *Oh Joy Sex Toy*. It's a historical collection of our educational greatest hits, a mishmash of the topics we wanted to cover each week. So, this is your reminder to go out and do your own independent research on any subjects catching your attention.

If you're looking for our top resources, they're listed below! At the very least, it'll be good reading material while you wait to get that Space-STI laser-treated.

Scarleteen.com
A free online curated sex education website. Inclusive, comprehensive and awesome.

S.E.X.: The All-You-Need-To-Know Sexuality Guide to Get You Through Your Teens and Twenties by Heather Corinna
Just an absolute UNIT of a book. This thing has it ALL.

PlannedParenthood.org
An incredible organization with a HUGE repository of up-to-date sex education material.

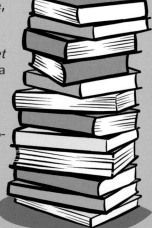

Wait, What? by Heather Corinna and Isabella Rotman
More delightlful sex education in comic book form!